"Rhonda PallasDowney has collected a great amount of material, skillfully blended together with case histories and personal experience, which demonstrates the spiritual and healing potential of plants. She shows us that homeopathy, herbalism, and flower essence therapy are interrelated disciplines. Most importantly, Rhonda gives the professional and the lay-person enough well-defined indications to make her work a practical guide book for therapeutic use."

— Matthew Wood, herbalist and homeopath, and author of *Seven Herbs,*
Plants as Teachers, The Magical Staff, and *The Book of Herbal Wisdom*

"The pioneering work of Rhonda PallasDowney and her book *The Complete Book of Flower Essences* is both timely and vastly important to the overall realm of natural healing. She leads us to a greater depth of knowledge to understand the vital role of plants and flowers in health and healing. Especially revealing and helpful are the insights gained from the information on the chakras, the flower essences and how to use them in our daily lives. For those health practitioners who use a holistic approach, this book is essential!"

— Charlie McGuire, M.A., R.N.C., H.N.C., founder of the American Holistic Nurses'
Association, co-founder of the Southwest Institute for Women's Healing,
and co-founder of the Buffalo Woman Ranch

"For those interested in flower remedies from an energetic medicine point of view, Rhonda PallasDowney's integration of herbs, homeopathy, and flower essences is superb. I know of no other source for this comprehensive approach."

— C. Norman Shealy, M.D., Ph.D., founder of the Shealy Institute,
founding president of American Holistic Medical Association,
president of Holos™ Institutes of Health, Inc.,
and author of *Sacred Healing*

the
complete
book of
flower
essences

the complete book of flower essences

48 Natural and Beautiful Ways to Heal Yourself and Your Life

Rhonda M. PallasDowney

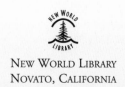

NEW WORLD LIBRARY
NOVATO, CALIFORNIA

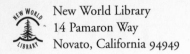

New World Library
14 Pamaron Way
Novato, California 94949

Edited by Katie Farnam Conolly and Carol Venolia
Front cover design by Mary Beth Salmon
Interior photographs by Rhonda M. PallasDowney
Text design by Mary Ann Casler
Typography by Tona Pearce Myers

The material in this book is intended for education. It is not meant to take the place of diagnosis and treatment by a qualified medical practitioner or therapist. No expressed or implied guarantee as to the effects of the use of the recommendations can be given nor liability taken.

Grateful acknowledgment is given to Llewellyn for permission to reprint excerpts from the Sound/Vibrations section of *A Healer's Manual* by Ted Andrews in chapter 4 of *The Complete Book of Flower Essences*. Copyright © 1998 by Ted Andrews. Reprinted by permission of Llewellyn.

Library of Congress Cataloging-in-Publication Data
PallasDowney, Rhonda M.
  The complete book of flower essences : 48 natural and beautiful ways to heal yourself and your life
/ by Rhonda M. PallasDowney.
      p.   cm.
Includes index.
  ISBN 1-57731-141-8
  1. Flowers—Therapeutic use. 2. Bach, Edward, 1886–1936. I. Title.
  RX615.F55 P35 2002
  615′.321—dc21   2002005910

First Printing, October 2002
ISBN 1-57731-141-8
Printed in Canada on acid-free, partially recycled paper
Distributed to the trade by Publishers Group West

10 9 8 7 6 5 4 3 2 1

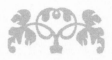

*To my mother, Bernice Reichenbach, and in loving memory
of my late father, Fred Reichenbach, for their love
of nature and flowers
and
to my family,
Curt, Sarah, Jenny, Nataraj,
Tanya, Cortney, and Heather
for their love and support*

CONTENTS

PREFACE
by Trevor Cook, Ph.D., H.M.D., R.C.S.

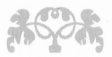

Throughout this excellent book, Rhonda PallasDowney emphasizes the relationship among herbs, homeopathy, and flower essences by describing them as a continuum. I have long held the belief that we tend to create barriers between natural methods of healing, when they should be seen as facets of a whole, continuous, overlapping spectrum that expresses the natural order of life. Rightly, Rhonda also stresses the continuum of plant healing effects, from the physical through the psychological to the spiritual.

What the plant healing methods have in common is that they may calm, activate, confront, resolve, relieve, regulate, remove, free, cleanse, comfort, strengthen, restore, stimulate, restrain, increase, cause, promote, drain, or expel symptoms in a truly holistic way — the whole treatment with the whole plant.

The section on making one's own flower essences gave me a feeling of embarking on an exciting adventure, and through Rhonda's writing I at last believe that I understand the chakra system.

Rhonda PallasDowney's inspired writing will stimulate you to seek a deeper understanding of our botanical heritage and encourage you to teach others.

I wish this book the success it deserves.

Trevor Cook, Ph.D., H.M.D., R.C.S.
Director and Principal of the British
Institute of Homoeopathy and former
Royal Warrant Holder as personal
supplier of homeopathic medicines
to Her Majesty Queen Elizabeth II
and the Queen Mother

FOREWORD

by Gladys Taylor McGarey, M.D., M.D.(H)

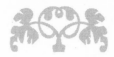

On a really hot day in July 2001, I was talking to a friend of mine about medicine — the way it's practiced, the way it's taught, and the way it's received by patients and professionals. I was telling my friend that it seemed to me that medicine had become a killing machine; its major purpose seemed to be a war on disease. The focus is on killing bacteria, eradicating AIDS, eliminating cancer, controlling diabetes, etcetera. Women are even talking about fighting osteoporosis as if they need to stage a war against their very bones. If we are going to be doing this killing, we need ammunition, and the ammunition in the field of medicine is primarily drugs. In 1955, the *Physicians' Desk Reference* was about half an inch thick, and now it is more than four inches thick.

Many people identify themselves with their disease process and lose their identity. We hear people saying, "I am an epileptic," or, "I am a diabetic." The disease has taken on so much reality that they actually, in their own minds, become the disease. If our focus in medicine is to destroy a disease, we frequently manage to destroy the person who has the disease.

Another part of the approach that medicine takes towards healing is that it is really geared towards fighting life itself. We talk about anti-depressants, antibiotics, anti-aging, and anti-fungal. Our whole focus is against the life force.

While I was talking to my friend about the confusion we have in medicine, I suddenly heard myself saying, "What we really need is living medicine, not killing medicine." And then I stopped and said to the divine universe, "Thank you very much. I've been waiting eighty-one years for this term."

The concept of living medicine is truly exciting because if we're alive, we're going to have illness, we're going to have pain, we're going to have all of the problems that go along with life, but we're going to be alive. Our focus needs to change from killing to helping enhance the life process within each individual. If we do this, we're going to need living materials, such as living air, living earth, living water, and living food.

Perhaps our focus in relation to surgery needs to shift and become more like pruning a tree. The tree is pruned, not just to remove the parts that are not serving the tree well, but primarily the tree is pruned so that the life force can be stronger and the tree can function better as a living organism. If we thought about surgery in this way, our focus would not be so much a matter of destroying the disease that needs to be eliminated, but enhancing the life force within the individual by eliminating the nonfunctional, or the aspects of the body that are preventing the life force from manifesting itself.

Many years ago I was waiting for a patient to deliver her baby at Doctor's Hospital in Phoenix. It was about three o'clock in the morning and a colleague of mine was also assisting a delivery, and we got into a discussion. His comment was, "The fun has all gone out of medicine." I thought a lot about that through the years and realized that if our whole focus is towards killing and destruction, there is no fun in medicine. The fun and joy will return to the practice of medicine when we accept the fact that we are working with living human beings who happen to have disease processes. We can then help the patients in their process of becoming more whole.

With *The Complete Book of Flower Essences,* Rhonda PallasDowney brings a living healing method to our attention. This type of healing truly is working with living medicine. The plants and the flowers have lived and they pass on their living essence to the person who uses the naturally derived product. Life enhances life, and as we involve ourselves in the healing process — with its joys and sorrows, its good times and hard times — I know that nothing makes this truth more clear than flower essences.

Gladys Taylor McGarey, M.D., M.D.(H)

GLADYS TAYLOR MCGAREY, M.D., M.D.(H), is internationally known for her pioneering work in holistic medicine. A founding member and past president of the American Holistic Medical Association, she also serves on a research committee of the Office of Alternative Medicine, National Institutes of Health. Dr. McGarey's work, through the Gladys T. McGarey Medical Foundation has helped to expand the knowledge and application of holistic principles through scientific research and education. A family physician for more than fifty years, she and her daughter have a joint practice, the Scottsdale Holistic Medical Group, in Scottsdale, Arizona. Dr. McGarey lectures internationally and is the author of numerous books and articles.

INTRODUCTION
Plants and Flowers: Our Friends and Helpers

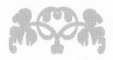

I have been a lover of nature and her plant kingdom for as long as I can remember. As a child, I used to walk to my Uncle Harley's woods, find a comfortable log or a soft grassy spot, and just sit and stare at the many wildflowers that seemed to gaze back at me. The flowers stirred my passion for living. Their gentle, eloquent beauty gave me hope and inspiration. They helped me believe in myself. I found peace, love, and nurturing among the flowers, and I knew they were my sacred friends.

Our family often went for drives in the country, looking for flowers and berries. My mother would gather them and create beautiful flower arrangements that often won first prize at local fairs. Sometimes she showed my sister and me how to make our own flower arrangements. My parents also had a flower garden that attracted neighbors, relatives, friends, and local townspeople.

As I grew older and walked through the meadows and forests and along the creeks, I always noticed the flowers and other plants. They stood by me, sang to me, embraced and welcomed me, and reminded me that they would always be back in their rich fullness in the spring. Their open invitation for me to adore their beauty and their memorable presence evoked tears of joy and sadness. How could a flower's presence be so pure, so gentle, so sacred, and so vulnerable?

In my late twenties, I began to study the use of plants and herbs at about the same time when I decided to simplify my lifestyle. In the summer of 1980, during a major life transition, I went on a personal retreat and set up a camp on some property owned by friends, nestled in the foothills of the Appalachian Mountains in southeastern Ohio. My camp was surrounded by a forest of enormous trees, as well as spotted joe-pye weeds, sassafras, wild grapevines, wild berries, many other wild plants, and bull snakes. There was even an old dilapidated shack where "white lightning" was once made.

I lived near a small rural town (population 200) and was often seen walking around with my plant books and asking questions about the local plants and herbs. Two middle-aged mountain men, who were brothers, offered to take me into the higher mountains to collect plants, including American ginseng and goldenseal. These two men were my first "plant gurus," and they taught me a lot about identifying, collecting, and cultivating plants. I appreciated their trustworthiness and their genuine relationship with the plant kingdom.

I found my first American ginseng plant on a field trip with these mountain men. American ginseng is easy to identify. The stem is simple and erect, and the leaves are distinguished by their whorls of three, with five leaflets in each whorl, shaped like an open palm. A bright red berry grows in the center of the three whorls, adding to the plant's attractiveness. Just seeing it gave me a rush of excitement. In gratitude, I gave a prayer and blessing and thanked the plant for showing itself to me. Excited, I reached for my hand shovel and dug to the bottom of its human-shaped roots. As I pulled the roots free, a root shaped like a little person with arms and legs presented itself to me. I felt as if a part of myself was connected to those ginseng roots. My mountain-men friends nodded and smiled in approval as they chewed on their own freshly dug roots.

All that day, I felt a surge of energy while gathering roots and plants. That night, lying in my sleeping bag, I snuggled against the sacred gunnysack that held my cherished findings as I traveled from one rich dream journey to another. I still treasure that day's experience in my heart.

Throughout that summer, I collected many plants. I particularly remember digging black cohosh; its root system is extremely entangled and challenging to dig up, and it brought out my anger while digging. At that time in my life, I was having a difficult time emotionally, and I found that digging up the black cohosh seemed to bring up my anger even more strongly. However, when I sucked on the black cohosh root or made a tea of the root, I almost immediately felt relaxed, grounded, and at ease. It seemed to help me step outside myself and observe my reactions to my anger and my digging. I could see and feel my entanglements with myself through the role of an observer. It helped me confront parts of myself in a way that I hadn't experienced before. Throughout the summer, I established an intimate relationship with this plant and a new relationship with myself.

By September, I was ready to leave my camp and begin a new phase of my life. Other mysteries awaited me.

In 1986, my awareness that I was stuck in a dysfunctional and abusive reliaionship led me to attend an herb workshop in Flagstaff, Arizona, presented by Dave Milgram and Matthew Wood. After taking one look at me, Matt gave me two flower essences: Monkeyflower and Black Cohosh. The Monkeyflower was to help me face my fears and free myself from the sticky situation I was in, and the Black Cohosh was to help me confront my shadow side and free me from entanglement.

This was the first time I had ever heard of flower essences. Matthew explained that the plant's flower blossoms had been placed in a clear bowl of purified water and placed in the sun — a process called "infusion." This infusion extracts the energy of the blossom into the water and creates a life-force pattern that reflects the character of the plant.

As the first few drops of the essences dissolved under my tongue, I felt an immediate, subtle connection with the plants and their flowers. It was as if the resonating frequency of the plants was talking to me. I felt that the plants were inter-kingdom partners in the way that they aligned my body, soul, nature, and spirit. A memory of my experiences in the Appalachian Mountains and my personal relationship with black cohosh reentered my mind. I remembered struggling with those roots and pulling them out of the ground. And there I was again, struggling with myself and my own roots and values, feeling stuck in the darkness of an unhealthy, dysfunctional situation.

The flower essences helped me feel grounded and peaceful. In a matter of seconds, a sense of relief and freedom swept through me. I felt more able to connect with my emotions and, at the same time, awaken an innate understanding of myself and the situation I was in. I gained insight,

strength, and a broader perspective on myself and my life.

That experience was also the beginning of a long and fruitful journey. I felt bonded with Matt from the first moment of meeting him. Thanks to an ongoing relationship with him as my mentor and friend, I have studied, researched, and continued to pursue my relationship with plants and their flowers.

Over the years, through my personal discoveries with plants, I have developed an ever-deepening relationship with myself and the earth. These plants have taught me to honor the sacredness of nature, including the divine nature of self and others.

Plants have helped me search more deeply into the meaning of life and the meaning of who I am in terms of the Self that is greater than my personality. They have enriched a part of me that will forever be dear to my heart. They have provided an opening from the depths of my soul that allows me to unfold throughout the cycles of the seasons and this great mystery of life.

Each time I make a flower essence, I experience a life lesson or story that seems in harmony with the personality of the plant. I remember finding a sacred sanctuary of yerba santa with my good friend Roby Nelson in April of 1986. Roby and I immediately felt a sense of reverence for this plant, and especially for the sacred and secluded area in which this particular grove of yerba santa lived. It was divine timing to experience yerba santa at this particular period in our lives. Through the process of being with this plant and its flower, we both experienced a natural receptivity toward a personal discovery of Self that had previously been hidden to us. Yerba santa offered a gentle yet persuasive character, giving us the guidance to sort out our inner impurities. Yerba santa gave us the spiritual and personal devotion to follow through on our intuitive insights. I gained great respect for yerba santa.

Later in our lives, Roby and I both had a confrontation with black-eyed Susan. Our families went on a camping trip together in the mountains near Jemez, New Mexico. It was a long drive, and I was very relieved when we arrived at our camping spot. However, my husband, Curt, decided that he needed to go back into town to get some supplies; I had no interest in going anywhere. We had a conflict over this, and I decided that I needed some personal space. He took our daughter Sarah, who was then one year old, and went to a nearby country store while I went on a walk to look for plants.

I soon came upon a black-eyed Susan in full bloom, with a comfortable, nice-sized rock next to it to sit on. I was amazed that this rock fit so well beside the plant. It was as if it were there just for me, though I felt resistance to being with it. When I sat on the rock and began studying the plant, I noticed how coarse, rough, and hairy the stems and leaves were. I became aware of how "rough" I was feeling in my mind and emotions, yet I felt a great reluctance about facing it. As I looked into the

dark center disk inside the flower, I felt and saw my own darkness. I struggled in the presence of this flower, wanting to resist the emotional pains I felt deep inside. Being with black-eyed Susan this way took me deeper into my own core.

As I allowed myself to feel the pain I had been avoiding, I felt a burden lift. The yellow halo around the disk in the black-eyed Susan reflected my own ability to embrace light, moving me toward a higher level of thinking. I felt a shift, and my criticism of Curt for leaving our new campsite began to dissolve. I experienced my shadow-self embracing the light, much like the dark disk that spread out into bright golden petals.

I sat on that rock for a long time. Just as I was ready to get up and move onward, Roby came by. She looked like I had felt before I sat on the rock. She took one searching look at the black-eyed Susan, waved her hand at it, and in a stern voice said, "I hope you don't think I should sit with this plant." I laughed and said, "Of course I do." Teary-eyed, she sat down on the rock and had an experience similar to mine.

Neither of us wanted to look at the mirror black-eyed Susan showed us. We both struggled in the plant's presence, resisting the emotional pains we felt deep inside. The journey into Self that we experienced with black-eyed Susan helped us release our emotional and mental bondage. We both felt freed up inside after working through our individual confrontations. With this release came freedom of thought and expression, giving us each a deeper sense of inner peace.

This is how plant medicine often works for me and for others whom I know. The characteristics and personalities of the plants offer a lesson or message at exactly the time when we need it the most, helping us to be in touch with our innermost nature.

Over the years, Curt and I have had many magical moments in nature together; our hikes, walks, ceremonies, and music inspired our budding relationship. Curt is a Western mystic who is deeply influenced by indigenous shamanism and who connects with the earth much like I do. Our first hike together took place in the evening in Sycamore Pass, near Sedona, Arizona. Curt was sensitive about my being a woman and concerned about whether I might walk into the nearby cacti. As darkness fell, he suggested that I stay close behind him, not knowing that I had taken many solo journeys under night skies and didn't need his guidance. Farther down the trail, Curt was amazed when he discovered that I wasn't right behind him. That's when he realized that he had a true hiking companion.

Several years later, we were married among the beautiful red rocks of Sycamore Pass, where we first hiked together. Curt is a patient nature companion for me, as I spend much of my time in nature contemplating and studying the wonders of the plant kingdom. The subtle nuances and messages from the nature kingdom continue to play a significant role in our journeys together, and we have spent countless hours exploring and experiencing plants and their flowers.

One adventure in the summer of 1995 is especially memorable. We were on a journey into the White Mountains in northern Arizona with our then two-year-old daughter Sarah when I told Curt that if I could find a wild rose bush I would be very thankful. On the third day of our trip, we were driving on an old mountain road into a ponderosa pine forest at about 8,000 feet elevation. I was feeling disappointed about not having found a wild rose. Suddenly, a flock of wild turkeys caught our attention. We were inspired by the powerful presence of thanksgiving and blessings that the turkeys represented to us. We stopped the car and watched them until they noticed us and quickly flew away. Only then did we realize that we had stopped beside a prolific wild rose bush in full bloom.

We walked over to where the turkeys had been roosting. The setting was absolutely pristine. Many wild rose bushes, all in their fullest bloom, were clustered near a small flowing mountain stream. The entire area was vibrant with life. We found ourselves feeling nurtured, loved, and protected in this special area. Sarah was delighted that we had finally found our "spot" for the day.

The wild rose flower had a sweet fragrance. Its pink petals opened broadly and its circle of yellow stamens were completely visible — a striking statement of the flower's simple beauty and vulnerable character. The wild rose always seems protected amidst its thorny branches. The thorns are the plant's expression of protection; to me, they represent our need to protect ourselves from life's disappointments, pain, and challenges. The flower's destiny is to live among the thorns, yet it holds a celebratory energy that expresses its compassion and joy for life.

Our day with the wild roses was gentle, soft, nurturing, and uplifting. It opened our hearts to the meaning of love and acceptance without emotional resistance or suffering. We were all greatly touched by the dynamic yet simple presence of wild rose. The day was also a testimonial of how nature takes care of me when I pay attention to her signs and honor her sacredness, even when I'm in doubt. It was indeed a day of thanksgiving.

I am deeply inspired by the powerful, profound healing qualities that can be accessed through whole-plant medicine and the essences of flowers. With plants and flower essences as my friends, helpers, and guides, I have grown greatly in my understanding of life.

I want to emphasize my belief, based in years of study of many great traditions, that all things are an expression of our Creator, Great Spirit, Father/Mother/God. Throughout this book I may use any of these terms; they all refer to the same Source who lives and breathes through every one of us.

I hope that this book will help deepen your relationship with and appreciation of plants and their flowers, and reveal to you unfolding discoveries, wisdom, and insights into your personal journeys of Self.

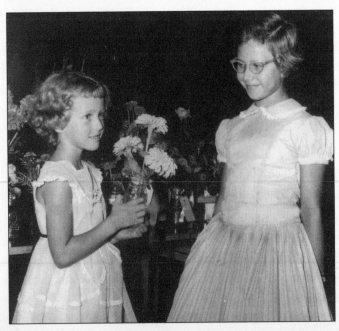

Rhonda, age 6, showing her prize flowers to her older sister, Linda.

PART I

The World of Flower Essences

Beyond the Floral Blanket

Silently I sit on soft grasslands
surrounded by Mother Earth's rainbow colored floral blanket,
I feel the warmth of the sun against my face and
observe the sunlight glistening through the crystal bowl at my feet.

An infusion of Air-Fire-Water-Earth sparks
a creation of Divine Alchemy,
bringing forth a mystery of Nature.

The flowers' fragrance beholds their secrets.
Their enriching colors behold their beauty.
Their unique signatures behold a personality and expression.
The taste of their nectar beholds their essence.
A whole plant journey with a flower beholds a silent presence that heals the Soul.

Oh subtle essence of the flowers,
my mind in silence listens to your prayers and voices
and seeks the wisdom that you share.

I am awakened to your secrets
through my senses.

You have touched me, a doorway opens.

By Rhonda PallasDowney

CHAPTER I
What Are Flower Essences?

Flower essences were first developed in England in the late 1920s and early 1930s by Dr. Edward Bach, who began his career as an orthodox physician and later became a homeopathic physician. As an intuitive healer and practitioner, Dr. Bach constantly sought a simpler, more natural way of healing that dealt with how people's personality traits related to their illnesses. (See Chapter 2 for a more detailed history of Dr. Bach's work.) He was inspired to spend time in nature studying plants: where they grew, what they looked like, and how they tasted. He spent many hours wandering the meadows of England.

After discovering that certain flowers seemed to affect him emotionally in various ways, he began sipping the dew that collected in their petals and leaves. The results were amazing. Bach found that the dew from each plant held a distinct power. He even discovered that just holding his hand over a particular flower would help him in some way — not because of its chemical composition, but because

of its vibrations, its individual nature, and its spiritual qualities.

Bach believed that emotions such as anger, hate, and fear wear down the immune system, leading to physical breakdown, stress, pain, and illness. He concluded that flowers have an energy that can balance human discord, reestablishing the link between body and soul, nature and spirit. He based his remedies on the theory that one should treat the patient, not the disease.

HOW ARE FLOWER ESSENCES MADE?

To extract a flower's unique energy pattern, the flower is picked and placed in a clear glass bowl filled with purified water. The bowl containing the water and the blossoms is then placed in direct sunlight or, in some cases, moonlight.

The energy of the light — sun or moon — transfers the energy of the blossom into the water, extracting a life-force pattern that embodies the character of that flower. This is called an infusion.

Flower essences are vibrational; they are charged with a particular frequency and special quality of a flower's subtle energetic life-force field. The subtle energy pattern is stored within the flower essence and can be used for physical, emotional, mental, and spiritual healing.

Are flower essences safe?

Flower essences are nonaddictive and generally safe. Our company, Living Flower Essences (LFE), prepares them in a formula with a base of brandy or apple cider vinegar, vegetable glycerin, and pure water. They can also be prepared by putting a few drops of the flower essence in hot water and the brandy will evaporate. These essences are highly diluted and are generally recognized as safe for most people. However, if you have any questions or doubts, please check with your health professional before and during use. People who have difficulties consuming alcohol should avoid the brandy base and request an apple cider vinegar base. Also, these products may not be safe for people who are diabetic.

Flower essences are usually safe for babies, children, animals, and the elderly, preferably in a base of apple cider vinegar or vegetable glycerin. If you are giving a flower essence to a small child or an animal, observe the effects and continue or discontinue use based on the response.

When taking a flower essence, you should know what the remedy is for and be clear about your intention. The clearer your intention, the more powerful your relationship with the flower essence will be and the stronger its effects on you.

To have a better understanding of flower essences, let's first review the history and the profundity of the roles between herbalism, homeopathy, and flower essences. All three of these natural forms of healing acknowledge our interde-pen-dence with all of life and honor the plant kingdom as part of our heritage and our environment. All three of these natural approaches have a history of interrelationship with each other, and they each offer a variety of therapeutic effects.

CHAPTER 2
How Herbalism, Homeopathy, and Flower Essences Interrelate

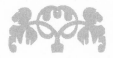

Herbal medicine, homeopathy, and the use of flower essences exist on a continuum. They all offer a natural method of healing and they come from the same source: plants. Plants heal in many ways, affecting us physically, spiritually, and psychologically (both emotionally and mentally).

A History of Folk Medicine and Herbalism

From the earliest days of life on this planet, animals and humans have been naturally dependent on the plant kingdom. Plants have served as a primary source of nourishment and replenishment, as well as being used to heal illness, from colds and coughs to tuberculosis and malaria. Plants were also used in rituals, and certain herbs were believed to contain sacred and magical powers in addition to their medicinal qualities. Folk medicine and herbalism are the oldest form of

health care and the first empirical science, recorded in the scrolls of ancient history.

Herbal remedies have not been selected by any particular individual or group of people. They are selected over generations, in a vast array of cultures, in different times and places. Herbal history is quite extensive. Ancient cultures, including the Greeks and Romans, the Aztec, Maya, and Inca peoples, Islamic, Ayurvedic, Asian, and early North American civilizations, have passed down their wisdom of medicinal plants, animals, and natural substances, some with written documentation. Indians throughout North America learned to treat their illnesses using plant medicine, which they saw as a gift of protection and medicine from Mother Earth.

The records and writings of ancient historians, doctors, alchemists, monks, prophets, philosophers, scientists, "witch" doctors, farmers, and even woodspeople have passed on herbal information, including descriptions of plants and remedies, herbal formulas, methods of preparation, methods of prescribing, symptom treatments, testimonials, and case histories.

The Egyptian Ebers papyrus of 1500 B.C. is the first written account of many medicinal plants and their uses along with incantations and spells. The Vedas, epic poems from India containing herbal lore, were also written in about 1500 B.C. A medical treatise called the *Charaka Samhita,* written in the Middle East in about 700 B.C., includes descriptions of about 350 herbal plants. In about A.D. 70, the Greek physician Dioscorides wrote the first European herbal manual, which included pictures of plants. It was called *De Materia Medica.* These are some of the earliest written accounts of herbal medicines that paved the way for an even greater and more extensive herbal history that exists today.

Other early leaders in the development of medicine include Hippocrates (460–350 B.C.), who is acknowledged for his systematic approach based on tradition and deductive reasoning. He believed that nature cures by itself when not interfered with, and he taught that fasting helped the body to heal. The Greek Empedocles introduced the belief that the universe was made of four elements: earth, water, fire, and air. Plato, who followed Empedocles, also held this belief. The Greek philosopher Aristotle (384–322 B.C.), a student of Plato, added the plant kingdom to the four elements. He also classified herbs into categories or qualities based on their hot, dry, cold, and moist properties. Aristotle's student Theophrastus attempted to classify all plants, animals, and minerals according to these four qualities. The Roman physician Galen (A.D. 131–201) made this approach into a system of medicine. He wrote many books on herbal plant medicines, expanding on the ideas of his predecessors.

Hildegard of Bingen was a twelfth-century German mystic recognized for her knowledge of herbs and spices. Our own English tradition follows in the footsteps of John Gerard, who wrote *The Herball* in 1597, and Nicholas Culpepper who, in 1652, wrote a practical reference book on herbal plants titled *The English Physician.*

The Doctrines of Herbal Medicine

Theophrastus Bombastus von Hohenheim, more widely known as Paracelsus or "the Swiss Hermes" (1493–1541), became a leading medical reformer in his time.[1] Paracelsus taught several key systems known as the "Doctrines," which are still in use by herbalists and homeopaths today. According to Paracelsus, the Doctrines suggest that there is an inherent essence in all of nature known as the "arcana," or hidden property, that is the origin of all natural forms or substances. This essence can only be seen and experienced through "the light of nature, the spiritual eye."[2]

THE DOCTRINE OF CORRESPONDENCE

Paracelsus has been credited with asserting that there is a remedy in nature that corresponds with each organ of the body. There is a correspondence between the microcosm (the individual) and the macrocosm (the whole world, the environment in which we live, the universe) so that the very essence of our organs correspond to the functions of the plant in nature. Therefore, the plants can be medicines for our organs. He called this the "Doctrine of Correspondence."

Paracelsus also asserted, as have many cultures and holistic health-care practitioners, that diseases often have psychological origins and that imbalances in the mind and emotions lead to imbalances in the body, causing ailments to occur. "Our emotions correspond to organs, and both correspond to plants, animals, and minerals of a similar essence or nature."[3] For example, he believed that emotional tension and stress corresponded with indigestion and problems of assimilation and elimination. The positive emotions that correspond with the heart are self-confidence and the love of life. Negative emotions associated with the heart include a tendency to be frightened and a lack of vitality, spirit, and love. The positive emotions that correspond with the kidney are truthfulness, perseverance, self-regulation, good judgment, and freedom from addiction. The negative side is addiction, self-criticism, fear, regrets, and lack of self-control. Matthew Wood offers an in-depth look at the Doctrine of Correspondence. "Each organ, tissue, or function is in correspondence to an underlying archetype or primordial part in the body of the Divine Human. Each disease correlates to a perversion in the function of the underlying archetype. For this reason, the archetypal configurations inherent in the macrocosm are the basis for an understanding of medical phenomena. If an organ is sick, the doctor appeals to the corresponding organ in the macrocosm. This will be personified in a mineral or vegetable which possesses the properties of that organ."[4]

This is to say that the makeup of the universe, above and below, the heavens and the earth, the source of all of creation interrelates with the characteristics of all nature. This includes the very essence of who we are in our human bodies, our virtues, and our powers, and how they are expressed in the world at large. For every created thing in the universe there is something that corresponds to it.

THE DOCTRINE OF SYMPATHIES
(ALSO KNOWN AS THE "LAW OF SIMILARS")

Paracelsus adopted the Latin phrase *similia simiibus curantur,* which means "like cures like." He believed that "the essence of the plant is similar to the essence of the disease, organ, or constitution to which it is suited as medicine. This similarity was, for Paracelsus, the Divine principle behind the cure."[5]

The word "sympathy" is made up of two Greek words and means "with suffering." It refers to self-acceptance and to selecting the plant that best sympathizes with the condition or inner turmoil of the person. It is about selecting the remedy that is most like the condition of the person, and matching the similarities based on the plant's qualities and traits — otherwise known as the "Doctrine of Signatures."

THE DOCTRINE OF SIGNATURES

The Doctrine of Signatures states that the personality and characteristics of a plant are a statement about its medicinal qualities and properties. This doctrine demonstrates the practical use of the Doctrine of Correspondence and plays an important role in gathering information about the plant. The plant's "signature" is an encompassing evaluation of the plant's parts — its leaves, root, stem, flowers, buds, seeds, pods, and fruits — as well as its constitution, shape, color, texture, and appearance and the environment in which it grows. In other words, it would be of interest whether a plant has long or shallow roots; whether its texture is hairy, smooth, fuzzy, or prickly; whether it likes the sun or shade, sandy soil or rich soil; and how it tastes and smells. These traits offer signatures of the plant, and these signatures offer suggestions as to the medicinal value and healing properties of the plant.

An example of the Doctrine of Signatures is given by the plant yarrow. One of this plant's signatures is the feathery, lacy, saw-toothed leaves. The signature of the leaves points to the plant's application as a wound remedy and for treating all the physical conditions that relate to cuts, wounds, burns, blood, and inflammatory conditions. The flowers also have a lacy appearance and are bone-white or sometimes pinkish; this signature also suggests bones and blood. These signatures also show the plant's vulnerability and yet its ability to thrive and heal. Yarrow is known as a remedy to stop nosebleeds, to bring on suppressed menses, to reduce excessive bleeding, and to help break up stagnant blood in the gynecological tract. The plant may also have characteristics that look like the organ. A good example of this is chilidonium for the liver because its yellow sap looks like bile.

The color of a plant is another important signature. For example, red plants such as red root, red lychee berries, and red ginseng root are stimulating and warming, and they revitalize the blood. Generally, blood-building remedies are burgundy in color. Examples are rehmannia root (a Chinese herb for the blood), beet root (a Western herb for the blood), and yellow dock root (the bright seeds are burgundy red). Red plants are associated with the sexual organs and the reproductive system. Orange plants revitalize the adrenal glands, spleen, stomach, bladder, and kidneys. Examples of orange plants are sassafras, California poppy, and pomegranate. Bile is yellow-orange and associated with the liver. Yellow plants invigorate, stimulate, and cleanse the adrenals, stomach, digestive system, assimilation process, liver, and gall bladder.

contemporary Herbalism

Herbalists today value the whole plant, using various parts including the roots, stem, seeds, bark, leaves, flowers, and fruits for specific purposes. There is a general understanding among Western herbal practitioners that the plant used as a whole, rather than as separate parts, has a more powerful therapeutic effect than the active constituents of its individual parts. Through scientific research, clinical observation, traditional hands-on experience with the whole plant, storytelling, and testimonials, we access a greater understanding of each plant as a whole and of its medicinal qualities.

The Western biomedical model and the Chinese herbal model generally offer two different systems for approaching herbal medicine. The Western approach is more analytical and quantitative, based on logic, and focused on isolated body parts or disease conditions. The Chinese approach is more qualitative and holistic, based on observation, integration, synthesis, and the treatment of whole patterns of disharmony.

Many modern Western herbalists combine the two approaches, utilizing the strengths of each and finding neither to be right or wrong. The two approaches are like the Chinese concepts of *yang* (the Western and more analytic, logical, masculine approach) and *yin* (the Chinese and more spatial, harmonious, integrative, and feminine approach). As opposites, they complement each other and form an integrated whole in the study and practice of herbal medicine.

Many herbs used commonly today — German chamomile, osha, echinacea, ephedra, goldenseal, ginseng, and hawthorn — were selected millennia ago. Knowledge about them has been passed down and built upon through generation and cultures. Herbs are the natural basis for nearly 25 percent of all prescription drugs on the market today. Almost 75 percent of these herb-based drugs are used consistently with their traditional use. Out of the approximately 500,000 plants on earth, it is estimated that about 10,000 are used regularly for medicinal purposes. Such plants include the opium poppy, which produces the powerful painkiller morphine; the Peruvian bark, cinchona, which has quinine — a cure for malaria — as an active constituent; foxglove, or digitalis, which contains cardiac glycosides that tone the heart and is made into a heart medicine called digoxin; and ephedra, which is an active component of many prescription drugs and over-the-counter medicines used to treat asthma, hay fever, colds, and flu.

Herbs are processed into various forms: the whole loose herb, teas, extracts and tinctures, capsules, tablets, essential oils, salves, balms, ointments, plasters, poultices, decoctions, infusions, medicated ghee, syrups, douches, inhalers, compresses, cosmetics, creams, lotions, liniments, floral waters, spices, oils, vinegars, butters, sachets, soaps, and incense.

Homeopathy

Many people who have experience with herbs find themselves opening to another healing avenue of the plant and mineral kingdoms: homeopathy. Concepts similar to those of homeopathy date back to as early as 460–350 B.C. in ancient Greece. At that time Hippocrates, known as the father of medicine, wrote: "By similar things a disease is produced and through the application of the like, it is cured,"[6] much like the Law of Similars. Hippocrates also believed, like homeopaths, that it was the nature of the organism that healed the patient. Hippocrates, Aristotle, Galen, and Paracelsus were also great contributors to the body of wisdom that became homeopathy. Unfortunately, they lacked the scientific evidence to back up some of their theories.

Dr. Samuel Hahnemann

Dr. Samuel Hahnemann (1755–1843), a German physician, is recognized as the founder of homeopathy. During Hahnemann's time, the medical field lacked humane treatment and was based on violent ways of ridding the human body of disease. Conditions such as whooping cough or pregnancy were often treated with a knife to rid a person of several pints of blood. Other conditions were treated with large doses of poison or with purgatives such as extensive enemas, violent laxatives, and nauseating emetics.

In 1778, Hahnemann wrote his first medical essay, "Directions for Curing Old Diseases." In it, he stressed the need for radical change in the medical field. He emphasized fundamental public hygiene needs, such as proper sewage, spaced housing, fresh air, and adequate diet, sleep, and exercise. He strove for a compassionate, humanitarian system of medicine. To Hahnemann, this included quick, permanent restoration of health with few or no side effects. It also meant treating the whole person and the whole disease, based on scientific principles.

While translating an English text — *A Treatise on Materia Medica,* by William Cullen — into German, Hahnemann discovered a type of experiment, which he later called a "proving," that would open the doorway to a new medical era and become the basis of what was later to be called homeopathy. Hahnemann found that by taking doses of cinchona, a Peruvian bark *(Cortex Peruvianus)* used to cure malaria, symptoms similar to those of malaria occurred. These symptoms, such as drowsiness, cold feet and fingertips, trembling, increased pulse and heart beat, thirst, and redness of the cheeks, recurred each time he took cinchona. He then administered cinchona to normal, healthy people and discovered that they experienced the same symptoms. Next, he gave cinchona to people who were stricken with malaria and observed improvement and recovery in many of these people's lives. Through this experiment, he "proved" that the remedy cinchona would cause the same symptoms as those of the disease it cured.

This experiment with cinchona led Hahnemann to adopt the principle of "like treats like," or the Law of Similars, as a globally effective therapeutic principle. In applying this approach, Hahnemann was the first person to substantiate the theory set forth by his predecessors, Hippocrates, Aristotle, Galen, Stahl, and Paracelsus.

Hahnemann continued to test substance after substance, experimenting with himself and others to understand and document how each one affected the human body. He called his new system of medicine "homeopathy," which was derived from the Greek words *homion* and *pathos,* meaning "the cure is like the disease." Later, the term *allopathy* — which means "the cure is unrelated to the disease" — was given to conventional medicine.

From 1791 to 1843, Hahnemann researched, experimented, documented, and proclaimed the primary principles of homeopathy: the Law of Similars, provings, posology (the infinitesimal dose), and treating the whole person. He believed, and demonstrated repeatedly, that by administering a specific remedy to healthy people, the remedy would cause the same symptoms as those of the disease it could cure.

Hahnemann gradually amassed a substantial knowledge base, known as a *materia medica* (a compilation of experimental data and literature about the effectiveness of numerous remedies in treating particular conditions) and repertory (the list of remedies included in the *materia medica).* Much of this *materia medica* was based on provings. A proving is a systematic method of testing substances on healthy people in order to clarify the symptoms that demonstrate the action of the substance. Provings provide the background information by which a particular remedy can be selected for a person. "In this way, the symptom manifestation of the patient and the symptom manifestation of the remedy are matched, thus enabling the principles of resonance to excite and

strengthen the defense mechanisms of the patient and bring about cure."7

The formulation of a *materia medica* also includes clinical experience, wherein a given remedy is administered to sick people according to the symptoms that occurred in the provings. Data collection includes documenting the symptoms that are cured during the healing process of the whole person. As a complete picture of a given remedy is gathered from various sources, including toxicological literature, provings, and clinical observations, the remedy is then ready to be included in the *materia medica.* A *materia medica* contains the results of such provings, as well as an entire symptom picture of a given remedy and its "essential personality."

Over time, Hahnemann and his volunteers showed that these remedies were a natural means to help the body heal itself — a method preferable to suppressing disease, which robs the body of its natural healing process. Through his provings, Hahnemann also found that infinitesimally small doses of substances were safe, free from side effects, and therapeutically effective; this became one of the bases (posology) of formulating homeopathic remedies. Hahnemann also learned that, while homeopathic remedies can be administered in powerful potencies, they are nonaddictive and nontoxic, making them far superior to the common treatments of the day.

The Hahnemann method of potentization and preparation of homeopathic remedies includes two unique steps. The first step is the serial (or sequential) dilution of the mother tincture, which is mixed with alcohol and water. The mother tincture is the most concentrated form of plant or animal substance. It is prepared by breaking down a fresh substance in various strengths of alcohol. The substance is then aged anywhere from one hour to one month; the solid particles, which have become suspended in the liquid, are then filtered out by gravity or compression. The strengths of the final alcohol mixture depend on the water content.

The second step is the "succussion" of the dilution, by which vigorous shaking creates a powerful effect known as "potentization." Hahnemann discovered that the more a remedy was diluted or "succussed" (vigorously tapped or shaken to release the molecular energy of the substance into an alcohol-and-water solution), the greater its potency. In preparing decimal series of potentizations, one part of the mother tincture and nine parts of a 20- or 30-percent mixture of alcohol and pure water is put in a glass container. The mixture is succussed, providing an initial potency of "1X." One part of this solution is then put into another glass container, and nine parts of the alcohol/water mixture are added. The solution is then succussed again, creating a potency of "2X." Further dilutions and succussions are repeated to produce successive potencies of "3X," "4X," and so on. Thus, the principle "less is more" came into homeopathy.

Hahnemann stressed that "the patient, not the disease" such as arthritis or leukemia, must be given attention. When a homeopathic diagnosis is given for an ailment, it includes an investigation and understanding of all the symptoms, integrating physical, mental, and emotional imbalances.

Hahnemann has written numerous essays and books about his discoveries in homeopathic medicine. The most popular are the *Organon of Medicine* and *Materia Medica Pura*. The *Organon* is still universally acknowledged as the substantiated document on the therapeutic practice of homeopathy. Six editions of the *Organon* have been published, and it has been translated into ten languages. The *Materia Medica Pura* is recognized as an established medical reference book for homeopaths around the world. It includes results of many scientific provings conducted by Hahnemann.

constantine Hering

Another great doctor of homeopathy is Constantine Hering, known for his law of healing called the "Law of Direction of Cure," or "Hering's Law." This law states that in order for true healing to take place, it must first begin at the deepest and most vital parts of the person, then proceed to the less vital parts. It is the process of sorting out impurities from within to without, from above downward, and allowing symptoms to leave the body in the reverse order of how they began. Since Hahnemann's time, numerous other homeopaths have contributed greatly to the base of knowledge in this field, including William Boericke, M.D., James Tyler Kent, A.M., M.D., John Henry Clarke, M.D., and Margaret Tyler, among many others (see the bibliography for their works).

flower essences

Dr. Edward Bach was a great British homeopathic physician and healer who trusted his intuition and inner knowledge. He followed his instincts and trusted his personal sense of self, his insights, and his understanding of the relationship between people and their diseases.

Bach had one goal in life: to find a safe, simple way to heal physical, mental, and emotional imbalance. His compassion for people and his love of nature led him to just such a cure: flower essences.

Bach began his career in 1915 at University College Hospital in London, England, as an orthodox physician specializing in bacteriology. Through his studies of vaccination, bacteriology, and immunology, he discovered certain types of bacteria in the gastrointestinal tract of people with chronic illnesses such as arthritis and rheumatoid disorders. Bach proved that by injecting people with vaccines made from intestinal bacteria, a cleansing of the system occurred, which created noticeable improvements in these chronic symptoms.

In 1917, Dr. Bach became ill from a severe hemorrhagic disease and resigned from University College Hospital the following year. In 1919, after his recovery, he joined the staff at the London Homeopathic Hospital as a pathologist and bacteriologist. Here Bach was given Dr.

Samuel Hahnemann's book, the *Organon of Medicine,* to help him better understand the philosophy of the hospital. Bach soon learned that his own discoveries in bacteriology were similar to those of Hahnemann.

Like Hahnemann, Bach believed that once a remedy was given to a patient, a second dose shouldn't be given until the first was no longer effective. Bach also believed in giving minute doses of toxic substances to cure illnesses, which was similar to Hahnemann's homeopathic theory.

Reading of Hahnemann's research and discoveries inspired Bach to adopt his concept of "treating the patient, not the disease." Bach then decided to abandon the vaccine concept, and instead prepared homeopathic remedies to treat illness related to intestinal bacteria by administering these remedies orally.

Dr. Bach's Bowel Nosodes

Bach categorized seven types of bacteria, all of which were related to chronic illnesses. He then found that each of these seven bacterial types were related to seven different personalities and their emotional expressions. He then developed treatments for each type, which he referred to as "bowel nosodes." Bowel nosodes may be considered as great cleansing powers that address specific intestinal bacteria within the human body. The nosodes were prepared as homeopathic remedies, based on the actual substance of the disease. This was a gentler approach than vaccines.

Although Bach's bowel nosodes were

successful in treating his patients, he was dissatisfied that they didn't cure all chronic diseases. Bach then endeavored to replace the substance of the disease with plants that were characteristic of each bacterial group in their effects.

In his clinical research, Bach found that patients in a given personality group reacted to their illnesses similarly to each other in their moods, behaviors, and states of mind. He began to identify the emotional and mental states of his patients in order to choose a remedy to cure the chronic illness. Again, the concept of "treating the person, not the disease," was emphasized. Bach's seven nosodes became known and used worldwide, both by homeopaths and allopaths.

Dr. Bach's Recognition in the Medical Field

In 1926, Dr. Bach published a book entitled *Chronic Disease: A Working Hypothesis,* written with his London Homeopathic Hospital colleague Dr. C. E. Wheeler. Bach also studied the effects of diet and vaccine in relation to disease and, in 1924, he addressed the British Homeopathic Congress with a paper entitled "Intestinal Toxemia in its Relation to Cancer."

In 1928, Dr. Bach wrote another paper, "An Effective Method of Combating Intestinal Toxaemia," which was printed in the journal *Medical World.* In January of 1929, he published a paper entitled "The Rediscovery of Psora" in the *British Homoeopathic Journal,* announcing a purer approach to medicine.[8]

Dr. Bach's Discovery of Flower Essences

Meanwhile, Bach yearned to develop an approach to healing that would be based in nature's plant kingdom; that would include identifying, understanding, and changing a disharmonious relationship with one's self; and that would replace mental, emotional, and spiritual anguish with balance, peace, belonging, and happiness.

His love of nature and the outdoors inspired Bach to seek plants with qualities that resembled human nature. Through his observations of people, he further identified certain human personality types and correlated them with particular plant expressions and personalities.

He found two particularly appropriate and beautiful plants — impatiens and mimulus — growing near a mountain stream in the English countryside. He returned to London and prepared them in a fashion similar to his oral vaccines. He then prescribed for each patient the flower that related to the patient's personality.

Later in the same year, he then found another appropriate plant, clematis. Bach found that impatiens was helpful for dealing with tension and irritability; mimulus helped people overcome fears and shyness; and clematis addressed daydreaming, inattentiveness, and indifference. These three flowers were the beginning of a new system that was to eventually comprise thirty-eight flower remedies.

Toward the end of 1929, Bach was so deeply inspired by the effects of these three plants and the purity of their extraction that he decided to replace the bowel nosodes with flower remedies and to further his exploration and study of plants. He felt that the intestinal flora in the bowel nosodes were not as pure as flower essences. He gave up preparing oral vaccines and all other methods of treatment to pursue more time in nature studying plants. He observed the moods, personalities, mannerisms, habits, characteristics, and every response of his patients to disease, then sought plants that matched the personality of the patient.

In 1930, Bach published an article entitled "Some New Remedies and Their Uses" in the journal *Homeopathic World*. He gave up all other forms of treatment and focused only on plants as healing agents. He left his prestigious medical practice at the height of his career, and he began to prepare for a new work that was guided by his intuition and wisdom. He was determined to let go of less natural ways of healing and to study a purer and simpler way of healing provided by nature.

Bach went to live in Cromer, a small village in Wales. He studied many kinds of plants and made observations of where they grew, the way they grew, the kind of soil they grew in, and the color, shape, and number of their petals. He tried to grasp the whole picture of the plant, its habits, and characteristics, working toward applying the Doctrine of Signatures.

By spending time in sitting with, studying, and imbibing plants, Bach became more finely attuned to the mysteries of nature, enhancing his sensory and intuitive awareness. Through this heightened internal development, he acquired the ability to perceive the plant's vibrations and the powers it emanated. Bach was so sensitive to subtle energies that he was able to feel the effects of a given flower by touching its petal or its morning dew to his tongue. Some flowers produced a positive, uplifting effect, while others produced a more negative, draining effect.

Dr. Bach's preparation of flower remedies

Dr. Bach concluded that the life force of the plant was held in its flower, which also carried the seed. He further believed that the flower was at its greatest potency when in full bloom in midsummer, when the days were the longest and the sun was at its peak. He selected flowers that were rich in character, colorful, and at their height of bloom.

While walking through a field in an early morning dew, Bach realized that the dewdrop embodied the properties of the plant on which it rested. The heat of the sun, energized through the fluid of the dewdrop, drew out the plant's properties into the dewdrop and exalted it with its power. Bach believed that this simple form of extracting the healing properties of the plant was profound. He began to collect the dew from flowers, shake the dewdrops into bottles, take them back to London to prepare as remedies, and give those remedies to his patients.

But collecting dew from flowers was a time-consuming process, and Bach sought a more direct method to extract a plant's qualities. He picked a few blossoms from several similar plants growing in the same area and placed them in a glass bowl filled with water from a clear stream. He covered the entire surface of the water with petals and left them in full sunlight for several hours or until the petals faded slightly, to make certain their medicinal properties had been released into the water.

Bach found that the water was energized by the power of the blossoms, creating a potent remedy and eliminating the need for homeopathic means of potentization or succussion. He then removed the petals from the glass bowl and preserved the liquid essence of the flower by adding it to brandy. Bach was pleased with this simple new method; it contained the four natural elements — earth, water, fire (the sun), and air — as well as the "essence" of the flower. Interestingly, this essence was earlier referred to by the Pythagoreans and Paracelsians as the "quintessence" or "fifth essence," an invisible spiritual energy source that is experienced as an expression of the soul. As a whole, the four elements and the "essence" produced a powerful, effective means of healing.

Bach also developed the "boiling method," in which various parts of a plant are boiled in water rather than using the "sun method." In 1930, he wrote about his new boiling method of preparation in a paper entitled "Some Fundamental Considerations of Disease and Cure," published in *The Homeopathic World*. Today, the Bach Flower Remedies are prepared by

the application of heat through either the sun method or the boiling method.

Dr. Bach's Link of the Human Personality to Flower Remedies

In 1931, Bach wrote a book called *Heal Thyself*, which described how certain emotions and moods can lead to illness. He then wrote another book in 1932 — *Free Thyself* — based on his belief that happiness is the foundation of good health. His assertion was that happiness is uplifting and helps us move beyond our barriers and challenges, while unhappiness drains our energy, brings us down, and leads to disease.

Bach continued to explore how people's personality traits could be grouped and correlated with disease states. He focused on treating his patients' moods and states of mind, seeking remedies that would cure the emotions as the underlying cause of illness. "Treat the patient's personality and not the disease" became his new principle.

As Dr. Bach progressed in his exploration and understanding of flower remedies, he further came to believe that, instead of treating or trying to aggravate the disease, it was more wholesome to introduce into the patient's life the positive virtue that would counteract the disease. He also observed that his flower remedies were more deeply effective and longer lasting than other methods for treating the emotional and mental imbalances of an individual.

Bach further noticed that the flower remedies heightened his patients' personal awareness and spiritual awakening. This became another avenue for physical healing through balancing and uplifting one's emotions, mind, and spirit. The higher vibrational pattern of the remedies provided a healing from the inner spark of a person's higher consciousness. The person thus became more in tune with and devoted to a deeper awareness and a higher path of living, which opened the doorway toward active participation in the healing process.

Dr. Edward Bach's Last Years

Bach treated many patients with his new system of flower remedies. He was especially fond of the fishermen and lifeboat men of Cromer, whom he treated in trade for fish, eggs, or vegetables. On one occasion, Bach treated a shipwrecked boatman who was unconscious, nearly frozen, and foaming at the mouth. Bach gave the man three flower essences: Rock Rose for terror and panic, Clematis to overcome fainting, and Impatiens to relieve tension. He administered doses of the remedies at frequent intervals, and the man regained consciousness within minutes.

This was the birth of the flower-essence formula known today as Rescue Remedy. Bach later added Cherry Plum (for fear of losing control) and Star of Bethlehem (for trauma and numbness). Rescue Remedy is known as the thirty-ninth Bach remedy and is used in emergencies as a first-aid treatment for such conditions as shock, trauma, terror, panic, tension, and passing out. It is also given to people who have witnessed a violent or traumatic incident or are about to undergo an operation.

In 1934, Bach left Cromer to search for a quiet village in England. In Oxfordshire, England, he found a small house that bore the name "Mount Vernon." There in the countryside, he found and prepared the Wild Oak remedy and continued to seek new plants that eventually made up Bach's thirty-eight individual remedies. He visited London weekly to test the remedies on his patients and to collect data for his research.

In 1936, Dr. Bach published another small book entitled *The Twelve Healers and Other Remedies*. In this book, he placed the thirty-eight remedies under seven descriptive headings:

- For Fear
- For Uncertainty
- For Insufficient Interest in Present Circumstances
- For Loneliness
- For Those Oversensitive to Influences and Ideas
- For Despondency or Despair
- For Over-Care for Welfare of Others

For example, under the heading "For Fear," Bach listed Mimulus (for treating known fears, such as fear of the dark, pain, accidents, and illness), Cherry Plum (for treating fear of doing harm to self and others), and Aspen (for treating fears of the unknown). Under the heading "For Insufficient Interest in Present Circumstances," he listed Clematis (to treat indifference, inattentiveness, daydreaming), Honeysuckle (to treat nostalgia and homesickness), and Wild Rose (to treat apathy and general lack of interest in life). Each particular character of the plant was then matched with a given patient's symptoms.

Around this time, Dr. Bach's health declined due to the physical stress of moving, house renovation, completing the research for the thirty-eight remedies, and completing his last book. He gradually became weaker, and on November 27, 1936, he died in his sleep.

Dr. Edward Bach accomplished a great deal in his fifty years of living, and he succeeded in his goal of finding gentle, simple ways to promote healing.

The Development of Flower Essences since Dr. Bach's Time

The Bach Flower Remedies continue to be an inspiration to many and are used by practitioners worldwide. Prior to Bach's death, he arranged for the Nelson Company to bottle his remedies and market them for sale. Today, the mother essence tinctures are prepared at the Dr. Edward Bach Centre at Mount Vernon, and A. Nelson & Co. Ltd., in Wimbledon, England, sells and distributes the Bach Flower Remedies. Today, Bach Flower Remedies are a familiar item in many health-food stores in the U.S., and they are known worldwide.

It was not until the late 1970s that a new series of flower essences was developed by Richard Katz and Patricia Kaminski, founders of the Flower Essence Society (FES) of Nevada City, California. FES began to introduce flower essences made according to Dr. Bach's method of preparation and using native plants of California. This inspired other flower essence practitioners to make flower essences from the native plants of their own geographic areas.

Dr. Bach himself may not have been satisfied with his thirty-eight single remedies. Had he lived longer, he might well have been guided to pursue new plants as remedies. The study and clinical use of flower essences is as unlimited as the number of flowers themselves. Exploring and experiencing native plants from various geographic regions can be helpful in the treatment of mind/body/soul/spirit. We have the freedom to evolve beyond any limitations set forth by one location or time period.

We are still pioneers in this wonderful exploration of healing with flower essences. As we continue to seek out new remedies, may we uphold the simplicity, purity, and beauty that Dr. Edward Bach has led us to understand. Dr. Bach himself implied that through the development of our individual expressions we serve our divine nature and highest good — and that through this divinity we can connect with our own divine power and free ourselves. Flower essences aid us in this connection and help us gain personal freedom and self-empowerment in our soul's journey.

Summary: Similarities and Differences

Now that we have reviewed the intertwined yet distinct histories of herbalism, homeopathy, and flower essences, we have a background for comparing how each is used in practice today.

Applying the Doctrine of Signatures

Examples are the best way to understand both the concept of plant signatures and the differences among herbalism, homeopathy, and flower essences. I've included a few illustrative cases here.

The onion's main signature is the odor and vapor that induce sneezing and cause the eyes and nose to water. Therefore, onion (Latin name *Allium cepa*) is a remedy given for head colds with symptoms of sneezing, watery nasal secretion, and mild tearing. An herbalist may recommend drinking cooked onion broth when the above symptoms occur. A homeopath may recommend taking *Allium cepa* to relieve the head cold and sneezing. A flower essence practitioner may recommend the Onion flower essence to help release suppressed feelings of grief and sadness by peeling off old emotional layers to get to the "heart" of the matter.

The chamomile flower's gentle appearance and sweet fragrance offer a light, sunny, peaceful, relaxed disposition. The plant contains a volatile blue oil that has a soothing, peaceful presence. Chamomile is used to treat irritability, nervousness, and tension, especially in children. An herbalist may recommend drinking chamomile as a tea to relieve a headache or to settle the stomach. A homeopath will check the "keynotes," or primary traits, of Chamo-

milla, which in the case of children's conditions is one cheek hot and flushed and the other cheek pale and cold. Teething, peevishness, restlessness, sleeplessness, crying uncontrollably, and colic give crucial indications for Chamomilla. Hot, green, watery stools are also a feature of the Chamomilla type. A homeopath will also look for "modalities," such as the child improves in warm, wet weather and from being carried or rocked; the child's condition worsens in tantrums, anger, open air, and at night from 9:00 P.M. to midnight. A flower essence practitioner may give a Chamomilla flower essence to release emotional tension and to restore emotional balance and relaxation. A Chamomilla flower essence given to an adult creates a peaceful, balanced emotional relationship to the illness through understanding and sympathizing with the underlying emotion that caused the illness.

Mullein has several powerful signatures. Its stalk is stout, thick, and tall and its base is especially strong. The entire plant is soft, fuzzy, and velvety, resembling the soft hairs of the mucous membranes. The plant's character of strength along with softness represents its ability to release coughing and bronchial spasms that damage the soft hairs lining the mucous membranes. The woolly earlike leaf resembles a donkey's ear and points to the plant's use as an ear oil made from the flower. The absorbent quality of mullein's leaves is also significant; they act as a relaxant and they promote absorption in cellular dropsy, chronic diseases, pleuritic effusions, and similar accumulations of fluid. On another level, this signature can be related to a person's process of assimilating certain emotional and mental states that no longer serve the individual. Through the process of assimilation, the individual is able to most effectively take in and incorporate what can be absorbed. Mullein is used both herbally and homeopathically to treat such conditions as earaches, catarrhs, colds, hoarseness, bronchitis, and coughs. On a subtler level, Mullein flower essence is used to promote strength with softness, enhancing intimacy and gentleness. The flower essence also assists in assimilating emotional and mental states that we no longer want to hold on to.

commonalities among Herbalism, Homeopathy, and flower essences

We can now see that these three healing modalities have a great deal in common.

1. All are natural methods of healing.
2. All are used to build up a person's vital force.
3. All include treatment based on acute and/or chronic disease.
4. All strive to treat the whole person, highlighting the uniqueness of each individual (this is not true of all herbalists, but it is typical of Western herbalists).
5. All may incorporate integrative thinking, embracing the interaction of inductive reasoning and intuitive spiritual insight.
6. All rely on quality of remedy, not quantity (however, herbalists regard quantity as important).
7. All may utilize the Doctrine of Signatures and integrate plant history, although the history of each of these areas is unique.
8. All may include a diagnostic procedure that describes the nature, location, origin, and progression of the disease.
9. All relate to the vital force as the principle by which the disease can be known. The symptoms, as a whole, suggest the means of transformation back to health or restoration of the vital force.
10. All offer remedies that may calm, activate, confront, resolve, relieve, regulate, remove, free, cleanse, comfort, strengthen, restore, stimulate, restrain, increase, cause, promote, drain, or expel symptoms.
11. All can incorporate the chakra system (described in part II).
12. All may offer a mindful and conscious journey into personal awareness, self-empowerment, and spiritual guidance.
13. All have an interwoven history, though the history of each is unique.
14. All offer a variety of therapeutic effects.
15. All acknowledge the contacts and the gifts of the plant kingdom.
16. All strive for balance, healing, natural body rhythm, and living life to its fullest.

17. All can incorporate the four ele-
    ments: earth, air, water, and fire.
18. All are most effective when a person
    is open to higher values and takes
    responsibility for personal growth
    and positive action.

significant differences in the practice of herbalism, homeopathy, and flower essences

While these natural healing practices have
a great deal in common, they are also distinguished from each other by a number
of features.

Herbalism

1. Commonly applied to the daily diet
   as a supplement and nutritive.
2. Taken mostly as the plant's physical
   parts: leaves, stem, root, berries or
   fruit, flowers.
3. Can be applied as a specific to act
   on an organ or tissue or as a tonic
   with general properties.
4. Includes numerous external uses
   (poultices, oils) as well as many
   internally ingestible forms (capsules,
   tablets, teas, infusions, tinctures).
5. Commonly applied as several herbs
   in combination.
6. May be mildly homeopathic due to
   the processes of diluting, shaking,
   triturating (producing potencies in
   a solid form), and boiling. The
   method of preparation varies
   according to the herb and its use.

7. Treats symptoms according to the
   organs of the body rather than the
   symptoms of the body, as in homeopathy.
8. Does not apply the principle "less is
   more."
9. Utilizes remedies derived from
   plants only, commonly from
   the plant's roots, leaves, and stems.
   The method of extraction and use
   of herbs is concentrated more on
   the physical level.
10. Based on methods of selection
    passed down over the millennia,
    from culture to culture, from gener-
    ation to generation, combining tra-
    ditional use, testimonials, and
    scientific research.
12. May include a diagnostic procedure
    that describes the nature, location,
    origin, and progression of the dis-
    ease.
13. Relates to the vital force as the
    principle by which the disease can
    be known. The symptoms as a
    whole suggest the means of trans-
    formation back to health, or
    restoration of the vital force.

Homeopathy

1. Evaluates the energetic or sympto-
   matic blueprint or matrix of the
   disease in great detail. The remedy
   is like a hologram; it gives all the
   representation of the disease without the substance and works
   with the totality of an organism.
2. Treats toxic symptoms, otherwise

described as the most serious underlying condition of a disease. Negative vibrations from the diseased state are transformed by the positive healing vibrations.

3. Because of the dilution and succussion process, the remedy goes to a higher vibrational state than the direct plant herbal form, producing a positive polarity. The higher vibration addresses greater extremes of emotional/mental disorders and can cure deep pathology in physical, emotional, and mental realms. When the emotional/mental body has been disturbed in addition to the physical body, a homeopathic remedy is advised over an herbal remedy.

4. Remedies are prepared from pure animal, vegetable, or mineral substances given in the form of granules or lactose-based tablets.

5. The primary principle is "like treats like."

6. The vital force of a given patient plays a significant role in determining potency for that person. There are certain cases in which low potencies should be given first: people with weak constitutions, the elderly, and hypersensitive people should initially be given potencies ranging from 6x to 30c. Higher potencies can overstimulate lowered or weak defense systems, which could cause unnecessary aggravations. Keep in mind that the guiding principle of selection and potency is the clarity of the symptom picture and the degree of certainty the homeopath has about the remedy.

7. Remedies are more sensitive and can be easily counteracted by certain herbs. A person needs to be aware of such interactions.

8. Once a constitutional remedy is given to a patient, a second dose shouldn't be given until the first is no longer effective.

9. Generally deals more with regions and symptoms of the body, as opposed to organs of the body as in herbalism.

10. Unlike herbs and flower essences, remedies are also made from diseased products and poisons, although many homeopathic remedies are derived from plants.

11. Departs from the use of root and leaves, though the "whole plant" concept is still valuable.

12. Remedies are selected based on Hahnemann's provings and similar provings since his time. The *Materia Medica* is based on what allopathic doctors were using as medicine; there aren't as many herbs used.

13. Remedies work directly and powerfully on the physical body, influencing the emotional and mental aspects of healing, thus affecting higher states of consciousness.

14. The remedy, especially a high dosage, may cause an agitation of

the symptoms. The vital force is provoked and stimulates the defense mechanism to cure itself.

FLOWER ESSENCES

1. Can be used with both herbal and homeopathic remedies.

2. Help us develop a direct relationship with the spirit of the plant, or the plant's quintessence (herbs especially and homeopathic remedies sometimes do this).

3. Are diluted, but the process differs from that used in herbalism or homeopathy. Flower essences are generally taken as liquid drops of brandy, water, and the mother tincture. The dilution process is much simpler than that used in homeopathy.

4. Are prepared by the application of heat, either through the sun method or the boiling method. The healing essence of the flower heads or plant parts is released through water. This method, according to Dr. Bach, potentizes the remedy or healing essence, and there is no need for the homeopathic means of potentization or succussion.

5. May employ the principle of "like treats like," or may involve remedies that confront or elevate.

6. Are known more as social/emotional/mental/spiritual remedies in which the source of the vibrational healing pattern begins in the higher consciousness of an individual. This higher vibrational pattern provides a healing from within the inner spark of a person's higher consciousness, heightening spirituality. Practitioners treat the emotional/mental symptoms in relation to the physical disease in a deep, gentle way that inspires the totality of an individual. Flower essences may be longer lasting, and they bring a person more in tune with and devoted to a deeper awareness and a higher path of living.

7. Are a subtle vibrational essence charged with a particular frequency and special quality influenced by a flower's energetic life force. Flower essences are stored in the purer and more easily accessed parts of plants and flowers, which allow their healing power to be readily released. Thus the goal of healing with flower essences is a more subtle, gentle, natural way of healing.

8. Can be given one at a time or in combination according to the intention, need, and desire of the recipient as well as the expertise of the practitioner.

9. Are generally administered on a repetitive basis, usually three or four drops, two to four times a day, for days, weeks, or even months according to individual needs. This allows time for inner growth and outward manifestations without agitation or side effects. The frequency of the dosage also creates a

devotion within the individual, which serves as a catalyst in overcoming the imbalances and negative aspects of the personality.

10. Are chosen mainly through people's attraction to certain flowers and their signatures.

11. Are considered by many to be a type of homeopathy, while herbs are not.

conclusion

There are many ways to conceptualize and work with herbs, homeopathy, or flower essences. Ultimately, what we do and how we relate to these forms of healing is up to each of us individually. Sometimes our symptoms may appear to be primarily spiritual, mental, emotional, or physical, yet our healing is an integration of all these levels. We can't always tell how we will react to a plant or flower until we are actually taking it and responding to it. The healing process is even more powerful when we become aware of what is going on with us at every level.

By establishing a new relationship with the sacred nature of a plant, we can come to recognize and acknowledge our own soul. The ignition of this sacred flame within the soul will spark our personality selves and help us realize and draw from the energy of our soul. This is what Gary Zukav refers to as "authentic empowerment — the alignment of the personality with the soul."[9] Every day brings new opportunities to align our personality selves with our soul. As we become more and more in touch with ourselves, we will discover a natural energy that utilizes our higher power and aligns us with the personality and the soul. We will find that our personality begins to embrace choices that offer evolutionary growth and a deeper understanding of ourselves and of living and loving life.

The choices we make to use an herb, a homeopathic remedy, or a flower essence may vary from time to time, from circumstance to circumstance, and from person to person. Understanding and experiencing the gifts that plants offer helps us to align this sacred relationship between plants, our soul, and our personality. This alignment awakens us to ourselves and to the plant kingdom, empowering our relationship with the earth.

PART II

Chakras and Flower Essences

The Language of Flowers

There is a language, little known,
Lovers claim it as their own.
Its symbols smile upon the land,
Wrought by Natures wondrous hand;
And in their silent beauty speak,
Of life and joy, to those who seek
For love divine, and sunny hours
In the language of the flowers.

By F. L. W.

CHAPTER 3
An Introduction to the Chakra System

In working with flower essences, it is valuable to understand and work with the chakra system — a network of subtle energy centers within the body. This energy system has been recognized throughout history by ancient spiritual traditions, from Eastern religions to Western mysticism. As we open our awareness to the chakra energy centers, we become more in touch with who we are. Each chakra is related to a different part of the physical body and its functions. Because each flower essence corresponds to a particular chakra, exploring the chakra system will increase the effectiveness of healing with flower essences.

Chakra is a Sanskrit word that means "wheel of light," or "circle and movement." In Tibetan literature, the word *khor-lo,* or "wheel," refers to the same subtle energy centers. In Sufi teachings, the energy centers are referred to as *latifas* or "subtle ones." Positions on the Native American medicine wheel represent energy centers in the body and the energy field of the earth itself; through these centers, the plant and animal kingdoms resonate with our being. In the *Metaphysical Bible Dictionary* of Unity Church, reference is made to the golden candlestick with its seven lamps of the tabernacle: "The tabernacle and the Temple represented the body of man, and the seven centers in the organism, through which intelligence is expressed."[1] In early Christianity, these centers were also referred to as "the seven centers in the soul of man."[2]

The chakras are also associated with the colors of the rainbow. In the Old Testament, God sent a rainbow at the end of the great flood as a sign of change, harmony, and union with God. "And God said, 'This is the sign of the covenant which I make between me and you and every living creature that is with you, for all future generations. I set my bow in the cloud, and it shall be a sign of the covenant between me and the earth.'"[3]

To this day, people are awed by the

sight of a rainbow; it offers a mystical light, energy, color, and hope. According to ancient traditions, rainbow energy patterns or centers exist around every living thing and are expressed in the chakras. Each chakra is associated with a different color of the rainbow, as we will explore more deeply in this and later chapters.

A Brief Historical perspective on chakras and the Human Energy field

Numerous esoteric teachings address the energy centers, including ancient Hindu Vedic writings as well as those of the Pythagoreans, Theosophists, Rosicrucians, Native American medicine people, Tibetan and Indian Buddhists, Chinese herbalists, and Western mystics. Scholars throughout the millennia also addressed subtle energy fields, including Boirac and Liebeault in the twelfth century; Paracelsus in the sixteenth century; and Helmont, Mesmer, and James Clark Maxwell in the nineteenth century.

In the mid-1800s, Count Wilhelm Von Reichenbach researched the properties of what he called the "odic" force for nearly thirty years. He discovered that in the odic energy field, or subtle life-force energy field, like poles attract each other, rather than opposite poles attracting each other as in electromagnetism (this is similar to the homeopathic principle of "like attracts like"). Von Reichenbach also found that people responded to colors; red colors produced a feeling of warmth and blue-violet colors produced a feeling of coolness. This finding correlates with both medicinal herbal discoveries and the ancient traditions of the chakras. Similar to the Chinese teachings of yin and yang, Von Reichenbach also found that the left side of the body is a negative pole (–) and the right side of the body is a positive pole (+).

In the early 1900s, Dr. William Kilner studied the human energy field, diseases, and psychological disturbances using colored screens and filters. He found that a glowing mist appeared around the whole body in three zones:

a) a quarter-inch dark layer closest to the skin, surrounded by b) a more vaporous layer an inch wide streaming perpendicularly from the body, and c) somewhat further out, a delicate exterior luminosity with indefinite contours about six inches across. Kilner found that the appearance of the "aura" (as he called it) differs considerably from subject to subject depending on age, sex, mental ability, and health. Certain diseases showed as patches or irregularities in the aura, which led Kilner to develop a system of diagnosis on the basis of color, texture, volume, and general appearance of the envelope. Some diseases he diagnosed in this way were liver infection, tumors, appendicitis, epilepsy, and psychological disturbances like hysteria.[4]

In 1927, Reverend Charles Leadbeater described the color system of the chakras in relation to emotional states and physical disease conditions. He depicted the chakra system as centers of conduction in which energy moves from one subtle layer to the next. These subtle layers form a sphere of energy around the body known as an "aura." Leadbeater also described the energy centers as continually rotating and receiving a higher energy through their open vortex. According to Leadbeater, the physical body must absorb higher energy into the chakras in order to exist.[5]

In the mid-1900s, Dr. Wilhelm Reich, a psychiatrist and colleague of Freud, studied the universal energy he called "orgone" using up-to-date medical and electronic equipment of that time. He explored the effects of the orgone energy field in the human body in relation to physical health and psychological disturbances. Reich developed a psychotherapeutic system for releasing energy barriers that could relieve mental and emotional dysfunctions.

In the past forty years, various medical doctors, health-care practitioners, and researchers have explored the human energy system. One scientific study, conducted by Dr. Valorie Hunt of UCLA, involved the effects of Rolfing (a type of bodywork) on the human energy field. During a series of Rolfing sessions, Dr. Hunt recorded the frequency of signals from the subject's body by placing electrodes on the subject's skin. Simultaneously, Rev. Rosalyn Bruyere (of the Healing Light Center in Glendale, California) observed the auras of both the Rolfer and the person being Rolfed. The report included color, size, and energy

movements of the chakras and the auras. The wave patterns (recorded by a Fourier analysis and a sonogram frequency analysis) were analyzed, and it was found that the auric colors correlated with the recorded wave patterns. This experiment was subsequently repeated with the other aura readers.[6]

color correspondences with the seven chakras

Most spiritual traditions recognize seven major chakras or energy centers within the body. These chakras function as an integrated system, relating and responding to each other. Each chakra is associated with a particular color of the rainbow. The color of the first chakra is red, the second chakra is orange, the third chakra is yellow, the fourth chakra is pink or green, the fifth chakra is blue, the sixth chakra is violet-purple, and the seventh chakra is white.

The lower three chakras relate to our personality selves, survival issues, and physical-emotional-mental concerns. The upper three chakras relate to living and being in the world through the awakening and transformation of our higher consciousness. The center chakra is the heart chakra, which is the bridge between the three lower chakras and the three higher chakras. The colors associated with the heart chakra are pink and green. Pink is the union of the first-chakra color (red) and the seventh-chakra color (white). Green is the bridge between the third-chakra color (yellow) and the sixth-chakra color (blue) and is associated with healing. Both pink and green represent love.

exploring the mystery of the chakras

When we harmonize with nature in silence, inquiry, and breath, the veil of illusion falls away like the peeling of an onion. We become more aware of and in harmony with this mystery, and through our awareness we gain wisdom, insight, and an understanding of our roles and responsibilities. By deepening your understanding of your chakra system, you will begin to realize the mystery of being within yourself and of your relationship with all of life. This awareness will bring to you an understanding of who you are in this moment and may open your awareness of where you came from (your genetic makeup, life patterns, and personal and family history), where you want to go from here, and all your relationships.

As you read about each chakra, notice how it relates to your own energy patterns. Doing so, you will form a new relationship with each area of your body while more deeply understanding how it relates to your whole being. By planting new seeds of awareness, you will naturally be drawn to create new life patterns and choices.

In your exploration of self, take the flower essences associated with each chakra and follow the exercises given for each plant later in this book. Soon you will discover the healing power of the chakras and the flower essences. May they empower you to live your life joyfully and at its fullest.

chakras energy chart	
First Chakra (Red/Physical)	The way we survive in the world
Second Chakra (Orange/Emotional)	The way we relate emotionally to ourselves and others
Third Chakra (Yellow/Mental)	The way we think and use our power
Fourth Chakra (Green/Pink/Heart)	Our ability to love
Fifth Chakra (Blue/Communication)	Our ability to to communicate and express ourselves
Sixth Chakra (Violet/Perception and Imagination)	Our ability to perceive and intuit
Seventh Chakra (White/Wisdom and Knowledge) contains all the colors in the spectrum	Our ability to think and have greater understanding

CHAPTER 4
The Seven Chakras

The chakras are more than energy centers of the body; they are also a comprehensive system that relates with the spirit, however you define it — God, Goddess, Mother-Father God, Great Spirit, the Omnipresent, the Divine Spirit, Our Creator as One — and human beings, animals, plants, nature, and all things as an expression of that One. In work with flower essences and plants for personal healing and growth, the chakras manifest that Oneness by incorporating qualities of Spirit and nature.

This chapter will explore in greater depth the particular aspects of the seven chakras. By becoming familiar with the qualities of each chakra, you will be better able to understand the needs of a given person and how to select the proper flower essence to deal with that person's imbalance. Each chakra has its own combination of qualities, which I will describe in relation to the following categories:

1. Seven colors and energy fields (red, orange, yellow, green, blue, violet-purple, and white). Each color is a function of particular wavelengths of light, and each chakra is associated with a specific color that indicates its vibration.

2. The four elements (earth, water, fire, and air). The first five chakras are each associated with an element; each element demonstrates its relationship to the human body through the chakras.

3. The senses (touch, taste, feeling, movement, smell, sound, sight, and psychic faculties). Each chakra is also associated with certain senses that relate directly to the functions of that chakra.

4. The eight principle patterns of Chinese herbal medicine (four pairs of polar opposites that aid in recognizing patterns of disharmony). Each principle is demonstrated in some manner by each chakra.

YIN/YANG: dark vs. light, female vs. male, passive vs. active, soft vs. hard, quiet and withdrawn vs. agitated and restless, shallow respiration vs. deep respiration, feminine appearance vs. masculine appearance, pulling energy in vs. pushing energy out, negative vs. positive, receptive vs. expressive, magnetic vs. electric. For example, yin chakras (the second, fourth, and sixth) pull energy in and have more feminine life-energy qualities. Yin and yang require each other for balance. Although they are opposite forces, they exist simultaneously and complement each other. They are the electro (yang)-magnetic (yin) polarities in the body that need each other in order to operate.

INTERIOR/EXTERIOR: chronic conditions vs. acute conditions; deep-seated emotional conditions vs. sudden onset of emotions; dealing with the deep interior emotional core of the issue vs. dealing with surface emotions; internal vs. external, such as the physical manifestation of symptoms. Each chakra relates to either deep-seated conditions or the sudden onset of conditions.

DEFICIENCY/EXCESS: weak movement vs. forceful movement; retreat or rest as a way to hide from a situation vs. covering up the situation or emotions; exhaustion of energy reserves vs. excess of energy. As we express ourselves through a particular chakra, a lack of energy or an excess of energy is demonstrated.

COLD/HOT: cold vs. hot; plants that grow in cold places vs. plants that grow in warmer places; slow deliberate movement vs. quick and more impulsive movement; pale, white face vs. red face; cold limbs vs. warm limbs; desire for heat vs. desire for cold. The body has to be invigorated or strengthened with warm colors when the physical emotions or sensations are cold and weak. When the body needs to be sedated and soothed from excess anxiety, restlessness, insomnia, or deficiency excess (such as feeling tired from being hyper), then soothing, cooling colors and plants are used. The chakras demonstrate their function in cooling or heating through their colors.

5. The law of cause and effect. In working with flower essences and chakras, one can relate to a cause, or one can relate to an effect. In treating with flower essences, the intention is to treat the underlying cause of the problem. A person may have a memory, image, or flash of the experience that set a problematic pattern in motion. That's the cause. The effect is the person's response to that particular experience. By becoming aware of and understanding the experience, they may be empowered to change the way they think, thus changing the way they feel.

first chakra: physical, root, or base chakra

ELEMENT: Earth
FOCUS: Survival and physical security
COLOR: Red
ENDOCRINE GLAND: Adrenals
SOUND/VIBRATIONS: Tone of middle C; long "u" or long "o" vowel sounds; *lam* or *lang* (Hindu) sound; bass-toned and percussion instruments

POLARITY: Yang

COLD/HOT: Hot to warming; most intense heat of all the chakras

SENSES: Kinesthetic sensations such as touch; physical feelings of pleasure or pain; movement that may include walking or deep breathing, as in meditation or relaxation techniques

FLOWER ESSENCES: Black-Eyed Susan, Blanketflower, Bouncing Bet, Century Plant, Crimson Monkeyflower, Desert Willow, Echinacea, Indian Paintbrush, Mexican Hat, Paloverde, Pinyon, Pomegranate, Peace Rose, Saguaro, Scarlet Penstemon, Strawberry Hedgehog, Yellow Monkeyflower

FUNCTIONS: The base chakra is located between the tailbone (the coccyx) and the pubic bone. It includes the functions of the anus, rectum, and circulatory system, and the lower extremities such as the feet, legs, and entire pelvic area. The base chakra is associated with the adrenal glands, which are located atop the kidneys and produce steroid hormones that regulate salt concentration in the blood, hydrocortisone, which assists the body in its response to physical stress, and small amounts of sex hormones — both male (androgens) and female (estrogens) — that augment the hormones secreted by the gonad.

positive Healing patterns

The root chakra has a grounding energy that connects us to the earth and helps us build our foundation. This is an innate primal energy and the vital root of our spiritual and soul heritage — where we have come from and how we will proceed with who we are. It is about survival, power, and sensuality. It includes our physical needs, such as food, shelter, clothing, exercise, and nutrition, yet it also includes a deeper awareness that takes us back to the roots from which we came. The earth takes us deep inside our darkness and helps us face the shadows of ourselves from the past to the present. Establishing an understanding of and a relationship with our root chakra initiates a deep internal journey into the discovery of the self. It is the turning point for knowing our true selves; it gives us the strength to choose our direction in life in the context of a greater picture of ourselves and our origins.

A conscious, healthy relationship with the root chakra empowers us to be who we need to be. With this grounding, we can create harmony in our homes and with our families, and choose friends, jobs, and situations that empower and nurture who we are. The root chakra is the seat of the *kundalini,* or life-force energy, and affects the way we breathe and move. Expression of the kundalini energy is represented by the serpent, which is associated with both masculine and feminine traits. A common symbol in the medical field is made up of two serpents (male and female) intertwined along the "caduceus," or staff, and topped by a pair of wings; it represents a mystical awakening of the hot, fiery kundalini energy. This energy rises from the base of the spine and aligns with the chakras all the way to the crown chakra at the top of the head. Experiencing the kundalini brings harmony, balance, and an incredible feeling of flowing life-force energy. The crown and root chakras are opposite in polarity and equal in value.

Partners who practice tantric sexuality can gracefully experience the kundalini. Deep meditation and relaxation — or even a rush of excitement and happiness — can also create a kundalini awakening experience.

symptoms and patterns of imbalance

DEFICIENCY: When we are weak and lack our physical life-force energy, we suppress ourselves (low energy, low vitality, lack of passion or motivation). Deep fears, especially those related to survival issues, and a sense of powerlessness may overwhelm us; we may withdraw or avoid our feelings. Our circulation becomes sluggish and our breathing becomes shallow. We allow ourselves to become disempowered, to fall into a victim or scapegoat consciousness, allowing ourselves to be bullied, manipulated, or taken advantage of, yearning for approval by others in order to feel good about who we are. We feel limited and therefore we give up on believing in ourselves. Since our identity is based on the condition of the first chakra, all other chakras are affected by it. First-chakra deficiencies can influence our memory, our sex drive, and our ability to tap into our higher consciousness.

Physical conditions may also include coldness in the limbs, especially the hands and feet, and an overall feeling of low body temperature (deficient yang). On the other hand, conditions may also include fever in the afternoon due to stress and fatigue (deficient yin). With deficient yin there is insomnia; with deficient yang there is oversleeping and the inability to wake up refreshed.

EXCESS: When we are overstimulated and misuse our power chakra or vital root chakra, we become belligerent, aggressive, manipulative, possessive, controlling, impulsive, and sexually obsessed. Physical conditions may also include a hyperactive sex drive, nervousness, and restlessness, leading to insomnia and overreaction to stimuli.

INTERIOR: Deep-seated emotional conditions associated with the first chakra include chronic fear, anger, and agitation or deep suppression. These conditions may manifest in obesity, nervous disorders, eating disorders, hemorrhoids, frequent urination, or constipation. They can also lead to chronic diseases such as adrenal disorders (Addison's disease or Cushing's syndrome), bone disorders, cancer, arthritis, or Alzheimer's disease.

EXTERIOR: Acute conditions related to the first chakra include the sudden onset of fear, anger, or agitation, or making an impulsive, unconsidered decision about something significant.

Physical conditions may include sexual dysfunction; iron deficiency causing anemia, especially related to women and their menses; adrenal imbalances; broken bones, cuts, or bruises; hernia; reproductive problems; paralysis; coma; and shock. Symptoms may also include spontaneous sweating and chills or frequent clear urination.

Treatment with Red plants

Red plants revitalize the weakened first chakra. They are stimulating and warming. For example, cayenne pepper energizes the whole system; red lychee berries (which are succulent and juicy) increase reproductive secretions in cases of hormonal deficiency and imbalance to allow healthier sexuality; red root cleans out toxicity in sexual glands, purifies blood, and clears lymph stagnation; and rose hips clear out toxicity, especially related to the kidneys, adrenal glands, and heart. Weak heart and kidneys are related to fluid stagnation in the body, which depresses sex drive and general energy level. Red ginseng root charges the physical body and helps to relieve stress. Hawthorn strengthens digestion and the heart simultaneously, allowing the body to be stronger; it soothes irregular and unstable heart conditions such as palpitations and irregular heartbeat. Red clover restores blood and nourishes the body, provides cleansing and clearing of toxins, and stimulates urination. Manjista, also known as Indian madder, has a bright, light-red bark that is used to treat gynecological disorders such as blood clotting, painful menses, and sexually transmitted diseases.

Treatment with Red flower essences

When the vital force of an individual is depressed, a root-chakra flower essence will help invigorate the person. But take care: If you treat a first-chakra condition with a flower essence over a long period of time, the result may be overwhelming instead of rejuvenating or uplifting; the person's reserves may become exhausted. Check for the conditions of imbalance associated with the root chakra (deficiency/excess, interior/exterior). If the individual's balance is not being restored by a red flower essence, you may want to use a pink flower essence associated with the heart chakra, which is the complement of the root chakra. Opening one's heart in love and compassion may simultaneously lift the vital force and restore balance to the root chakra.

For example, you may want to take Scarlet Penstemon if you feel you are lacking courage and you have no energy to carry out an activity for which you want courage. But you need to be careful of becoming overbearing in your confidence. If a man is impotent yet craves sex, he may take Scarlet Penstemon to give him the courage to express himself in a creative, positive sexual way that is not overbearing or forceful to his mate. If he finds himself exhibiting excessive energy, he may need to back off the Scarlet Penstemon. There is no wrong or right here. It's a matter of connecting with the plant's resonance and how it serves who and where you are in the moment. If your intention is to gather your courage and faith, and if you are willing to make positive life changes, Scarlet Penstemon is a good choice. When you feel you have found your courage, perhaps in relation to a particular situation, stop taking Scarlet Penstemon and choose an essence in the pink or white realm to maintain the balance. On the other hand, if you have taken Scarlet Penstemon for a few weeks without any results, you may want to choose a different flower essence. Tune in to yourself or get help from someone else, and ask what you really want guidance with. You may decide to resonate with a different color scheme.

Indian Paintbrush flower essence relates specifically to both the first and second chakras; it stirs creative, passionate, visionary, and artistic self-expression, while allowing one to feel grounded and connected to one's roots. Crimson Monkeyflower is a bright crimson-red to reddish orange flower. Crimson Monkeyflower essence takes us back to our roots or our past to heal emotional bitterness such as anger, addictions, impulsiveness, sexual obsessions, bullying, and an overall feeling of fear and powerlessness at a core level. Crimson Monkeyflower flower essence helps us let go of sticky relationships or situations, and helps us work with our core emotions to regain our personal power. Through claiming our power, we become compassionate, strong, courageous, and full of passion for life.

---

second chakra: emotional, spleen, or regenerative chakra

ELEMENT: Water
FOCUS: Sexuality, procreation, emotions

COLOR: Orange
ENDOCRINE GLAND: Gonad
SOUND/VIBRATIONS: Tone of D above and next to middle C; "oo" vowel sound; *vam* or *vang* (Hindu) sound; bass-toned, percussion, brass, and woodwind instruments
POLARITY: Yin
COLD/HOT: Warming
SENSES: Sensations connected with the emotions of anger, fear, sadness, grief, shame, guilt, joy
FLOWER ESSENCES: Blanketflower, Calendula, California Poppy, Century Plant, Crimson Monkeyflower, Echinacea, Indian Paintbrush, Mexican Hat, Mullein, Paloverde, Pomegranate, Scarlet Penstemon, and Yellow Monkeyflower
FUNCTION: The second chakra is located in the gonad and includes the reproductive system (the prostate gland and sex organs; the testes in the male and the ovaries in the female); the production of estrogen, progesterone, sperm, and testosterone; the lower back; and the body's muscular system. This energy center also includes some of the functions of the adrenal glands, the lymphatic glands, the spleen, bladder, pancreas, and kidneys, which are also covered by the first and third chakras. The second chakra also has an effect on the process of elimination and the detoxification of the body.

positive healing patterns

The second chakra, or emotional center, is the driving force that gives us the incentive to get where we want to go and to help us get in touch with how we feel about who we are. This chakra is the actual expression that we choose to act out in our lives. John Bradshaw describes emotion as "E-Motion": "E = energy or life force, M = the means or fuel we use to get where we are going. E-Motion = Energy in Motion."[1] I see emotion as the expression of our soul drama or soul pattern that we have learned to develop and feel over our lifetime — or even lifetimes.

Emotions such as fear, anger, grief, and guilt need to be understood and put into their proper perspective. Learning how powerful our emotions are — and how strong an energetic impact they have on us and others — can help us use our emotions as effective tools and as lessons in who we are or who we want to become. Our emotions flow like a river, depending upon the driving force of energy moving through us. We learn to yield as the tide and to flow as the river, continually releasing, cleansing, changing, and evolving. We are constantly pulled between release (letting go of old feelings and emotions that limit us, prevent personal growth, and possibly cause us to blame others for our suffering) and moving forward in a new way that frees us from the bondage of old feelings and stuck patterns while requiring a new identity.

We experience our gut-level emotions as physical sensations. How often have you heard yourself or someone else say: "I felt it coming," "I felt this would happen," "I sensed my mother's death before anyone called me," or "I could feel it in my bones"? The awakening of our emotions is an awakening to our consciousness.

When we come to terms with the emotional attachments that have held us in bondage, we are preparing ourselves for a new future. Any control issues, victim or abuse issues, competition issues, deaths, or severe traumas in our lives that have prevented us from releasing stagnant emotions will come to the forefront of our conscious awakening when we are ready to make such changes. We will then have to face those things — in our lives, ourselves, or in our relationships with other people — that are unfinished or unresolved. By confronting our fear, anger, sadness, guilt, grief, and shame, and possibly by reexperiencing events or images to help us release them, we can then move on.

The second chakra holds the key to our personal investment in ourselves, to our creativity and the birth of new emotional patterns and ideas, and to our ability to take care of and nurture ourselves and others. By discovering ourselves through our emotional realms, we can receive our own inner treasures of harmony, balance, and peace. And, most importantly, we can feel a new sense of trusting and knowing who we are. We develop confidence, endurance, and emotional security.

The second chakra is the center of sexuality and sensation. As we come into a new identity, our new sense of freedom includes the freedom and balance of our own sexuality. We learn new steps in the dance of life that stir our passion and excitement for living. We have accepted and embraced life's setbacks, and we are evolving a new style of living that supports who we are and what we have established in the foundation of our being.

symptoms and patterns of imbalance

DEFICIENCY: When we are emotionally exhausted and overwhelmed, we lack the energy that gives us a feeling of worth. Although we crave love, nurturing, and belonging, we lack the inner emotional strength to feed the very things that we want most. Instead of nurturing ourselves, we become disempowered. We lose emotional trust in ourselves as well as in others. Our attention becomes focused on what others think, and we lack the ability to fit in socially. We give power to emotional reactions and emotional patterns that drain our energy and deplete our emotional energy resources. Our emotional deficiency results in a lack of true self-expression and a lack of creativity.

The emotional state of the second chakra is affected by our attitudes toward sex and our own sexuality. We may suppress who we are as sexual beings or experience a lack of ambition and sex drive. We also may experience an overall feeling of helplessness. We might tend to use drugs or alcohol in privacy as a way to avoid or withdraw from our feelings.

A deficiency of the gonadal hormones may cause infertility, delayed or premature puberty, the development of mixed gender characteristics, and menstruation problems in women.

EXCESS: When we are emotionally overstimulated or feel that we have to prove ourselves, we tend to live out an emotional personality that is influenced by pride, conflict, power struggles, confrontational tendencies, emotional insensitivity, lack of respect for others, dishonoring others' boundaries, misuse or excess of sexual stimulation, drugs, alcoholism, and social addictions. Feelings of excess can lead to denial as a way to avoid confrontation with our core issues.

By choosing to live in intense emotionally overstimulated states, we become oblivious to the ability to "go with the flow." Therefore, our energies become rapidly dispersed and drained. Emotionally blocked energies may interfere with first- and second-chakra sexual and excretory functions. This can block the natural energy exchange with the higher-frequency vibrations or the higher chakras. Another aspect of this blockage is sexual impotence or constipation when energy is not moving through the first and second chakras.

An excess of gonadal hormones can also cause infertility, delayed or premature puberty, menstruation problems in females, and development of mixed gender characteristics.

INTERIOR: Deep-seated emotional conditions associated with the second chakra include chronic states of fear, anger, sadness, grief, shame, guilt, and an overall deep suppression of these emotions.

As with the first chakra, these conditions may lead to obesity, eating disorders, or sexually transmitted diseases such as AIDS or venereal disease. They may also cause diseases linked to the spleen, pancreas, kidneys, intestines, and bladder, such as a weak immune system (as in chronic fatigue syndrome), candida, poor digestion, low or high blood-sugar levels, colon cancer, or kidney stones. When these conditions exist in the body, there are usually insufficient enzymes in the pancreas and intestines. Hormone imbalances can cause a variety of problems, in women especially.

EXTERIOR: Acute conditions related to the second chakra can cause the sudden onset of any emotion. Just when we think we have made a breakthrough in a certain soul pattern, look out! Doubts and worries may creep in when we least expect them. External symptoms of imbalance may include a lack of creativity or the inability to stay in a committed intimate relationship. We may become more easily distracted by new ideas without the tools or incentive for follow-through.

Our emotions don't ever go away; what changes is our response to our emotional state. It is a learning process to transform our more challenging and lower-frequency emotions, such as anger and fear, into higher-frequency emotions such as happiness and love. Our conscious awareness of emotional patterns gives us the ability to redirect our emotional energy in a way that promotes health, allowing higher-frequency energies to expand throughout our bodies and auric fields.

EXTERIOR TO INTERIOR: Sometimes an exterior, or superficial, condition can move into the interior. For example, when there is a superficial condition such as a stomach virus, there can be clamminess and sweatiness of the abdomen and a feeling of heat. When this feeling goes deeper and moves into the interior, there can be nausea, intestinal or stomach cramping, and dizziness. Other conditions may include irregular menses and abdominal pains.

Treatment with orange plants

Orange plants revitalize the adrenal glands, gonad, spleen, pancreas, stomach, bladder, and kidneys. For example, sassafras deals with the glandular aspect and offers a rejuvenating effect during illness. Sassafras has a naturally sweet, refreshing taste that is soothing, relaxing, and uplifting. It also helps clear physical stagnation. California poppy is used as a sedative to treat tension and imbalance of the nerves, especially in the second and third chakras. It is also known to relieve pain and is used in the treatment of colic and gall-bladder problems and as an antispasmodic. Pomegranate root bark, which is red-orange, has been used as a purgative or to expel worms from the intestinal tract. The powdered fruit rind of the pomegranate is used as an astringent and has been used to treat dysentery, diarrhea, intermittent fever, and excessive perspiration, and as a gargle for sore throats.

Red root has an orange-red root used to treat chronic blood congestion and venereal infections. Red root also stimulates and removes toxins in the liver and the lungs. Manzanita has a reddish orange bark and reddish berries. The berries of the manzanita are used to treat mild urinary infections, water retention, bladder gravel, and chronic kidney inflammations.

Treatment with the orange flower essences

When a person's emotions are depressed, second-chakra flower essences will help emotionally stimulate them. As with the first-chakra description, if you rely energetically on a flower essence to treat an emotional condition over a long period of time, the emotional body may become overwhelmed; instead of being rejuvenating or uplifting, it may exhaust one's reserves. If you feel emotionally imbalanced, stop taking the flower essence. You may need to choose another orange flower essence or its complement, a blue flower essence that provides a more soothing and uplifting quality.

California Poppy flower essence has a cleansing effect and acts as a purifier for emotional toxins or emotional buildup. It heightens our sensitivity and helps us tap into the sensations of our inner knowing. It also opens us to the spark of fire deep within our sensuality and sexuality. A person may take California Poppy to help release certain unwanted dysfunctional emotional patterns. California Poppy may offer immediate charges of energy that help one release emotional baggage.

Blanketflower essence is a mixture of golden-yellow and orange-red colors. I call it the "fire dance" because of the flower's bright flame-like colors and incredible force of energy. Blanketflower serves as the fire that melts the ice, instilling warmth, vitality, exuberance, and joy for life when feeling shut down.

Calendula is a golden yellow-orange flower used as an essence for those who need deep emotional and mental healing in a soothing, calming way. Calendula flower essence calms nervousness and brings a quiet centering to the abdomen and solar plexus, which also helps build confidence. Calendula flower essence provides an inner warmth and radiance that extends outward and upward.

Third chakra: Mental, personal power, or solar plexus chakra

ELEMENT: Fire
FOCUS: Will, purpose, power, self-empowerment, self-honor
COLOR: Yellow
ENDOCRINE GLAND: Pancreas
SOUND/VIBRATIONS: Tone of E above middle C; "ah" sound (as in father); *ram* or *rang* (Hindu) sound; flutes, woodwinds, strings, and piano instruments
POLARITY: Yang
COLD/HOT: Warming

SENSES: Intuition or inner knowing

FLOWER ESSENCES: Aster, Black-Eyed Susan, Blanketflower, Blue Flag, Calendula, Century Plant, Chamomile, Cliff Rose, Columbine, Comfrey, Desert Marigold, Desert Willow, Honeysuckle, Mexican Hat, Mullein, Ox-Eye Daisy, Palmer's Penstemon, Paloverde, Purple Robe, Scarlet Penstemon, Strawberry Hedgehog, Sunflower, Wild Rose, and Yellow Monkeyflower

LOCATION AND PHYSICAL FUNCTIONS: The third chakra is related to the solar plexus area and includes the functions located there: the adrenals, pancreas, stomach, digestive system, assimilation process, liver, and gall bladder; some of these functions are shared with the second chakra. The pancreas is the endocrine gland associated with the third chakra. As a digestive organ, the pancreas produces enzymes that aid in the digestion of food, breaking down protein, fats, and carbohydrates. As an endocrine gland, the pancreas secretes insulin and glucagon to regulate blood sugar. This energy center is also associated with the left hemisphere of the brain and its activities; while the brain is located in the sixth-chakra area of the body, it influences the functioning of the lower chakra areas. Mental imbalance, psychosomatic illnesses, ulcers, and intestinal/digestive malfunctions can be relieved by healing work or therapies applied through this center.

positive Healing patterns

The third chakra gives us our ability to think and reason, to find purpose and desire in life, and to empower ourselves to be who we need to be. It helps us understand our thought dialogues in relation to our feelings. It strengthens our mind to pursue a state of stableness, courage, positive faith, hope, humor, and joy. This energy center brings about a balanced mental state of responsibility, mental objectivity, and wisdom. It teaches us to surrender the mind when needed and it's also the link of the rational mind to psychic energies and enhanced intuition. It gives us the courage and faith to trust and act upon our intuition. The third chakra reveals a higher consciousness within the lower three chakras and an innate capability to understand self and others. It is the bond between the lower chakras and the heart, uniting love and harmony to empower the process of dissolving or decrystalizing old patterns.

By loving ourselves and taking personal risks in our best interest, we develop honor, dignity, and self-esteem. In the third chakra, we come to terms with who we are, why we are here, what we have learned, and what we desire. This journey with and as our true selves leads to dignity and self-empowerment.

By working with this chakra, we can dissolve our prejudices, judgments, and criticisms; learn how to effectively deal with anger; understand our hatred and its roots; and dissolve and unplug from our fears, both rational and irrational.

A conscious, healthy relationship with the solar plexus chakra helps us trust our intuition and the higher guidance we may receive from the higher chakras. The third chakra is complemented by the violet-purple ray of the sixth chakra, which indicates our ability to receive higher aspirations and allow spiritual guidance and vision to flow through us.

symptoms and patterns of imbalance

DEFICIENCY: When we are deficient in the third chakra, our emotions cloud our mental judgment. We lack mental clarity and the ability to focus. We lack mind power in relation to courage, fear, panic, hopelessness, despair, guilt, unworthiness, nostalgia, uncertainty, worry, anger, hatred, and prejudice. We may have lots of great ideas but lack the intention and ability to follow through with them. We tend to become bogged down with what others think about us and, in addition to our own self-criticism, we lack a feeling of recognition and self-esteem.

These deficiencies act as a violation against ourselves. It is as if we have allowed someone or something to take our spirit away from us, leaving us empty-handed or empty-bellied with no internal resources. We have lost our connection to our intuitive selves, which is reflective of our desperate need to just survive. Our energy levels become depleted and withdrawn. We are losing our power, our purpose, and the will to be our creative, expressive, empowering selves!

Prolonged stress affects the function of the pancreas and the adrenal glands. Diabetes mellitus or high blood sugar is common among people with endocrine disorders. Type 1 diabetes occurs especially in young people when the pancreas in unable to produce insulin. Type 2 diabetes generally occurs in people over forty who have an insufficient insulin output for the body's needs.

EXCESS: When we invest our energy in judgment, criticism, dishonesty, and control of others, we lose our power. When we try to force things to happen, rather than allowing them to happen according to their own time and place, we lose our power. When we buy into the emotional outbursts or patterns of others, we also lose our power. This kind of overstimulation uses up energy in ways that don't replenish our reserves; in other words, it depletes our energy. We use up all our energy on destructive forces, and we lack the foundation of stable emotional patterns that build upon positive or constructive energies.

Excess stress and a lack of stress management affect the endocrine system and the body's ability to regulate blood-sugar levels.

INTERIOR: Deep-seated emotional and mental conditions associated with the third chakra lead to chronic states of fear, worry, anxiety, nervousness, anger, sadness, grief, shame, or guilt, and an overall deep suppression of these emotions and thoughts. These conditions may lead to digestive problems, immune deficiencies, and problems or diseases related to the solar plexus, adrenals, stomach, liver, and gall bladder, such as hepatitis, gallstones, gastritis, and appendicitis.

Internal physical symptoms may include hot or cold internal organs, depending on the condition. For example, a person with deficient chi would feel coldness in these areas. The conflict of emotion can also create heat in the middle chakras that can lead to disease. When anger, frustration, or depression weaken our thoughts and emotions, we become depleted in our digestive processes and our blood-sugar level is also affected. Both diabetes types 1 and 2, as mentioned previously, can occur due to the lack of insulin production.

EXTERIOR: Acute conditions related to the third chakra include the ongoing internal and mental dialogues and irrational thought processes that drain our energy and make poor investments of our time. These excessive thoughts, opinions, judgments, and criticisms hold us back from connecting with our heart chakra, limiting our personality selves from gaining their true power. When we invest in negative mental states, we are affected emotionally and physically. We are drawing lower energy-frequency rates into our body/minds, making it difficult to receive the higher frequencies of the upper chakras. By becoming conscious of our mental/emotional patterns, we begin to understand that we no longer need to invest ourselves in people or situations that don't support us. Instead of giving negative power to these people or circumstances, we can now release them, bless them, and go on our way. We now have the ability to redirect our mental/emotional energy to a way of living that promotes health and vibrantly higher-frequency energies throughout our bodies and auric fields.

External physical third-chakra conditions could include sweating, rashes, heat, or fever in the middle part of the body. A general feeling of being run down is associated with imbalance in this energy center.

Treatment with Yellow Plants

Yellow plants invigorate and stimulate. For example, mullein roots can be used as a diuretic, to treat incontinence, and to tone the bladder after childbirth. Mullein invigorates and releases lymphatic congestion and promotes lymphatic drainage of the ear. Mullein provides a feeling of heat and dryness, and can be smoked to relieve chest complaints and to treat asthma. Calendula treats skin problems, cuts, inflammations, bruises, and minor burns. Calendula also strengthens the eyesight and heart as well as alleviates digestive inflammations, gastric and duodenal ulcers, liver and gall-bladder problems, jaundice, water retention, cramps, fever, and stomach-aches.

Chamomile (white and yellow) treats nervous conditions such as colic, irritability, and impatience, especially in babies. Chamomile is also used as an antispasmodic for the treatment of such conditions as indigestion, upset stomach, heartburn, flatulence, tension related to the liver, and menstrual cramps. Chamomile is an anti-infective for conditions such as fevers, asthma, bronchitis, and colds.

Yellow dock clears toxins, cleanses, and releases congestion in the kidneys, liver, and intestines. Yellow dock also promotes bowel movement and urination and restores blood deficiencies, especially related to weakness and fatigue.

The boiled leaves and root of yellow columbine have been used to treat scurvy, plague, fever, and bladder problems.

Treatment with the Yellow Flower Essences

When a person's mental activity is either deficient or excessive, a yellow flower essence may help to either stimulate or soothe, depending on the flower essence. A yellow flower essence such as the Black-Eyed Susan will help us confront traumatic or painful past experiences. For some people, such memories may have been repressed. Black-Eyed Susan can help bring these experiences to the forefront in order to face them and allow healing to occur. Columbine flower essence, on the other hand, is a loving and gentle essence that helps us discover our hidden treasures and inner beauty. It would make sense for the Columbine essence to be a follow-up to a Black-Eyed Susan essence, since we may first need to confront and face the pain so that we can then see and experience our inner worth and beauty. Columbine flower essence is more soothing and nonconfrontational, especially when compared to the Black-Eyed Susan.

Century Plant has a yellow blossom that promotes the inner and outer strength necessary to survive in a harsh environment. It is about taking time to nurture and empower ourselves. Century Plant also helps us stay focused on our goals and helps us to make breakthroughs in replacing an old pattern with a renewal of energy.

Fourth Chakra: Heart Chakra

ELEMENT: Air

FOCUS: Love, compassion, and forgiveness

COLOR: Green or pink

ENDOCRINE GLAND: Thymus

SOUND/VIBRATIONS: Tone of F above middle C; long "a" vowel sound, as in "ray"; *yam* or *yang* (Hindu) sound; harps, organs, flutes, wind chimes, and string instruments

POLARITY: Yin

COLD/HOT: Lukewarm sensation, neither cold nor hot

SENSES: A feeling of love

FLOWER ESSENCES: Bells-of-Ireland, Bouncing Bet, Desert Willow, Indian Paintbrush, Morning Glory, Onion, Palmer's Penstemon, Peace Rose, Pinyon, Strawberry Hedgehog, Sweet Pea, Thistle, Wild Rose, and Willow

LOCATION AND PHYSICAL FUNCTIONS: The heart chakra includes the functions of the heart, thymus gland, immune system, and circulatory system. The thymus gland is located in front of and above the heart, beneath the breastbone. The thymus secretes thymosin and other hormones that regulate the immune system. It is believed that the thymus is related to nutrition and growth in childhood. This center is also associated with the right hemisphere of the brain and with tissue regeneration.

positive Healing patterns

The heart chakra is the link between the three upper and the three lower chakras. It is here at the center where spirit, vision, light, wisdom, and communication from above meet with matter, survival, procreation, knowledge, and personality from below. When the upper and lower chakras are balanced and their energy currents are flowing freely, the heart chakra radiates its creative energy and power. The merging of sexuality with the true expression of sexual love is generated, and passions of mystical awakening are stirred and experienced.

The heart center is the place within us where our personal development reaches a new level. This growth is experienced and demonstrated by our ability to let our heart dictate who we are and the choices we make. Our heart center awakens to a higher expression of love, compassion, and willpower. We become open to unconditional love of self and others in a universal way that expands well beyond our families and friends.

We begin to embody a balance of physical power with spiritual guidance and wisdom. Through this balance we become aware of what it means to invest in both spirit and matter. We develop the passion to live by a new honor system — to trust that Spirit, divine inspiration, and the mastery of Self will lead us down our path. Our path becomes one of integrity,

honesty, respect, forgiveness, compassion, and understanding. We learn to honor all things for who or what they are without judgment or criticism.

The life aspect of the soul is rooted in the heart center. Here we can heal our heart wounds that may date back to our earliest memories and beyond, deep in our soul record. In our heart chakra we offer healing, forgiveness, and love of others. We come to realize that we no longer need to feed negative energies or limitations in relation to ourselves or others, and that we can bless and love others while staying on our path. This awareness and growth enables us to decrystalize or dissolve the old patterns.

symptoms and patterns of imbalance

DEFICIENCY: Lack of meditation and prayer — not making time for sacred space — shuts down our heart center and slows the energy connection between the upper and lower chakras. We become weary and lacking in vitality, breath (especially conscious deep breathing), love, and the joy of living. We become disinterested in life and in ourselves, thus losing our personal power and closing down our hearts. When our hearts are shut down or disassociated, we also tend to withdraw from others or seek approval by others. We may experience self-doubt, mistrust, neediness, and a lack of "belongingness." Old wounds of the heart may seem hopeless and depressing. We may be faced with our own death, the death of a loved one, or a part of ourselves that is dying. We lack courage and faith, and we dwell on our pain and suffering.

EXCESS: Excess of misery and suffering is the opposite of denial of misery and suffering (a deficiency condition), but both lead to disease. Excess can lead to a lack of compassion or tolerance for self and others that may become abusive. This lack of concern may be shown by blaming others, possession or control of others, jealousy, anger, or inappropriately forcing one's personal will. Or it may express itself in a seemingly contradictory fashion, such as giving too much attention to others, trying to love others in superficial ways, or trying too hard to gain recognition by others.

INTERIOR: Deep-seated fourth-chakra conditions lead to chronic states of sadness, grief, shame, guilt, and an overall deep suppression of these emotions. These conditions may include digestive problems, immune deficiencies, hiatal hernia, heart diseases (chest pain, angina, or cardiac disorders), and problems or diseases related to the thymus, circulation, and tissue deficiencies. Physical symptoms can include heat-based hiatal hernia, palpitations of the heart, and emotionally induced asthma, such as a breathing difficulty after a stressful event (an argument, a death in the family). Grief and sadness would worsen those symptoms.

EXTERIOR: Acute conditions related to the fourth chakra include the ongoing patterns of living that emotionally close down the heart and its ability to bond between the upper and lower chakras.

When we are suffering in the heart chakra, we generally don't want to face our lessons in life. We may not take personal responsibility for our thoughts, making others our problem, and we may feel easily threatened and quick to blame; we are not taking charge of our lives.

The way to take charge is through forgiveness and compassion, first with ourselves and then with others. As we allow forgiveness, we no longer blame the other person and we forgive ourselves for the choices we made. The quality of our relationship to self and others improves immeasurably. Our heart center opens, and we become more responsible to ourselves and all our relations. The real connection is realizing that the Higher Self loves unconditionally.

Exterior physical conditions include light wheezing, sweating, or a rash on the surface of the chest. Other conditions may include insomnia or hysteria.

Treatment with fourth-chakra plants

Green and pink are the fourth-chakra colors. Green plants tend to be slightly cooling and pink plants tend to be slightly warming; together they offer a lukewarm sensation. They are a balance of heat and cold, yin and yang. The color green tempers emotional imbalances such as anger, frustration, and depression. Pink is a blend of the first chakra color (red) and seventh chakra color (white).

Many plants have green parts, especially in their stems and leaves. I generally refer to pink flowers for the heart chakra. However, in a recent conversation with Dr. Vassant Merchant, a friend and follower of Sri Aurobindo, I learned that the bougainvillea flower grows in every color of the rainbow, including the color green (at Coimbatore, South India, at about 2,000 feet altitude). I don't know of any other plant that has a green flower.

Many plants are used to treat various heart problems: garlic (white and green), foxglove, lily of the valley (white and green), valerian, American ginseng, bloodroot (red root, white flower), lobelia, milk thistle, hawthorn, willow, evening primrose (green with white flower), and immortelle (commonly called everlasting). Ephedra is used to treat allergic or asthmatic reactions; it opens the breathing passages and increases the heart rate to accelerate circulation and compensate for stress. Longan fruit is a Chinese remedy for unblocking heart energy and emotions related to the heart.

Treatment with pink flower essences

The rose family is one of my favorites in dealing with the heart chakra. The Wild Rose flower essence teaches us to love ourselves, others, and all life forms. It is especially good for those who are indifferent toward themselves and their life circumstances. It is for those who are weary and lack vitality, love, and joy in living. The Peace Rose is a gentle, soft rose with incredibly pure colors of cream and pink. It is for those whose hearts are closed due to depression (possibly related to a death), for those who lack courage or faith, and for those who tend to reside in their pains and miseries. Both the Peace Rose and the Wild Rose flower essences help us come to terms with our heart wounds and activate the opening of the heart chakra by releasing judgments, unforgivingness, sadness, and grief.

fifth chakra: Throat chakra

ELEMENT: Ether
FOCUS: Communication, sound, vibration
COLOR: Blue
ENDOCRINE GLAND: Thyroid
SOUND/VIBRATIONS: Tone of G above middle C; short vowels (e, i, a, u); *ham* or *hang* (Hindu) sound; harps, organs, pianos, and high-pitched instruments (flutes, pennywhistles, violins)
POLARITY: Yang
COLD/HOT: Cooling sensation
SENSES: Taste, smell, hearing, vocalizing
FLOWER ESSENCES: Blue Flag, Chicory, Comfrey, Crimson Monkeyflower, Desert Larkspur, Desert Willow, Palmer's Penstemon, Sage, Scarlet Penstemon, and Yellow Monkeyflower
LOCATION AND PHYSICAL FUNCTIONS: The throat chakra includes the throat, larynx, tongue, mouth, lips, teeth, esophagus, upper lungs, voice, bronchial tubes, thyroid, and parathyroid glands. The thyroid gland is located at the base of the throat and is wrapped around the windpipe. The thyroid secretes thyroxin, which regulates the body's metabolic rate. Attached to the

back of the thyroid are four or five small glands known as the parathyroids, which control the concentration and balance of calcium and phosphorus in the blood. The thyroid is known as a lubricator of energy transformation.

The throat energy center also includes the activities of the respiratory system, bronchial and vocal functions, and the processing and absorption of food and other nutrients. The throat chakra is also associated with the upper extremities: neck, shoulder, arms, and hands.

positive healing patterns

The throat chakra is the link between the upper two chakras and the heart; it is where we receive the higher vibratory frequencies of the sixth and seventh chakras and connect those frequencies with the heart. The throat chakra is the chakra of creativity and spiritual willpower, rather than the power related to the emotions and the personality self. I define spiritual willpower as "the will to do Thy Will." Having the willpower to face our fears, our anger, our barriers, or our blockages every day means having the ability to call upon Spirit to help us reach for and live in the Light rather than the darkness. As we become more open to embracing the Light and the higher energy currents within ourselves, we spontaneously bring spiritual guidance, creativity, and vision into our cognitive minds, thoughts, and images; we are better able to bring in positive thought-forms and attitudes. An opening or awakening of the throat

chakra is indicated by our ability to speak our truths from an inner depth of awareness, creativity, spiritual guidance, and compassion within our hearts. Communication takes place not only through vocal exchange, but through creative art forms such as dance, sculpture, painting, singing, chanting, and playing instruments.

Communication is the expression of our inner selves (our voice, its sounds and vibrations, our thoughts, our inner truths and insights) to the outside world and the responses that are returned to us. We become more aware of ourselves and even get to know ourselves better by observing and listening to the ways we communicate and the ways others respond to our communication.

One form of communication that we don't always access is a subliminal communication that goes beyond time and space. This type of communication, known as telepathy, involves exchanging nonphysical energy signals or information from the "ether." Through inner listening and a calm mind, we have the ability to channel communication through a subtle vibratory exchange of energy. An example of telepathy is when we think about someone we haven't seen or talked to in years, and we subsequently receive a letter or phone call from that person. Another example is when we feel that someone close to us needs our help or is in danger. Most of us have experienced telepathy at some time in our lives. This, too, is related to the fifth chakra.

symptoms and patterns
of imbalance

DEFICIENCY: Deficiency in the throat chakra is the lack of willpower and creativity needed to face ourselves and be strong in who we are. Deficiency especially occurs when we have been denied our expression or told to keep secrets. When we feel closed down, tense, weak, and lacking in willpower, we have difficulty expressing ourselves from our heart and our inner depths. When overwhelmed by depression, we are unable to reflect upon the emotions of grief, sadness, and melancholy enough to understand their underlying causes, and we have difficulty releasing emotions and feelings related to the need to cry or sigh. Crying releases fluids, and sighing expels toxic air. Deficiency means loss of creativity, of communication, and of our very spirit.

Physical conditions may include the inability to communicate, such as the inability to form moisture in the throat. Deficiency in the throat leads to dryness and soreness. An underactive thyroid burns food too slowly and may cause weight gain, lethargy, and an overall feeling of exhaustion. A thyroid hormone deficiency or a lack of iodine in childhood can impede physical and mental growth and cause other complications.

EXCESS: When we tend to preach to others, tell others how to live, and try to force our opinions and thoughts onto others, we have lost the connection between the higher will and the personality's will. Excess comes in various forms: excessive complaining; dumping negative words, feelings, and emotions onto others; talking a lot but saying nothing; or dwelling on melancholic states and overcrying. On the other hand, excess may include being highly unmotivated or uninspired to be creative and to speak for ourselves.

Physical conditions may include the Chinese concept of "plum-stuck chi," when overwhelming emotion, such as grief or sadness, closes down the throat chakra. A person in this condition may feel swelling or blockage — a "frog in the throat."

Overstimulation of the thyroid and parathyroid glands causes excess production of thyroid hormones, resulting in increased metabolism, overactivity, and restlessness within the mind and body.

INTERIOR: Deep-seated conditions that prevent us from expressing our true selves can lead to chronic states of fear, worry, anxiety, nervousness, anger, sadness, grief, shame, guilt, and an overall deep suppression of these emotions. These states may result in the physical conditions listed in relation to the first four chakras, as well as problems in the respiratory system, thyroid, parathyroids, ears, hypothalamus, and neck. Other conditions may include chronic bronchitis, chronic sore throat, asthma, hypothyroid or hyperthyroid, chronic post-nasal drip, or chronic dry throat.

EXTERIOR: Acute conditions related to the fifth chakra include patterns of living that close down effective communication and creative means of self-expression.

Physical symptoms may include acute toothache, sore throat, loss of appetite or increased appetite, loss of energy, fever, influenza, hot flushed skin, chest discomfort, difficult breathing, rapid heart rate, tremor, mucus production in digestion, diarrhea or constipation, weight loss or weight gain, or intolerance to cold.

Treatment with Blue plants

The blue color of the throat chakra is cooling and soothing. Blue plants cool hot emotions (anxiety, anger, pent-up feelings) and channel their release. Blue can help tone down a person's workaholic or addictive patterns. Blue plants can also tone down excessive sexual energy. For those who are overstimulated most of the time, blue plants will help them to regenerate and recharge rather than to continue pushing. Blue plants will also help lift us out of our deep emotions and can energize us in a quiet, soothing way. They can also serve as an antidepressant.

Blue vervain is an example of a plant that works on the throat to clear colds and viruses. It cools fever, relieves restlessness, and relaxes muscle tension. Rosemary generates warmth by dispelling cold, stimulates the heart and circulation, and restores and invigorates the lungs. Rosemary is a good remedy for anemia, low blood pressure, bronchitis, lack of speech, and painful menses. Rosemary has long been known for its ability to lift the spirits. Sage is used to treat hoarseness or inflamed throat. Fresh sage leaves can be rubbed on the teeth and gums to cleanse the mouth and strengthen the gums. Sage is also used to treat venereal diseases, epilepsy, insomnia, lung congestion, sinus congestion, and many other illnesses.

Treatment with the Blue flower essences

Treatment with blue flower essences has a quietly soothing yet energetic effect. For example, Desert Larkspur flower essence offers gracefulness in the ways we communicate and helps us to ease into life transitions. Desert Larkspur flower essence enhances our power to use imagination and clarity of thought in our communication.

Vervain flower essence encourages us to communicate our strengths and abilities to others; through our creative expression we can obtain the achievements we strive for. Blue Flag (Wild Iris) flower essence helps us to embellish creative communications; it inspires creativity and artistic imaginative talents. It can be helpful for artists, writers, speakers, or anyone working to fulfill creative interests. Sage flower essence helps us be conscientious of the sounds we make, the words we choose, and the way we communicate with others. It guides us toward conscious choice of words and voice tones, and increases our inclination to speak with kindness and gentleness.

Although their flowers are not necessarily blue, the Snapdragon family (including Palmer's Penstemon, Scarlet Penstemon, and Yellow and Crimson Monkeyflowers) also includes wonderful remedies for creative and positive self-expression due to their Doctrine of Signatures. Almost any-one can benefit from members of the snap-dragon family when their communication seems stuck or misused.

sixth chakra: third eye, eye of wisdom, or brow chakra

ELEMENT: Radium
FOCUS: Seeing, visualization, clairvoyance, light, psychic perception, intuition, and imagination
COLOR: Violet-purple
ENDOCRINE GLAND: Pituitary
SOUND/VIBRATIONS: Tone of A above middle C; long "e" vowel sound, "mmm-mmmmmmmmmm," or "nnnnnnnnnnnn"; *ohm* (Hindu) sound; harps, organs, pianos, wind chimes, and high-pitched string instruments
POLARITY: Yin
COLD/HOT: Soothing and cooling
SENSES: Intuitive seeing, visualization, clairvoyance
FLOWER ESSENCES: Aster, Blue Flag, Chicory, Desert Larkspur, Desert Willow, Echinacea, Indian Paintbrush, Lupine, Morning Glory, Palmer's Penstemon, Pinyon, Purple Robe, Sage, Thistle, and Vervain
LOCATION AND PHYSICAL FUNCTIONS: The third eye or brow chakra is located slightly above the eyes and in the center of the forehead. The brow chakra is associated with the pituitary gland and the entire endocrine system. The pituitary gland is a peanut-sized organ located at the base of the brain. It is also known as the "master gland" because it secretes nine hormones that affect the functioning of the five lower endocrine glands, keeping them in balance and harmony with each other. The pituitary hormones serve many functions, including regulating the body's growth, assisting the kidneys to regulate urine excretion, increasing the production of pigment cells in the skin, causing contractions in the womb at childbirth, and stimulating the breast to start milk production. Pituitary hormones also act upon the gonads, thyroid, and adrenal glands. The pituitary may also be related to memory and sleep patterns.

The hypothalamus is located directly above the pituitary gland. It serves as a primary coordinator of the endocrine glands and the nervous system, as well as monitoring and regulating the autonomic nervous system. The hypothalamus influences the timing and concentration of pituitary hormones that help regulate appetite, body temperature, sleep, and the menstrual cycle. Along with the pituitary, the hypothalamus secretes hormones that induce contractions and produce breast milk.

The brow chakra is also associated with the immune system, the synapses of the brain, and the face, eyes, ears, and sinuses. This energy center helps provide the balance between the left and right hemispheres of the brain, stimulating the brain cells and impacting the personality.

positive healing patterns

The third eye or brow chakra is the visionary chakra that gives us wisdom, balance, and spiritual insight. This is why it is referred to as the "eye of wisdom" or the "inner eye." On a more personal level, the brow chakra teaches us about judgment, truth, honesty, harmony, and integrity and how our minds respond to the truths that we know. This center empowers us to acknowledge and identify our wisdom and to act according to the wisdom we receive. It frees stagnation and helps us define purpose and spiritual understanding. It also enables us to literally allow Light to come through our third eye and to receive the messages that the Light brings. The third eye is the vibrational point where the darkness from the center of the earth and the light from the center of the sun merge as one. The light and darkness together create a balanced sixth chakra. This energy center works with the mental aspects of the third chakra and allows a higher vision and spiritual aspiration to direct our mental thought-forms.

The third eye gives us the ability to internally see our memories, dreams, thought-forms, and imagination. At this center we take in, hold, clarify, create, and manifest visual information. This chakra opens the gateway to step beyond ourselves and to access the higher power that is already inherently within us. It opens us to clairvoyance and psychic awareness — the ability to see beyond time and space. It helps us access information and perception from within our mind's eye that tells us about a person, place, or event. We may see lights, color, images, our own emotions, or the emotions or energy fields of others. Through the sixth chakra, we gain access to long-distance vibrational healing by sending our prayers and healing to others in their physical absence.

This energy center awakens our intuition and our insights at a deep level. It gives us the power to tap into a higher vibrational frequency that is linked with the collective unconscious. It is through this powerful connection with the collective unconscious that our energy is shared and united.

symptoms and patterns of imbalance

DEFICIENCY: Deficiency in the sixth chakra causes an inability to access spiritual vision, intuitive perception, psychic awareness, clairvoyance, or higher wisdom. Deficiency can also result in inability to internally see memories, dreams, ideas, or insights. Due to these deficiencies, a person may have difficulty expanding into new ideas and gaining access to higher spiritual understandings. Deficiency may also cause stagnation and a lack of interest in a higher purpose, in spiritual vision and guidance, or in cohesiveness of thought, planning, and inspiration.

Physical symptoms may include low melatonin production (related to skin pigmentation), sensitivity to light, frontal sinus infections (thick white phlegm-like mucus infections), insomnia, and fever due to overexhaustion or overwork. Deficiency also alters normal sleep patterns and cycles.

Deficient production of pituitary hormones can contribute to tumors and to imbalances in the thyroid, adrenal, and gonad glands. Lack of growth hormone can lead to dwarfism.

EXCESS: Excess in the sixth chakra manifests as an inability to receive or clearly understand psychic or intuitive messages. Excess is also experienced through nightmares, paranoia, hallucinations, and being psychically overstimulated (being so sensitive that one lacks boundaries or balance in receiving incoming messages). A person who experiences these excesses may need help in understanding them. Excess also includes a tendency to be too theoretical, idealistic, and ungrounded.

Physical symptoms of excess may also include frontal sinus infections (thick yellow-green mucus conditions), oversleeping or needing too much rest, and getting chilled easily.

Too much growth hormone in children can cause gigantism, and excessive secretion of pituitary hormones can also contribute to tumors.

INTERIOR: Deep-seated sixth-chakra conditions can prevent us from tapping into our psychic intuitive perception, deeper wisdom, and higher spiritual values of trust, integrity, and honesty. Other deep-seated conditions are expressed as unusual or extreme behavior, such as paranoia, hallucinations, and nightmares. Any of these conditions can lead to chronic states of fear, worry, anxiety, nervousness, anger, sadness, grief, shame, guilt, and an overall deep suppression of these emotions. These states may be associated with the conditions listed in relation to the first five chakras.

Physical conditions include chronic dream-disturbed sleep, chronic pain, inability to focus, mental confusion, inability to begin labor contractions, and difficulty in producing breast milk.

EXTERIOR: Acute conditions related to the sixth chakra include occasional hallucinations, nightmares, and psychic disturbances. Physical conditions may include light sensitivity, inability to maintain a normal body temperature, irregular sleep, and inability to control blood pressure.

Treatment with violet-purple plants

Violet-purple plants free up stagnation in the body, especially related to blood. Echinacea is a wonderful example of a plant that has the ability to clear stagnation and to work as a blood purifier, removing toxic stagnation of the blood. Spirituality is enhanced because of the clearing of the heavy toxic condition. Sage (blue-violet) has estrogenic properties — hormone precursors that help treat irregular menses and symptoms of menopause. Sage can also lower blood-sugar levels in diabetics. Sage has been used to treat diseases of the liver and to energize or enrich the blood. Platycodon, or balloon flower, is used to treat sinusitis or rhinitis in the frontal sinuses. As it physically clears out the sinuses, it lessens the physical pressure and induces mental clarity.

Treatment with violet/lavender/purple flower essences

The violet/lavender/purple flowers prepared as flower essences offer spiritual vision and guidance and enhance imagination, creative visualization, perception, intuition, higher awareness, and deeper understanding. Lupine flower essence brings a sense of balance, insight, and creativity that helps us actualize both internal and external changes guided by our higher vision. It also helps us bring resolution and completion to the unfinished aspects of ourselves and our lives in a down-to-earth way. Lupine flower essence connects us with our higher mind and our creativity from deep within.

Aster flower essence helps us to embrace a higher community and planetary awareness that is united with the collective unconscious. Aster also helps us follow through with higher spiritual principles in ordinary ways of living, working, and being in the world. Offering a boost to depression, Aster flower essence guides us toward spiritual truths in an accepting, positive way. Sage flower essence also teaches whole-life balance, integrating spiritual principles with practical applications of daily living. Sage flower essence helps us demonstrate our spiritual self through our personality self in how we behave in the world.

Seventh Chakra: The Crown Chakra

Element: Magentum
Focus: "The thousand-petaled lotus,"
bliss, understanding, oneness with the Infinite, peace, expanded consciousness, communion with the Divine
Color: White/gold
Endocrine Gland: Pineal
Sound/Vibrations: Tone of B above middle C; there is no sound to chant except for the sound of the universe coming through us; harps, organs, pianos, wind chimes, and high-pitched string instruments.
Polarity: Yang
Cold/Hot: Lightly cooling energy
Senses: Receiving, understanding, and knowing a concept that includes all the senses previously listed, yet that goes beyond and is more expansive than all these senses
Flower Essences: Bells-of-Ireland, Black-Eyed Susan, Blue Flag, Bouncing Bet, Chamomile, Cliff Rose, Columbine, Comfrey, Desert Willow, Evening Primrose, Honeysuckle, Lupine, Morning Glory, Onion, Ox-Eye Daisy, Peace Rose, Sage, Saguaro, Thistle, Vervain, Willow, Yarrow, Yerba Santa, and Yucca
Location and Physical Functions: The crown chakra is located at the top of the head. It is associated with the cerebral cortex, the central nervous system, the pineal gland, and all the pathways of the nerves and electrical synapses within the body. Like the sixth chakra, the seventh chakra represents the balance of the two hemispheres of the brain.

The pineal gland is a small ovoid body about the size of a pea, situated centrally in the brain and attached to the third ventricle of the brain. The biological role of the pineal gland is not well understood. Its primary hormone is probably melatonin, which regulates the cerebrum, the hypothalamus, and the body's sleep/wake cycle. Experiments have shown that the pineal gland consists of vestiges of optic tissue in which nerve impulses occur in response to light.

positive Healing patterns

The seventh chakra is associated with both conscious and unconscious thoughts. These thoughts include our belief systems, how we see ourselves, how we see others, and how we view events in our lives. This energy center is associated with the "thread of consciousness"[2] that is anchored near the pineal gland.

The actual passage into the seventh chakra occurs spontaneously and effortlessly, aligning us with our spiritual essence and an intrinsic knowing that is linked to our higher consciousness. Higher consciousness relates to a broader relationship with ourselves and with the Divine Power that is bigger than, yet inclusive of, the physical world and our experiences in it. Higher consciousness includes our ability to live in the here and now, to plant the seeds of our thoughts with Divine Intelligence, and to nurture these seeds so they will be made manifest. This consciousness comes from an inner place that allows us to reach for and obtain our knowledge.

According to Anodea Judith and Selene Vega, "A single human brain contains some thirteen billion interconnected nerve cells capable of making more connections among themselves than the number of atoms in the universe. This staggering comparison presents us with a remarkable instrument. As there are 100 million sensory receptors in the body and 10 trillion synapses in the nervous system, we find that the mind is 100,000 times more sensitive to its internal environment than the external. It is truly from a place within that we acquire and process our knowledge."[3] Our brains, as vehicles to the mind, are infinite and unlimited.

As we gain access to the crown chakra, we find an infinite reservoir with a wave of infinite speed that allows us to be nowhere yet everywhere all at once. The crown chakra is where we explore, study, and experience our infinite reservoir of information that gives us reruns of the way we receive information, the way we interact with the world at large, our systems of belief and value, the way we view ourselves and our internal patterns, and the way we evolve into our spirituality.

By working with the seventh chakra, we become more aware of our relationship with God. We consciously begin to devote time each day toward the sacred, which may include prayer, meditation, writing in dream journals, healing work, flower essences, or other practices. We become the purpose of our life's work, and through our awareness the bond between the heart and the sixth chakra becomes more evident. We feel a vibrant energy flow throughout all the chakras and throughout our being. We become conscious of all the chakras and how they work together to create our biological existence. We learn to see ourselves as a system of energy, being mindful of every situation we find ourselves in and the way we hold or give away our power.

We are awakening to that which has no words; only experience can be felt. We are thankful for our life's journey and the blessings we receive along the way. Carolyn Myss, PH.D., refers to the seventh chakra as "the spiritual bank account where we store Grace.... The more we unplug ourselves from the illusion of the mind, the more we can interpret and receive the Grace in our lives."4

The power and significance of the white and gold colors of the seventh chakra is illustrated in Jerusalem's Church of the Holy Sepulcher, which recently underwent a major renovation. A beautifully restored dome above the traditional site of Jesus' tomb reveals golden rays of light bursting from a backdrop of pearly white radiant light. Ara Normart, the designer, represents his work of art as "the glory of God enveloping the risen Christ."5

symptoms and patterns of imbalance

DEFICIENCY: Deficiency in the seventh chakra relates to a lack of flexibility in our outlook toward life. Whatever holds us back from expanding our consciousness, from exploring the depths of our internal storage banks, from identifying and understanding our belief systems, or from seeking and gaining higher spiritual awareness leads to deficiency.

Physical symptoms of seventh-chakra deficiency may include neurological conditions, such as multiple sclerosis, Parkinson's disease, or diseases of the digestive system (hemorrhoids, anal fissures). Another symptom is the inability to concentrate.

EXCESS: Excess in the seventh chakra is exemplified by "spiritual" people who talk about spirituality in a way that is authoritative and controlling. They seem to know it all, and they are obsessed with the topic of spirituality. Often these people are not grounded in the world, and they tend to exaggerate the higher chakras to make up for their lack of development in the lower chakras. There is a lack of physical/emotional/mental balance to support their spiritual goals. Their spiritual talk tends to be intense and burdensome to others, causing discomfort.

Physical conditions of excess include seizure activity, hyperactivity, and headaches. Headaches are referred to as "liver toxicity headaches," wherein pressure and stagnation create headaches or visual problems.

People with excess seventh-chakra energy tend to be emotionally cool, lacking warmth and affection, and they have difficulty connecting with others. An example is the spiritual hermit who floats in his own cave, unwilling to look at his lack of integration in other parts of his life.

Excess is also demonstrated by people who become obsessed with their diet, fasting or cleansing excessively in order to advance spiritually.

INTERIOR: Deep-seated seventh-chakra conditions prevent us from receiving or tapping into our higher consciousness and higher awareness. Physical conditions may include insomnia, dream-disturbed sleep, and short attention span.

EXTERIOR: Acute conditions related to the seventh chakra include headaches, mental confusion, nervousness, restlessness, and anxiety. Disorientation and dizziness are also exterior symptoms.

Treatment with white plants

Plants that are white or cream-colored promote cleansing and release toxic buildup, stagnation, and tension at all levels throughout the body. They help us to restore, stretch, and expand, reaching beyond any self-imposed limitations and allowing our Higher Source to be our guide. For example, kudzu root releases physical muscle tension, and the white peony is used in Chinese medicine to release liver chi stagnation. Yarrow restores the liver, stomach, spleen, kidneys, bladder, and bone marrow. Yarrow also reduces inflammation, aids in cleansing, stimulates the liver, removes kidney toxins, and promotes urination and the menses. Yarrow also causes sweating, resolves fever, relaxes nerves, and relieves spasms.

Yerba santa, known as the "sacred herb," guards our psychic space and our physical inner linings. Yerba santa is used as an expectorant and bronchial dilator, and is used to treat colds, bronchitis, asthma, hay fever, chronic alcoholism, and even some forms of tuberculosis. Yucca has a high saponin (soap-like) content that allows joints to stretch and expand. Yucca also helps the colon eliminate built-up bile or toxic wastes. Yucca is used to treat arthritis, strengthen immunity, relieve stress, reduce inflammation and swelling, eliminate mucus, get rid of harmful microbes, and promote overall health and hygiene.

It takes the opening and fluid energy flow of all the chakras to effectively resonate and operate throughout the body system. By eliminating toxic wastes — physical, emotional, and mental — we open the doorways of our internal walls and stretch ourselves to become the infinitely conscious beings that we inherently are.

Treatment with white flower essences

Flower essences made with white or cream-colored flowers offer psychic cleansing, protection, release, insight, and an overall lightness and spiritual elevation. Sometimes I like to give people a white flower essence before doing a consultation or healing treatment because it helps calm and center them; it is an effective tool for getting to deeper core issues.

Yarrow flower essence is a wonderful, much-needed essence for those who feel vulnerable, run-down, and stressed out. It is a great healer that offers a shield of protection, harmony, and insight that keeps one from being drained by others.

Yerba Santa flower essence is also a great healer and teacher that helps us sort out our inner and outer impurities. Yerba

Santa helps build strength of character — the acceptance, willingness, and determination to work from within in order to heal the whole person. Yerba Santa helps us get rid of "psychic toxins" — elements of our lives that no longer support who we are. It works as a cleanser and purifier, and gives us spiritual guidance in our ability to follow through with tasks and intuition.

Yucca flower essence offers a powerful cleansing effect. This plant has great strength and endurance, and teaches us the determination needed to stay focused, grounded, and centered while making wise choices. Yucca essence reminds us to surrender and, when necessary, to protect ourselves.

Ox-Eye Daisy flower essence helps us open the wisdom chakra at the crown of the head, acknowledging and tapping into our innate knowing and understanding. The white ray-flowers represent purification and cleansing of the entire energy system, and in particular, the crown chakra. The depressed yellow disk in the center resembles an eye; hence, the flower offers a balance between intellect and intuition, providing understanding, vision, insight, and clarity about the whole picture.

summary

Chakras have been symbolized by the lotus flower, the petals of which unfold as it emerges into full bloom. The lotus is a sacred and beautiful flower, precious in India. The transformation of the flower's opening can be compared to the opening of a chakra. The lotus emerges from the muddy ground, symbolizing a journey from the earth's darkness, and evolves into a thousand petals (the "thousand-petaled lotus") that glow with radiant light out of the crown of the head. The lotus has completed its evolution and has now reached its highest peak of manifestation, of infinite bliss, expanded consciousness, and Divine communion.

Flowers, like chakras, have a root system that grows from the darkness of the earth. The developmental process of a plant is like the evolution of a chakra. The plant begins as a tiny seed from within the earth, then forms a root to stabilize and grow. The plant requires the earth, water, fire (sun or light), air, and sound vibrations to help it develop. The plant forms a stem (spine) and leaves, emerging into its unique individuality and its own energetic vibrational frequency. Finally, the plant produces a beautiful flower at the crown, or the top of its head. The flower emerges into its own special identity, and it reaches its fullest peak of blossoming while merging the darkness of the earth with the radiant light of consciousness. The flower has evolved, completed its cycle, and surrendered to the Infinite.

Both plants and the chakras have cycles of growth and development, closing or opening to expand into their fullest blossom and experiencing the process of budding life followed by death.

The Seven Chakras and Their Corresponding Flowers

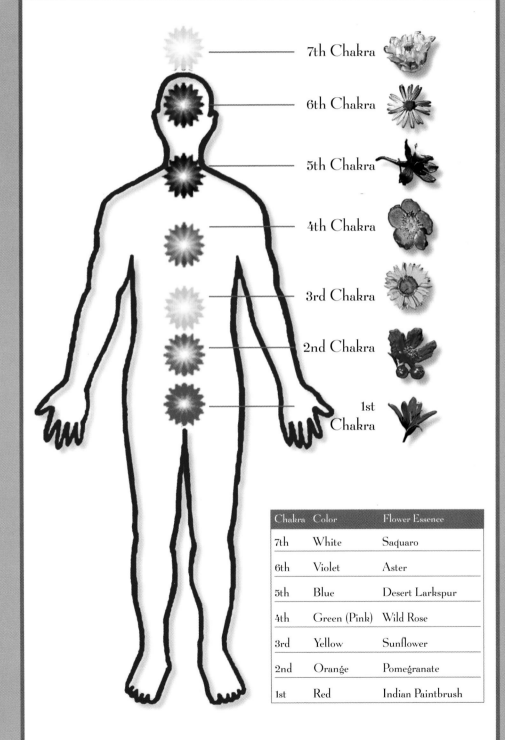

7th Chakra

6th Chakra

5th Chakra

4th Chakra

3rd Chakra

2nd Chakra

1st Chakra

Chakra	Color	Flower Essence
7th	White	Saguaro
6th	Violet	Aster
5th	Blue	Desert Larkspur
4th	Green (Pink)	Wild Rose
3rd	Yellow	Sunflower
2nd	Orange	Pomegranate
1st	Red	Indian Paintbrush

CHAPTER 5
Reflections on Chakras, Color, and Healing with Flower Essences

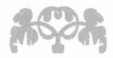

You may be wondering what all of this has to do with flower essences and why I brought the history and science of the human energy field and the chakra system into this book. The answers will gradually unfold as you continue to read. It is useful to begin by understanding the history and validity of the chakras. This subject is quite extensive, and I encourage readers to further their knowledge about the chakras and refer to the bibliography in the back of this book.

The vast amount of information written about the chakras is challenging. I do not present myself as an expert on the chakra system, but for years I have been naturally drawn to study the energy centers within the body. Through receiving treatments in various healing arts — massage, polarity, acupuncture, acupressure, chiropractic, homeopathy, herbal therapy, flower essences, myofascial release, Reiki, and laying on of hands — I have experienced the power of the chakras and the role they play in my relationship with myself. In giving healing treatments, I have also experienced how deeply I am affected by the energy exchange between giver and receiver that works through Spirit. While meditating or performing conscious exercises such as Tai Chi, yoga, and even hiking or walking, I have felt a balance from the first through seventh chakras throughout my body. I feel the same balance when I am making flower essences or when I am in nature with the earth, air, sun, and water.

I have studied and responded to the colors of the chakras for quite some time, and I have felt the effects that the colors of flowers have on the chakras physically, emotionally, mentally, and spiritually. These experiences have greatly inspired my personal growth and understanding. I have witnessed these profound effects not only with myself but with my family, friends, research participants, and clients. I am amazed by the truths that continue to be revealed by using flower essences, particularly in relation to the chakras.

Our chakras serve as a doorway to the infinite and give us access to the spirit of all life forms. Like the chakras, flowers have colors and vibrations of sound and light. Plant spirits speak to us through the color and sound vibration specific to each chakra. The more we become aware of how each chakra affects who we are, the more internally harmonious we will be and the better we'll understand ourselves.

In my experience, by becoming aware of the essence of the whole plant, I am tuning into its creative power, the innate intelligence and electromagnetism of its being. With this comes wisdom, insight, grace, strength, even pain, and all the things that are represented in the power of healing.

Just as plants and flowers have innate wisdom, so does the human body. Our innate wisdom is expressed through the seven chakras, from the root chakra to the crown chakra, by subtle vibrations or energy fields.

chakras, colors, and plants

When I meditate with a plant, I begin to resonate with the plant's wisdom and healing properties. This includes an awareness and identification of the Doctrine of Signatures, such as color, shape, touch, taste, and other properties. I also gain information from the plant intuitively, as a voice or an image. Through this I receive guidance as to what chakra the plant resonates with. I have found over and over that the colors of the flowers have direct correlations with the colors of the chakras, as well as with the integration of the whole chakra system. I have also found that the Doctrine of Signatures plays a vital role in showing us relationships between plants and chakras that may not be directly associated with a particular color but, instead, with the vibrational frequency of the chakra. In the case of Indian Paintbrush, for example, the plant's visionary qualities relate it to the sixth chakra as well as to the lower chakras. The sixth chakra is not indicated by color, but by Indian Paintbrush's ability to enhance imagination, insight, and vision.

Indian paintbrush is a fiery reddish orange plant that is semiparasitic because it lacks a well-developed root system. Its roots penetrate and depend on tissues of host plants, such as sagebrush or oak, to supply water and nutrients. Indian paintbrush's dependence on other plants is a demonstration of its low vitality, physical weakness, and depletion of energy. The host plants don't seem to suffer greatly from sharing their nutrients. Once the Indian paintbrush's vital force is "grounded" by burrowing its root system into the roots of the host plant, it has made a breakthrough from survival to the freedom of growing into its own creative and vibrant form. The significance of the roots of Indian paintbrush burrowing into the roots of other plants and of the reddish orange color of the leaf-like bracts (representing both the first chakra and second chakras) draws us to understand and identify the roots that connect us to our own spiritual heritage. From this vantage point, an awareness of dysfunctional patterns from this and past lives may surface for examination and decrystalization.

A conscious awareness of who we really are and how to manage our power may arise, and we are then able to interpret life's challenges in a new light and act accordingly. The brightly colored reddish orange bracts are highly artistic and give an incredible sense of emergence, creativity, inspiration, warmth, and vitality. By resonating with the essence of the Indian paintbrush, I feel energy at the base of my spine as if my own roots were growing into the roots of another plant and into Mother Earth. You may choose to take this energy as support for survival and for eliminating any parasitic relationships you may have with others; Indian paintbrush increases our awareness of any relationships in which one person is too dependent on another.

If I am a child who has become a teenager or adult, I may want to strive for liberation and to forge a new identity without codependency or attachment to my parents. By choosing to resonate with Indian paintbrush and its gifts, I will not allow myself to be taken over by another or to be a victim at my own expense; I realize that I need to become strong enough to depend on myself so that I can create my own destiny. There is a sense of a vital force coming through my feet, legs, and tailbone. It gives me a feeling of having the power to be and express who I am

without concern for what others think. A subtle sensation that leads to an opening in my tailbone comes from deep inside; it allows me the freedom to be creative without force or resistance.

I absorb the color of the Indian paintbrush and allow it to fill my entire being. With my eyes closed, I see the gentle face of a Native American medicine woman before me. She hands me a basket of corn and invites me to sit with her. In return, I give her the pouch of cornmeal that I'm wearing around my neck. We look deeply into each other's eyes and exchange an understanding that sends a tingling sensation of energy all the way down to my toes. Internally, a great shift of energy has occurred. The image of the medicine woman disappears and I open my eyes, feeling a new strength and empowerment to be who I am. Indian paintbrush has opened my sixth chakra; it is a visionary guide that helped me see and experience my own power and strength.

working with flower essences and chakras for Healing

I see the chakras — the subtle life-force energy centers within each of us — as playing an important role in who we are and who we are becoming. The power of the chakras, the uniqueness of what each chakra represents, the effectiveness of the color of each chakra, the way each chakra affects us, and what we can learn from our chakras can give us deeper understanding, the power of personal growth, and fluidity within ourselves. The chakras are the means by which we understand our responsibility to ourselves, others, and the world. As we form a relationship with the subtle intelligence of our energy centers, we become aware of the imbalances — the harmony or disharmony — that is projected outward from a specific center.

For example, if a man has prostate problems, he can inquire into his first or second chakra to help him understand his relationship with the disharmony of that chakra. He will learn that the first and second chakras are partially linked to the function of the adrenal glands, sexual function, and excretory functions. He will also learn that the first and second chakras greatly influence sexuality and the reproductive system, the entire muscular system, the eliminative system, and the functions of the spleen, bladder, pancreas, and kidneys. In addition, the first and second chakras relate to detoxification of the body. The second chakra is the energy center of sensation and emotion. Disharmony of emotions and personality dysfunctions can lead to imbalances in the second chakra. By increasing his awareness and consciousness of the second chakra, he may be able to identify what he needs to eliminate in his life, such as a blockage in sexual awareness.

By identifying and accepting the dys-function or blockage, he will better understand the flower essence that matches his disharmony and that will help him overcome his blockage. As he finds the flower that harmonizes with the blockage, the essence (with its resonance of sound, light, and vibration) will dissolve the disharmony in his auric field or in his second chakra. Emotional bondage is released. Where there was a lack of awareness, there will now be awareness. He can become empowered to do something about the problem. Where there was a blockage, there can now be an opening.

The flower essence and its vibrational influence on the chakra help us to align with ourselves, to understand our dysfunctions, and to make conscious choices about changes in our lives. Most important, this relationship with the flower essence helps us connect with the One who lives and breathes through us and as us.

Through prayer, meditation, and forming a relationship and an understanding of our energy centers, we can consciously learn to heal and evolve in ways we never have before. The power of our healing in these sometimes subtle ways is encompassing and harmonizing. The chakras are vibratory frequencies in which the power of Creation utilizes manifesting agents, such as flower essences, to create true and long-lasting changes in our lives that promote healing and well-being.

PART III

Healing with Flower Essences

Freedom's Reflections

Having climbed to a distant mountain meadow,
Resting among the myriad wildflowers,
And green, green grasses.

Breathing in and breathing out,
Taking in the fresh aromas
I feel relaxed.

I gaze intently across this rolling meadow,
To the horizon.
Mountain and sky
Become One.

A bird of prey settles on a
distant crag.

Wind no longer on the wing,
Touches my face.

Above, a swallow tail glides and dashes,
And all of Nature sings.

Right now, while feasting on this
Grand Earth Mother
And time has lots its throne,
Sensations flood a mind to stupor.

A body becomes a fountain of youth.
A heart is soaring
And a soul is free!

By Curt PallasDowney

CHAPTER 6
Breaking through the Veil:
Flower Essences and Personal Growth

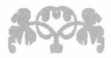

We are each born with a unique genetic code and our own set of past-life experiences and present-life circumstances. Our soul carries the record of our past experiences and chooses our current situation, setting forth our life's curriculum. The challenges and pitfalls we experience in our lives are merely tests in that curriculum, allowing us to learn and grow. By working through such setbacks and blockages, the mystery of why we came here reveals itself.

These challenges also present the first step in our healing. As we become aware of the core issue at the root of each blockage, we discover an opening deep within ourselves that brings release, decrystalization of old patterns, and new opportunities for personal growth. We experience renewed awareness of our soul's purpose; we feel on track in exploring the mystery of our soul's journey.

The soul as Resource

The soul has numerous functions. It is the breath of life and the original spark of our spiritual evolution as human beings. Most importantly for our healing process, the soul carries the record of our eternal life. At birth, we forget that we are one with the Divine; we forget that we are cocreators of our lives and the world. The soul creates this veil of illusion — this belief in our separateness from the Divine — as a stage in our learning process.

Our bodies are mirrors of our soul record and expressions of our eternal lives. Our chakras are the reservoir of soul dramas that need to be healed. As we deeply explore different parts of the body, each chakra reveals information about who we are through the historic patterns and blockages stored within.

This is the basis of the Eastern concept of karma. These records or dramas are established when energy is set in motion that is not in harmony with cosmic law or with our vital force. The soul is the record keeper from which these karmic patterns emerge.

We do not need to remain stuck in these stored patterns. They can be the beginning of a transformational journey. The greatest healing occurs, not by treating only the physical manifestations of these blockages, but by working at the spiritual level. Because our vital force, or spirit, is an aspect of the Divine mind, the mental/emotional/astral (soul) body is a more powerful resource in the healing process than is the physical body.

Healing our Blocked Energy patterns

A phenomenal transformation can occur when we realize that what we think is what we are creating in our lives. Our thoughts are an internal dialogue, often fed by our old dramas and blockages — imbalanced thoughts that originate in the soul record, either from this life or past lives. When we experience disharmony in our lives, it is often because the events around us are aligning with our subconscious dysfunctional energy patterns. This energy may surface in the form of worry, greed, anger, hate, or guilt, gaining momentum until it is released through the emotional body and expressed as inappropriate behavior. As this process repeats itself, a negative pattern becomes entrenched in the human organism. These negative patterns show up externally as physical or mental illness and dysfunctional relationships.

In short, our thoughts create what happens in our body and in the world around us. If we think a given thought for long enough, we will manifest it. That

action is energy in motion. An imbalance in the mental field will create an imbalance in the emotional and physical fields.

For example, if a woman was in an automobile collision, and the driver in the other vehicle was at fault, when she remembers that collision she may feel blame leading to anger. When an image of the collision comes up, she may say, "Why did that person pull out in front of me?" and "How could they have done this to me?" If these thoughts continue for a day, a year, or a lifetime, she is staying in the same pattern of blame. As this happens, her heart center closes down; instead of acting from love and compassion, she begins to act from anger and blame for what she feels is an injustice. This is the fertile ground for illness. The muscles in her neck and shoulders may become tense, her heart center shuts down from the failure to forgive, and energy is held in her solar plexus. Chronic states may lead to digestive problems, immune deficiencies, or other diseases related to the adrenals, stomach, liver, and gall bladder (gallstones or gastritis). This experience and its healing is the soul drama.

As another example, if your mind is holding a limiting fear — such as "How will I pay the rent?" — this is a projection from your subconscious memory and a reflection of your survival fears and/or family heritage. If you're following a subconscious memory pattern, you are on the path of an old drama; you're reliving history instead of recovering and living in the presence of Divine mind. If you don't overcome that negative pattern, it devours you. You live it until you successfully dissolve the soul pattern.

If you act out of fear ("How will I pay the rent?") instead of finding a way to make the money, a negative emotional pattern is formed. This pattern involves a loss of control and may be acted out in depression, alcoholism, or abusive behavior. These behaviors then re-create the old pattern, intensifying the lack of direction and the feeling of being stuck with no forward movement.

It may appear from this discussion that the subconscious mind is bad, but it really isn't; it's just giving us our curriculum. Each of us has patterns, history, and core issues to unravel and make peace with. When we choose to live exclusively in our rational mind, receiving information only through our senses, we may feel that the subconscious mind diverts us from our path. However, the enlightened approach is to allow our subconscious and conscious minds to work in harmony, not in conflict.

The Healing Process

How do we heal and change these patterns? The soul body is what holds them. When we embark upon healing, we must harmonize and balance the relationship between the physical, emotional, mental, and soul bodies.

In healing, we are working with the vital force, which has been described as "life force," "life energy," or "bioenergy." It helps us to understand the vital force as a spiritual field that encompasses the whole person — body, mind, and spirit — and includes the healing power of the body. Identifying, observing, and experiencing the presence of the vital force is the process by which the disease can be known. The symptoms, as a whole, suggest the means of transformation back to health or restoration of the vital force.

Both Hahnemann and Bach stressed that it is "the patient — the whole person, not the disease" — that must be given attention. A homeopathic diagnosis or the selection of a flower essence involves investigating and understanding all the patient's symptoms, physical, emotional, mental, and spiritual.

For every emotion there is a corresponding physical organ or region that is affected when that emotion is activated. When the emotion becomes blocked or stagnant, the corresponding physical organ and its functions also eventually become stagnant, leading to disease.

For example, the kidneys are related to deep-seated grief and fear, and the liver is associated with anger. If a person has unexpressed grief and holds the grief for a long time, the kidneys may be affected. An angry alcoholic may eventually have deficiencies and blocked energy in the liver. By quitting drinking and by resolving the cause of the anger, the alcoholic can release the stagnant energy held in the liver.

A particular plant may correspond with an organ or region in the body, which in turn corresponds to the emotions that stimulate it. It is the presence or core essence of the plant that communicates to the essence or spirit of the person. This innate communication allows healing to take place by tapping into the person's subconscious and uniting with his or her spirit. This energy connection affects the mind, presenting an opportunity for the person to understand the impact of certain thought patterns. Through this illumination, the person may better understand the blockage and may change how he or she thinks and feels about a past experience.

For example, a man with chest pains or cardiac disorder may come to understand the need to forgive instead of to blame. As he consciously forgives, feelings of blame and anger give way to feelings of acceptance and compassion. As he then changes his thoughts, this energy connection affects his emotions and imagination, highlighting the cause of the physical condition and helping him overcome it.

Flower essences help us dissolve the patterns formed by our past experiences. Flower essences can actually help create the emotion necessary to dissolve the soul blockages or soul patterns. In other words, flower essences help a person embrace the unconscious memory or pattern rather than resist it.

going beyond bach

I would like to take the study and use of flower essences a step farther than Dr. Bach took it. I believe we must go beyond

matching flower essences with physical symptoms and negative emotional states. We can more deeply explore what each plant has to offer by identifying the positive states we wish to uplift and by focusing on key words of affirmation that help us elevate those states.

How do we discover the underlying cause of a particular emotion?

True flower essence medicine works in ways that capture the medicine or gifts of the whole plant's spirit. This means sincerely understanding the whole plant's properties, including smells, tastes, colors, and shapes, and going beyond them to embrace its essence and spirit.

Each plant offers a Divine spiritual presence for us to connect with. This gift reveals itself when we take time to give thanks, pray, meditate on our breathing, observe the plant and its surroundings, and wait. The plant will express itself in some way, perhaps through movement, wind, imagery, stillness, or voice. It will show you something about yourself. You will feel its presence. You can ask the plant for guidance, for the spirit of the plant to share with you its healing qualities (if you need suggestions about how to do this, refer to the section on "The Plant Journey" in chapter 8).

Each flower or plant has a specific makeup that relates to a certain chakra or chakras. At the core of the flower's chemistry is a particular alchemical formula that consists of the actual flower essence and the energy it produces. That alchemical formula can dissolve the blockages in a particular chakra. At this deepest level within us, new patterns of thought and energy are given an opportunity to break through our illusion of separateness from the Divine. The alchemical power of the flower essence works with the human energy system to regenerate the chakras and provides a path for soul and spirit to reunite.

As this healing takes place, a renewed mental and emotional balance reinforces the physical healing and wellness of the whole person. As a person begins to dissolve old patterns and memories, the cosmic body becomes anchored in the Divine Self for longer periods of time, rebalancing the conscious and unconscious mind. Through this process, we are able to consciously plant the seeds of Divine awareness in our energy pattern. We learn to quiet the mind and bring balance and peace from within to without.

Our subconscious mind becomes fertile ground in which Divine thoughts can arise. These Divine thoughts and feelings serve as seeds for new growth in our bodies, minds, and spirits. As we plant these seeds of cosmic consciousness, our cellular structure becomes lighter — more transmutable and fluid in relation to its environment. Thoughts of limitation melt away. We begin to live, think, and act in an entirely new way. We learn that we are one with the Divine and with all of life. Working with flower essences enhances this transformation.

CHAPTER 7
How to Select Flower Essence Remedies

There are several methods for selecting a flower essence. One common way is to simply choose an essence or essences that one is naturally drawn to. There is no "wrong" choice when using flower essences; if the selected essence doesn't produce results, you can simply choose another essence. There are no negative side effects.

It would be to your benefit to acquire the flower essences listed in this book and take them as you work with the flowers. This experience will allow you to create a more powerful union with the plant and to gain a deeper understanding of its effects.

Here is a simple step-by-step guide to selecting among the flower essences listed in this book (later in this chapter, you will find several more in-depth approaches you may wish to use):

1. Gather your intention. Begin by focusing on a key issue that you (or another person) need help with. You may already know what this issue is, or you may need to take time to silence your mind. Ask yourself what you want to heal in your life. Is there something about yourself you would like to change? Later in this chapter, you will find more details about how to ask opening questions.

2. Look at the photos of the flowers in this book and notice which ones "speak" to you. If you connect with a particular flower, notice its color, shape, and anything about it that you are drawn to. Take some time to sit with that and observe how the flower affects you.

3. Take time to review the Key Rubrics Guide. Begin with each flower's primary quality. Allow yourself to capture a feeling of any particular quality that stands out for you. Take some time to bring the word/thought/feeling of the quality deep inside yourself.

4. In the Key Rubrics Guide, read the Key Rubrics for Positive Healing

Patterns and the Key Rubrics for Symptoms and Patterns of Imbalance. The sections are designed to help you pinpoint key words that directly relate to your intention and that match the qualities of a given flower. Look for your own patterns of imbalance (or those of another) that match the key words or phrases given. Also, look for the positive healing patterns you or another wish to achieve or experience.

5. Review the Quick Reference Chart for Flower Essences and Chakras (see chapter 10), and notice the chakra that corresponds with the chosen flower(s). You can look over the words on the chart that briefly describe each chakra, or you can more deeply review information about a chakra in part II of this book. Another method is to begin by reviewing the chakras as a guide to selecting the flower.

6. In chapter 11, read the in-depth description of the flower(s) you have chosen, and and try to imagine its Doctrine of Signatures.

7. Read the Helpful Suggestions section about your flower(s) in chapter 11. This is an exercise that will help you experience the flower or plant even more deeply. Each exercise is unique and will awaken your awareness of the plant and yourself. Allow yourself to surrender to the exercise and simply experience where it takes you. You are beginning a new relationship with the flowers as well as with yourself, and this relationship will only deepen as it unfolds further.

8. Read the Affirmations related to your flower(s) in chapter 11. Read them one at a time. You may want to repeat each one and read it out loud. You also may choose to write them down and place them on a mirror or in a special spot so that you can be reminded of them throughout the day. Use the affirmations as often as you wish; if you have the essence, take it throughout the day and before you go to bed.

You have the freedom to choose any flower, any time, and follow your heart's desire about what works best for you. You will find similarities among the flowers and affirmations; repetition and the power of words and thoughts will become seeded in your memory. This kind of power allows you to manifest a state of consciousness that will alter your life forever. The flowers, like all of life, come from One Source. May you find reverence with the flowers and trust your process.

The Clinical Approach

The clinical approach is a relatively formal means of selecting a flower essence for oneself or another person. The purpose is to gain basic information about the recipient that will aid in selecting the appropriate flower essence. Such a formal approach is not always needed, but it may be especially useful to health-care practitioners.

Gathering Information

There are several possible levels of information gathering. For the sake of simplicity, I will offer some general questions to ask the client. There are, of course, many other questions that can be asked throughout the consultation process. I generally select my questions based on the recipient's intention and the chakras that he or she is focusing on, whether consciously or subconsciously (a person may not be consciously aware of the chakra system, but symptoms and word choices provide indications). There are many ways to gather basic information, however, and none are right or wrong in themselves.

The main thing to keep in mind, as with any type of healing work, is our conscious intention: to release energy blocks and stagnation on any level and to allow energy to flow. When selecting a flower essence, base your choice on what is needed at the moment to release energy stagnation and appropriately direct its flow. I also find that flower essences are most effective when the recipient has a conscious intention when taking them.

Observation is one of the greatest skills of a healer. How a person speaks (fast or slow), the presenting tone of voice, the posture, any significant behaviors or physical conditions, dullness or brightness of the eyes, body language, and emotional expression while talking (nervousness, frustration, sadness, anger) are some of the things we observe as practitioners. Keen observation is an informative guide in the flower essence selection process.

Flower Essence Case-Taking Guidelines

During a consultation, remain mindful of the whole person. Ask open-ended questions and allow the person to express him- or herself without interruption. Let the person's behavior confirm all the information he or she provides.

GENERAL QUESTIONS TO ASK THE RECIPIENT:

1. What is the presenting issue? Why are you here? How can I help you? What is it you would like to heal? When did it begin? If known, why did it become an issue? Allow the person to describe the presenting issue and circumstances with as few interruptions as possible, using his or her own words.

2. Do you have specific fears? If so, what are they?

3. How well do you sleep at night? What is your dream activity like? Do you have nightmares? If so, what are they like?

4. Do you need constant approval from others? Do you feel unrecognized for who you are? If so, explain this.

5. What is your overall emotional state, and how do you usually deal with daily challenges? How do you respond to a crisis?

6. Do you have any addictions, such as alcohol, drugs, or abusive relationships? If so, please describe.

7. How would you describe yourself? How would a friend describe you?

8. Do you have specific concerns about yourself? If so, please describe them.

9. What is your medical history? How is/was your relationship with your parents, siblings? How would you briefly describe your childhood? Is there something significant in your childhood that stands out? If so, please share it with me.

CHAKRA-RELATED OBSERVATIONS

Determine what chakra is most affected. Where does the person tend to hold his or her energy?

Is the person's energy predominantly related to physical issues (first chakra)? (Typified by a high degree of activity or inactivity; chronic illness such as cancer, arthritis, poor circulation, or physical discomfort; deep-seated emotional conditions that lead to chronic fear, anger, agitation, or deep suppression; significant survival, security, or financial issues; a condition such as obesity, constipation, frequent urination, or a sexually transmitted disease.)

Is the person's energy predominantly related to emotional issues (second chakra)? (High-strung, fearful, emotionally exhausted, overwhelmed; lacking self-worth or creativity; being overly confrontational or insensitive toward others; having a weak immune system or sexual imbalances.)

Is the person predominantly of a mental nature (third chakra)? (Tends to overanalyze or worry; is highly critical, judgmental, or perfectionistic; lacks trust in his or her intuition; lacks mental clarity and the ability to focus; tends toward fear, panic, hopelessness, despair, guilt, unworthiness, nostalgia, uncertainty, anger, hatred, or prejudice.)

Does the person carry issues related to love, compassion, and the heart (fourth chakra)? (Lacks love or the joy in living; heart is shut down; experiences self-doubt and neediness; dwells on heart-related sufferings and pains such as the death of a loved one; is withdrawn, resentful, or unwilling to love others unconditionally.)

Does the person have issues related to communication (fifth chakra)? (Expression feels denied; has been told to keep "secrets"; lacks willpower in self-expression and communication; has difficulty releasing emotions by crying, sighing, or laughing; complains excessively and forces opinions and thoughts on others; "dumps" negative words and feelings onto others; talks a lot but says nothing.)

Does the person have difficulty imagining, visualizing, intuiting, or tapping into higher wisdom and insights (sixth chakra)? (Inability to access spiritual vision or intuitive perceptions; difficulty remembering dreams, ideas, or insights; lack of spiritual vision and guidance; no cohesiveness of thought and inspiration.)

Is the person disconnected from higher consciousness (seventh chakra)? (Lack of flexibility in her or his outlook toward life;

holds back from expanding consciousness or exploring the depths of values and belief systems; lacks a higher spiritual awareness and knowledge; talks about spirituality in an overly authoritative way or is obsessed with the topic of spirituality; lacks balance internally or in the world to support spiritual goals.)

PATTERNS OF IMBALANCE

Compare the recipient's symptoms, or patterns of imbalance, with the Patterns of Imbalance section for each flower essence shown in chapter 11. Find the plant or plants that best match the recipient's symptoms. For example, if you are a woman and you are overly moody, especially in relation to your menses; if you have lost your sense of creativity, including your sexuality, passion, and overall feminine nature; and if you find yourself struggling with your identity and how you relate to the world, your family, and yourself, your symptoms and patterns of imbalance match the Pomegranate's patterns of imbalance. Or let's say you've simply lost your sense of creativity and inspiration and you feel stuck; these symptoms and patterns of imbalance match Blue Flag (Wild Iris). You might also want to consider Indian Paintbrush, depending on which plant qualities most closely match your condition.

PATTERNS OF BALANCE (POSITIVE HEALING PATTERNS)

Compare the recipient's intention or positive healing patterns — what they want to achieve from taking a flower essence — with the plant descriptions in chapter 11. You will find that the positive healing patterns are the opposite of the patterns of imbalance. If a female recipient has an intention to stir passion, sexuality, and creative awareness of her feminine energy; if she wants to feel emotionally balanced during menses or through menopause; and if she has an urge to express her inner joys and freedom, Pomegranate's positive healing patterns make a good match.

However, if a recipient tends to burn out quickly and needs guidance with skillful pacing, is an artist, writer, or speaker, or wants artistic inspiration, that intention compares well with the Blue Flag's positive healing patterns.

On the other hand, if the recipient seeks higher visionary guidance, has difficulty meeting survival needs, and wants to uncover hereditary roots and work out family or past issues that block creativity, inspiration, and self-expression, you may decide to choose Indian Paintbrush.

THE DOCTRINE OF SIGNATURES

Next read about the plant's physical makeup and its Doctrine of Signatures. The recipient may share some characteristics with the plant; this can increase self-awareness. Take note of how the plant holds itself, what color it is, what its flowers look like, and where it likes to grow. Notice in what ways the recipient is attracted or repelled by the plant and its flowers. For example, Comfrey flowers droop toward the ground, making a statement of protection, surrender, and sacrifice; the protruding tongue-like center of the flower symbolizes our inner voice and the taste of our sweet essence that comes from deep inside. The lavender color represents higher visionary guidance and a clearer understanding of the sacrifices we make in life. The structure of the veins in the leaves represents an ability to put things into perspective. The fuzzy surface of the leaves and their rough, prickly underside symbolize the union of opposites, building a bridge of healing from within to without. If the recipient has similarities with the Comfrey's signatures — a need to make a personal sacrifice or offer service for the good of the whole, a need for clarity about the situation or the required service, and a need for guidance to speak the truth from a place of inner knowing — then Comfrey flower essence may be the right one.

Confrontation or Elevation

You may want to ask the recipient if the intention in taking a flower essence is to confront an issue or to get a spiritual boost. There are times when we need to confront a part of ourselves that requires change in order to release the energy, let go of old patterns, and face what we tend to resist. There are other times when we have faced and worked with the parts of ourselves we want to change, and we just need an energy boost instead of continuing to work through the confrontations. For example, flower essences such as Black-Eyed Susan or Mexican Hat take us through our pains and help us face the parts of ourselves that require confrontation, yet both of these bring inner peace and release as a result of the confrontation. On the other hand, if we have become weary from the confrontations and worked hard at those issues, we may choose essences such as Lupine, Echinacea, or Desert Larkspur to uplift us.

Color and the Chakras

The recipient's intention and symptoms will also guide you in selecting the appropriate flower color in an essence. When you work with the chakras, there comes a crossroad of deciding when to use a color that pertains to a certain chakra and when to use the complementary color associated with that chakra. For example, if a person has extreme anger, the color red may intensify the anger. On the other hand, red may reveal the love or passion that lies beneath the blocked anger. Depending on the person and the situation, a red flower essence may help identify the core issue of where the anger is coming from and support the process of understanding and expressing the anger. A red flower would be especially useful if the recipient has had little experience in processing anger.

On the other hand, if the person has identified the core issue of the anger and has a history of working with that anger, it may be more healing for that person to resonate with a more soothing pink flower. The pink flower essence would bring calmness, compassion, and balance to an otherwise fiery personality. As always, remember to also take the entire Doctrine of Signatures into consideration when selecting the flower essence.

Here is another example of how to select an appropriate color of flower essence. A man is seeking help for being overly mental and analytical; he has a rampant internal dialogue and a mind that never seems to slow down. He also shows symptoms of nervousness, anxiety, and worry and he lacks trust in his intuitions. A yellow flower essence might intensify his symptoms, but it's possible that a softer yellow flower may have a subtler effect, depending on its Doctrine of Signatures and its overall resonance. In this case, a good choice might be a violet-purple flower essence to soothe or soften his overstimulated third-chakra area. The violet-purple flower essence resonates at a higher level that would uplift and guide the third-chakra energy field to a more inspirational level. This approach may also help him open his third eye and spontaneously release and open his solar plexus energy as well.

As an example of the opposite condition, another man thrives on spiritual visions and spiritual guidance and isn't very grounded. He talks about spiritual life but doesn't apply spiritual values in his daily life. He may need to "come down" and learn to apply spirituality in practical ways. In this case, it may be helpful to give a yellow flower essence (because yellow is the color complement associated with the sixth chakra; see chapter 3) or a lower-chakra essence (to ground him in his body; see chapter 11 for essence/chakra correspondences), according to the Doctrine of Signatures and his core issues.

Yet another example would be a woman experiencing an emotionally painful crisis, such as the death of a loved one, being in a collision, or losing a large sum of money. Giving her a blue or lavender flower essence will help bring balance and calmness. It would also be soothing and cooling to the lower chakras. Pink flowers such as the Roses would also be helpful. On the other hand, if her ability to express herself is shut down, if she resists confrontation, or if she is suppressed emotionally, it may be helpful to give her an orange flower essence that would help her confront the emotion, express it, and release it.

Giving someone a white flower essence helps balance out the emotions and simultaneously offers protection and spiritual transformation. I like to give Yarrow (white flower) or the Yarrow formula (which consists of pink, yellow, and white flowers) in cases of shock or trauma because it offers a shield of protection around an individual and aids in the relief of fatigue and exhaustion. Also, many times I like to begin with a white flower essence to help a person center and open up to a higher power.

Another example of selecting a flower essence by the color of its flower would be a choice of California Poppy. As an orange, second-chakra flower, California Poppy essence offers a cleansing effect and acts as a purifier for emotional toxins. It heightens our sensitivity and helps us tap into our inner knowing. It also opens us up to the spark of fire deep within our sensuality and sexuality. A person may take California Poppy to help release emotional toxins or dysfunctional emotional patterns. California Poppy may offer immediate charges of energy that help in releasing this emotional baggage. If California Poppy is used for a month or longer, its effectiveness will wear off. At that time, a different essence would be needed to resonate with the person's energy field. A blue flower essence such as Chicory may be useful as a way to uplift and soothe the emotions. Chicory is an especially effective remedy for those who are self-centered, possessive, demanding, and emotionally irresponsible, yet have a deep desire to release their toxic emotional patterns. Chicory helps us create and express inner security, sharing, selfless love, sensitivity toward others, and a higher vision.

INTERIOR (CHRONIC) CONDITIONS OR EXTERIOR (ACUTE) CONDITIONS

It is also helpful to know whether a person's symptoms arise from underlying chronic conditions, such as childhood abuse, traumas, addictions, or abandonment. If the intention is to work with core issues, it is most effective to choose flower essences that help the recipient face and work out these issues. If the person's relationship with a particular issue has not changed even after confronting and working with it, then a flower essence that offers a boost may be useful. If a person's intention is to work with more acute conditions, such as increased stress, a sudden emotional dynamic with a family member, a change in career, or peeling off emotional layers that have been hidden for many years, then we may choose a flower essence that either confronts or uplifts, depending on the individual's needs.

The Intuitive Approach

Some people feel comfortable simply using their intuition to select a flower essence. There are several intuitive methods from which to choose, or you may develop your own approach.

An intuitive approach differs from a clinical approach in its reliance on feelings, guidance, imagery, and/or a plant journey (described later in this section) with the recipient. For me, this usually takes place in silence, with little verbal communication between myself and the recipient. I find that the more finely tuned I am, the less I need the clinical approach. By trusting my inner awareness, observations, and experience with the recipient, the appropriate plants often come to me spontaneously through their Doctrine of Signatures, color, message, image, environment in which they live, or other features. When that happens, that is without a doubt the flower essence remedy I select.

Visualization and Imagery

A simple way to select a flower essence is by looking at the colored photos in this book.

It's helpful to look at both the full-size plant photo and the close-up of the flower in bloom. If you are selecting a flower essence for yourself, you will probably feel a resonance and perhaps even a familiar feeling with certain plants. Without question, tune into those plants further and experiment with their flower essences.

Meditation

One of my key mottoes is: "If you don't know what to do, don't do it." The most effective way I've found for dealing with uncertainty is to enter the inner world of silence and pray about the matter. Silence is a profound way to connect with our inner light and to realize that we are all an expression of the same Source. Experience of the inner light through silence brings profound messages and insights that we may not otherwise pay attention to.

If you want inner guidance about selecting a flower essence, take some time to look at the pictures of the flowers, then close your eyes and find your inner silence. Follow your own inner guidance, its messages, images, and sounds when making your choice.

Muscle Testing or Applied Kinesiology

The use of muscle testing (also known as applied kinesiology) requires skill and experience, and primarily applies to selecting a flower essence for another person. This method activates the muscles to test for strength or weakness in relation to a given flower essence. It has been used for many years by chiropractors, physical therapists, and kinesiologists to evaluate muscle strength in response to a number of types of stimulation. In muscle testing, the recipient stands with his or her stronger arm extended out to the side and parallel to the ground. With an open palm facing down, the practitioner applies the three middle fingers of his or her right hand near the recipient's wrist and gently pushes the recipient's arm downward. This gives the practitioner a sense of the recipient's muscle strength. It's helpful to test the muscle strength at least one more time for accuracy.

When I use muscle testing to select a flower essence, I have the recipient hold a bottle of a given flower essence in his or her nondominate hand and hold that hand close to the navel. I then gently push the extended arm again. If the recipient's arm becomes stronger, that essence has tested positive. If the recipient's arm becomes weaker, the essence has tested negative. If the recipient's arm strength stays the same, I put the bottle aside and test other essences. I may come back to it later and test it again. For accurate results, it's important to avoid too much muscle testing during one session and to allow the recipient to take a break in between tests or to switch arms.

Pendulum Dowsing

Dowsing with a pendulum can also aid in the selection of flower essences.[1] This method requires experience, intuitive awareness, and good perceptual skills. When using a pendulum for testing, we are communicating subconsciously with the nervous system.

An ideal pendulum is a symmetrical object — generally lightweight, perhaps 1 to 2 inches long, and narrow ($1/4$ inch) — that is attached to the end of a thread or chain.

It takes time and experience to find out how to interpret the swing of the pendulum, which differs for each dowser. A simple method of finding out what works for you as a dowser is to draw a circle on a piece of paper, placing vertical and horizontal lines through the circle. Hold the chain or string of the pendulum between your thumb and index finger; let the pendulum dangle and watch how it moves. If the pendulum swings left to right (along the "horizontal" line through the circle), ask yourself if that means a negative or positive response to you. If the pendulum swings along the "vertical" line through the circle, ask yourself the meaning of that direction. Or the pendulum may move in a circle, clockwise or counterclockwise; ask yourself which direction is positive (yes); and which is negative (no). Whatever pendulum movements mean positive (yes) or negative (no) for you, go by that from now on whenever you use your pendulum. It is important that you remain consistent with the meaning of the direction of the pendulum each time you use it. For a right-handed dowser, common directions and meanings are

- No: Back and forth horizontally or counterclockwise in a circle
- Yes: Back and forth vertically or clockwise in a circle

I seldom use a pendulum because I rely on more direct intuition. When I do use the pendulum, I check to make sure that it swings accurately over both the left and right hands. I then have the recipient hold a flower essence bottle in the left hand near the belly while I hold the pendulum above the recipient's right hand. If the pendulum continues to move either clockwise or "vertically," the essence has tested positive. If the pendulum moves counterclockwise, moves left to right, or stops, the essence has tested negative.

Pendulum dowsing can be a good way to learn to trust your intuition, and it's an interesting experiment to try. Of course, you have to believe in it for the pendulum to be effective for you, but it's worth trying; then you can decide on the validity of the pendulum for yourself. It works better for some people than for others.

If you want to use the pendulum to select flower essences for yourself, holding a flower essence bottle in your left hand close to your belly, then hold the pendulum over the bottle and watch the direction in which it moves.

connecting souls through a journey

Sometimes when a person comes to me for a flower essence consultation, I see an image of a plant or flower in my mind. I may even spontaneously envision the person as a plant or a flower. When this occurs, it is clear that I should give the person a remedy of this plant's flower essence.

Usually, after gathering information

in a verbal consultation, I engage in a "journey" with the person. This process invites the connection of my soul with the recipient's soul, allowing our higher selves to exchange energy and act as one.

I always begin a journey with a prayer of protection and guidance for both myself and the recipient. I may decide to give the person a white flower essence prior to the journey (usually Evening Primrose or Yarrow), depending on the person's characteristics and situation. This choice is usually based on intuition, but if a person is exhausted and energetically drained I tend to give Yarrow, whereas if someone lacks inner strength my choice is usually Evening Primrose.

In the journey, the person lies face up on a massage table and I stand to his or her left side. I scan the person's body in my mind's eye, beginning with the feet. Then I sense the person's energy field by passing my hands about three inches above the body, beginning at the right foot and moving in a clockwise direction all around the body to the left foot. Next, using the same technique, I follow the chakra energy system beginning at the base chakra and moving up to the top of the head. The sensations in my hands tell me where the energy is blocked, where the energy is moving, locations of heat, and possibly locations of pain. I sometimes use a pendulum to verify the perceptions of my hands.

While I am doing this hands-on process, I may experience a variety of energy exchanges. Often I see colors or images of particular plants or flowers. I may even become the plant, similar to taking a plant journey as described in chapter 8. As the plant, I talk out loud to the person about his or her healing process as it relates to color, signatures, chakras, and so on. I may take the person on a plant journey or guided meditation so they can experience the plant and its flower. In addition to relating with the plant, I may do some type of massage, polarity work, or laying on of hands to support the healing process. A plant journey can take numerous forms; this is a process of flowing with intuition, resonance, perceptual skill, an understanding and relationship with the plant kingdom, and the trust in myself and the plant kingdom that allows me to do this.

When the journey is complete, I allow the recipient to remain lying down. I wash my hands in cold water, both to cleanse the recipient's energy from my energy field and for hygiene purposes. Then I go to my laboratory to select the flower essences that were chosen during the journey, and I combine them in a flower essence bottle as a personalized combination formula. I then give the recipient three to four drops of the flower essence formula and I place the flower essence bottle on the recipient's belly to form a connection. With the recipient's eyes closed, I guide a journey back to each flower as a simple meditation that helps the recipient reconnect with the whole plant, its flower, and its essence.

Usually I give no more than four

flower essences per session so that the recipient can establish a relationship with each flower without being overwhelmed. In some circumstances, I may give only one flower essence at a time to allow the recipient to establish a relationship with a given plant for at least two to four weeks.

When the recipient has had time to assimilate the flower essence(s) and the journey, I give thanks to Spirit for guiding us both. Then I gently help the recipient sit up, allowing time to share the experience and give each other feedback.

Integrating Both Approaches

A combination of the clinical and intuitive approaches works best for me. I strive for simplicity in gathering the information that helps me understand the whole person. As a trainer in neuro-linguistic programming (a method of identifying and understanding personality types, the way we receive and express ourselves through body language, and the way our brains receive and express information), I have learned to observe people's responses to various modes of healing. Also, through doing laying on of hands, polarity, kinesiology, and reiki, I have learned to access the body language of others and the parts of the body that ask for attention. Plants naturally guide me in all these modes of healing. I believe that the Spirit who lives and breathes in us will show me what I need to do and help my soul connect with the souls of others.

In general, people who are interested

in self-improvement will benefit from taking flower essences. As a practitioner, I don't advise flower essences as a "cure" for severe physical health problems, for people with psychosomatic illnesses, for people who aren't ready to change, for hypochondriacs and people who use their disease to gain attention, or for people who take powerful tranquilizers, drugs, or antidepressants. In such cases, there clearly is a need for a stronger physical treatment than a flower essence can offer. In any case, a flower essence, by itself, is really not a "cure." Flower essences are helpers or guides; they are used as a tool to enhance personal awareness. However, flower essences can help people who have a severe chronic health condition by increasing their awareness of their relationship with their con-dition. By establishing a new relationship to their health conditions, people may be able to transform the way they view their condition; the flower essence may open a new avenue for learning about themselves.

Flower essences are most effective for people who truly desire change and personal growth, and who want to take personal responsibility in their actions, emotions, and spiritual awareness.

selecting flower essences for pets

Selecting essences for animals is similar to choosing essences for people. Just check the animal's symptoms and look for similar symptoms in the repertory of essences in chapter 11 (for formulas listed below, see the appendix). Muscle testing is also effective with animals.

- What can be given to animals that are grieving the loss of their owners? Depression Formula, Yarrow Formula.
- What can you give to an ill-tempered bird who bites or who plucks feathers — or to the fierce dog who attacks or bites? Chamomile, Calendula, Crimson Monkeyflower, Stress Formula.
- Which essences can you give to animals that are afraid of loud noises such as thunderstorms, blenders, or vacuum cleaners, or afraid of unknown visitors? Century Plant, Yellow Monkeyflower, or Stress Formula.
- What can you give to a high-strung, nervous animal that may be restless and moody? Calendula, Chamomile, or Vervain.
- What can you give to an animal that has experienced a trauma? Stress Formula, Yarrow Formula.
- What can you give to an animal that is tired and withdrawn? Fatigue Formula, Stress Formula, or Yarrow Formula.
- What is a good remedy for an animal in heat? Calendula or Chamomile.
- What remedy would you give to a possessive or demanding animal? Chicory or Willow.
- What would you give to an animal that has difficulty sleeping or napping? Night Freedom Formula.

In giving flower essences to animals, the signs will be evident when the flower essence is effective. Generally, you will notice in a matter of minutes or a few hours if a flower essence is working. In some cases, you may need to wait for two or three days. In my experience, most animals have a fairly quick response to the therapeutic effect of flower essences and you will know if a particular essence is working or whether you want to try another essence.

If you feel the essence is working, continue to give the animal the essence for a minimum of three days for an acute condition and a minimum of fourteen days for a chronic condition.

If you feel the essence isn't working, then try another essence and observe the results.

CHAPTER 8
How to Make and Use Your Own Flower Essences

There is extraordinary value in honoring the life of a plant, its personality, its treasures, and its healing powers, and in partaking of its substance and essence. A given plant's botanical heritage, chemical constituents, personality, and spirit or medicine all present a picture of who the plant is. Sitting quietly with a plant and journeying with it — a form of meditation — is equally important in coming to know its gifts. In a journey meditation, the spirit of the plant comes through in many ways, and I find the most profound way is through the silence of my own mind and body.

In this chapter, you will learn how to make a flower essence, including data collection, plant identification, journeying with the plant, and bottling the essence. You will also learn how to choose the right dosage of flower essence to take or recommend. Remember that the more quality time you give to this process, the more you will receive from doing so.

It's best to make your essence under a sunny sky with no clouds. However, you may choose to make certain flower essences under partially cloudy skies or during rainstorms to experience different effects, or during a full moon, especially for night-blooming flowers such as yucca.

step one: Gather Your Tools

Making a flower essence is simple. First you need to gather the following items:

- Cornmeal or tobacco
- A clear glass bowl at least 5 inches in diameter and 3 inches deep
- Purified or natural fresh spring water (you can carry it with you in a bottle)
- Two sharp-edged stones (such as flint or sandstone) or two crystals that can be used for separating the flower from the flower stem
- A 4-inch square of untreated cotton muslin cloth
- A small funnel

- Labels
- A pen
- Colored pencils
- A notepad
- Brandy or grain alcohol (do not use methyl alcohol or rubbing alcohol!), or apple cider vinegar for those who don't want to consume alcohol
- A 1- or 2-ounce amber or cobalt bottle with a dropper for each essence you plan to make. If you want to preserve more flower essence, a second bottle with a lid is preferable (if you store flower essences in bottles with droppers for long periods of times, the essence may acquire a rubbery taste from the dropper). Each bottle should be one-third full of brandy, grain alcohol, or apple cider vinegar as a preservative before making the flower essence.
- One or more plant or wildflower identification books

step two:
choosing your flower

When you look for a flower with which to make a flower essence, it is best to find a group of the same flower growing in an area. You may already have your own special flower that you are drawn to, or you may come upon an unfamiliar flower that you feel attracted to. Either way, you want to use flowers that are in their fullest stage

of blooming. A flower in full bloom highlights the plant's most powerful energies and personality expression.

You may use flowers from your garden, from along a roadside field, from a pasture, a woodland, or any other place in nature where you are drawn, as long as it is free of toxins and not growing near heavily traveled roads. When appropriate, please ask permission of landowners prior to making a flower essence.

Locate a fully blooming plant that appeals strongly to you. Go near the plant, but don't touch it at first. Quietly notice where you are and sit down beside the plant. Take a few moments to feel the warmth of the sun, breathe in the fresh air, listen to nature's sounds, and consciously set all worldly and personal concerns behind you. Be fully in the moment with this precious flowering plant you have chosen.

Take out your cornmeal or tobacco and, with reverence for the plant, the earth, the sky, and the Great Spirit, gently sprinkle it on the ground near the plant and give thanks. Giving cornmeal or tobacco is a Native American tradition of giving thanks to the earth and to the plant. If you feel uncomfortable using cornmeal or tobacco, simply give thanks in your own way.

step three:
capturing the essence

Fill the glass bowl with purified water to about 1 inch from the top and place the bowl on the ground near or underneath your chosen blooming plant. Locate a fully blooming flower on the plant that appeals strongly to you and, using two sharp-edged stones or crystals, gently cut the bloom from the stem of the plant. By not touching the flower with your hands, you avoid disturbing its purity. If the plant has large leaves, you can use two leaves to remove the flower instead. Without touching the flower with your hands or body, place the blossom on the water in the glass bowl. This process assures that only the flower's vibration goes into the water and not your own energy and personality.

Depending on the size of the plant, you may take several more blooms and then go to another similar plant nearby and take a few blossoms from that plant, and so on. Cover the surface of the water with flowers and let it sit in the sun for about 2 or 3 hours until the flowers begin to wilt. You can also prepare essences in the moonlight by leaving them out for 3 to 4 hours or all night long. During this time, follow Steps Four and Five.

step four: gathering data: the doctrine of signatures

I call this step the left-brained part, and I always like to do it first so that I don't have to come back to it after the plant journey (Step Five). During and after the journey, I am better able to retain the plant's gifts and teachings when I can just be with its energy without thinking about anything else.

Gathering data is an important part of making a flower essence; we learn about the personality of the plant and the conditions under which it grows. The Doctrine of Signatures plays an important role in gathering information about the plant. Collecting this information is central to understanding, experiencing, and relating to the plant as a whole. All of the plant's parts play vital roles and have an influence on the whole plant. The following is a step-by-step process that is helpful in collecting objective information about the plant.

1. Identify the plant and write down its common name. It is helpful to have two or more plant identification books with you that are appropriate to your climate and geographical location. Often there is more than one species of a given plant, so be sure to correctly identify your plant, or you may become confused later when you need to know the precise plant you used.

2. Write down the Latin name of the plant. This will also help you later for identification purposes if needed.

3. Write down the date and time when you prepared the essence.

4. List any significant astrological occurrences on this date (you may choose to do this part at home later).

5. Write down whether the essence was prepared in full sun, in partial sun (sometimes clouds appear unexpectedly), in the rain or a thunderstorm, or in the moonlight.

6. Write down the location where the essence was made.

7. The Doctrine of Signatures: Plant Description (Consult the glossary at the back of this book.)

    a. Write a description of the environment where the plant grows. Does it like sun or shade, dry or moist soil? Does it grow at higher mountainous elevations (8,000 feet and higher), moderate elevations (4,000 to 8,000 feet), or in the desert or lower elevations (4,000 feet and below)? Does it grow in wooded areas or clearings? Does it like to be near or grow in the water? If so, does it like swampy, stagnant water or moving water? Are there other like plants around or does it seem to grow alone?

    b. What does the plant look like? Write down any significant shape or appearance.

    c. Root: What is the root like? Is it long, short, stubby, hairy, or smooth? Is it tough or easy to pull up? What color is it? Is it dry, brittle, milky, hollow? What does it smell like?

    d. Stem: Pick one stem with a flower or flowers to use as a specimen. What does the stem look like? Is it smooth or hairy? Is it rigid or flexible? Is it square or round? Does it make a sound in the wind or is it silent? Is it dry and brittle or somewhat moist? What color is it? Is there one stem or many stems? Does it have a smell? If it is a tree or a shrub, what is the bark like? Is it rugged or smooth, thick or thin? What color is the bark?

    e. Leaves/Leaflets: What do the leaves look like? How do they grow on the stem? Do they alternate, grow in opposites, grow in whorls, or grow in a basal rosette near the ground? What are they shaped like — are they linear, lance-shaped, oblong, heart-shaped, kidney-shaped, or arrow-shaped?

       Are the leaves lobed, toothed, toothless, or dissected? Do they have a leafstalk or are they stalkless? Do they clasp onto the stem or do they grow right through the stem? Do they appear like a feather, having parts on each side of the axis?

       Are the leaves fuzzy/hairy or smooth? What color are the leaves? Are they shiny or dull? What do their veins look like? What do they smell like? How do they taste?

8. The Doctrine of Signatures: Flower Description (Consult the glossary at the back of this book.)

    a. Color: What color or colors is the flower? What chakra does it correspond with based on its color?

    b. Petals: What shape is the flower? Is it a composite flower? Are the flower petals regular or irregular? Is the flower stalkless or does it have a stalk? Do the petals form a head, do they grow in a spike, or do they form an umbel? What impression do they give you?

c. Stamens: What do the stamens look like? Are they stiff or are they threadlike? Are they visible or are they hiding? Can you count them or are there too many to count? What color are they?

d. Pistil: Can you see the pistil? What does it look like? What color is it?

e. Sepal: Is there a sepal? What does it look like? How many parts or petals does it have?

9. Drawing: Take some time to draw the flower or plant if you wish. Use your colored pencils and your creativity!

step five: the plant journey: nature's spirits speak

The plant journey is a merging of your spirit with a plant's spirit. Each plant is an expression of the Divine Spirit, guiding us on a sacred journey. There is no right or wrong way to journey with a plant; every journey is different. The purpose is to be accurate and to trust your perceptions to take you to a place of inner knowing that brings clarity and understanding. A plant journey is a different kind of truth that isn't based on scientific fact. It is based instead on the truth of witnessing, experience, and testimony. By joining in relationship with the plant and the Divine Spirit, you can find and honor the plant's true expression.

Plants are multifaceted and offer many gifts. One person may receive a certain part of a plant's gift while another may receive a different part. When I sit with a group of people to study and journey with a plant, we usually all tap into the plant's central theme. Some people may experience more of the challenging aspects of the plant while others experience the spiritual elevation that it offers. Studying, experiencing, and being with the whole plant helps us absorb its fullest nature.

The purpose of the plant journey is to become the plant and to experience it without any expectations. You will take on how it feels, grows, moves, breathes, lives, touches, responds, communicates, gives, and receives. You will listen for the plant's messages, which generally come from the flower itself. The flower is the highest glory of the plant; when you reach the flower in the journey and become one with it, the messages and teachings you receive will affect you deeply. They will probably change the way you view and experience life.

The plant journey can be as deep and profound as you are with yourself. In fact, it is an intimate journey with yourself. Experiencing oneness with the plant is a sign that you have reached a high level of intimacy with yourself that is further opening and deepening. This level of personal growth creates an inner availability that allows you to unite the sacred nature spirit of the plant with your own spirit. As you embrace the spirit of the plant, you may experience energetic vibrations, openings, releases, and teachings of wisdom.

If you feel uncomfortable undertaking a plant journey, then just sit quietly and observe the plant. You can still learn something about the plant, and perhaps yourself, in your own way.

The flower almost always has verbal messages to give you that may even continue after the journey. When you take time to write down your journey afterward, you may find yourself writing as the plant. The Pinyon might say, "I offer you the freedom to be who you are without shame or guilt. Develop your foundation. Be strong and hold your own. Focus on your desires that serve the whole." Or the Wild Rose might say, "I invite you to come to me as you seek devotion. Open your heart to receive the love that is already within you. May you come to love the gift of being alive, to embrace the opportunity to face your challenges and your pains, and to find release from your miseries."

Journeying with a plant and experiencing union with it is an incredibly powerful, energizing experience. Every plant holds its own unique power and identity. The heightened level of power that you may experience with the nature spirit of the plant can deepen your relationship with yourself and help you use your power in creative ways. A plant journey may show you how you lose your power to yourself or others, or how to gain your power and be true to your own spirit. It may take days for all of these gifts of understanding to surface, but you probably will be subconsciously energized with their power while journeying with the plant.

The Journey

After gathering data (Step Four), put away your books, colored pencils, pen, paper, and any miscellaneous items. Sit near your chosen plant, get into a comfortable position, and quiet your thoughts.

Begin the journey by again asking the plant for permission to receive its blessings. You will need to trust your intuition about whether you have received permission. I have never been denied permission to journey with a plant; they are usually willing to share their teachings and gifts. However, I have learned that, in general, if something doesn't feel right, it's best not to do it. Perhaps there's a part of you that isn't ready to engage the gifts and teachings of the plant, leading to a tendency to misuse them. If so, find another plant, ask permission of that plant, and see where it takes you. It could be that you simply aren't ready to take such a journey.

Upon receiving permission from the plant, close your eyes and take several long, deep breaths. Inhale through your nose, taking the breath down through your throat, lungs, heart, stomach, spleen, genitals, and tailbone. Imagine long roots growing from your tailbone deep into the earth. Take your breath through the roots and into the earth until you feel that you are breathing into the earth. Then slowly release your breath out of your mouth and imagine that you are giving back the earth energy to the air. Repeat this exercise several times until you feel totally relaxed, comfortable, and mindless.

Now imagine your roots intertwining

deep in the earth with the roots of the plant you will journey with. As the roots get closer to the surface of the earth, your roots merge with the plant's roots. Notice how you feel as the roots of the plant — how you grow and move in the earth. Notice what color you are. Notice your odor.

Notice how the earth feels as you make your way up the roots and become the stem of the plant. How does it feel to be the stem? Imagine yourself standing up and stretching as the stem. Notice your temperature, your moistness or dryness. Notice the ease with which you extend your stem. Notice if you have branches or if you grow straight up as a single stem. Follow the stem. Notice whether you bend with the wind and how that feels. Explore one branch further. How does it feel? What do you see? What color is the branch? Does it have a certain smell? Find the places where the leaves attach to you as the stem. Imagine yourself getting continually larger and extending upward, allowing the walls of the stem and the leaves to determine your size and shape. Imagine the leaves hanging onto your arms and hands.

Go into a leaf and explore your texture and how you feel. How do you hold onto the plant? What is your shape? Follow your veins. Notice the top and the underside, the similarities and differences between them. Notice how you taste. Go back to the stem and explore another leaf. Notice your feelings and observations again. Notice the position of the leaves in relation to each other. Explore as many leaves as you wish, and then return to the central stem.

Follow the stem upward. Explore any other branches or leaves you are drawn to. Allow yourself to be gracefully led by the union of your spirit with the plant's nature spirit. Go where Spirit takes you. Be with the nature spirit of the plant. Let your body stretch and flow with the branches and leaves.

Find your way to a flower blossom that is in its peak of glory. Enter from the stem into the center of the flower. Explore the inner depths of the flower. Notice what colors you see. Touch the inside of your flower petal. Notice your shape. Then move to the outer center of the flower; depending on the type of flower, this may mean emerging from the mouth of the flower or onto the edge of the flower's central disk. Notice how your face appears and the direction it is facing. Notice your petals — how many you have and what they look like. Lick or taste your petals and notice how that makes you feel. Notice the color and appearance of your stamens.

Imagine your own head as the head of the flower blossom; your arms are the leaves of the plant, the stem is your spine and legs, and the roots are your feet. Notice any unique features of yourself as the plant. Notice how you smell. Notice your vibration and the kind of energy you emanate. Notice how you feel.

Listen for your inner nature spirit voice; hear what it is saying. Absorb the words, the way you feel, your smells, your touch, and the energy of this experience into your body, soul, and mind. Allow this energy to fill your entire being. Capture the essence of this energy and hold it. Breathe into it and then release your breath. Take another deep, long breath and follow it into the center of the flower to the stem. Follow the stem down to the earth. See yourself moving with your breath. If you want to, you can give thanks to other parts of the plants and say good-bye. Continue to move down the stem to the earth. Follow the stem to the roots and follow the roots until you find your own roots. Gently untangle your roots from the plant's roots and gradually release your long, deep breath.

Give thanks to the plant's roots for their powerful foundation in leading you on your journey. Continue to take long, deep breaths as you separate your roots from the plant's roots and follow them up to the base of your tailbone. Breathe in the energy of the plant through your tailbone, to your genitals, spleen, stomach, heart, lungs, throat, mouth, and third eye, then release your breath out through the crown of your head. Repeat this breathing cycle several times while holding the energy of the plant throughout your body.

Gradually open your eyes. Continue to sit quietly. Pick up your paper and pen and write the experience of your journey. Take time to connect with the experience of the plant's nature spirit and the messages you received. Write down any messages or teachings the plant gave you.

Notice how you feel and whether there are particular places in your body or your chakras where you feel an energy impact. Write down those feelings.

Based on the messages you received from the plant and its flower, list any patterns of imbalance or challenges that the plant may have presented. Then list positive healing patterns that the plant and its flower may have offered you.

Write one to three affirmations that the plant gave you on your journey. Read the affirmations out loud, or sing or chant them.

step six: preparation of the mother tincture

Usually by the time Steps Four and Five are completed, the bowl of water that contains the blossoms has been in direct sunlight for about two to three hours. Some flowers require more time than others, and the amount of time required varies with temperature, so check to see if the flowers show signs of wilting. If so, the flower essence has been captured. Otherwise you'll need to follow your own instinct and judgment; often the essence has been captured even if the flower shows little wilting. When the essence has been captured, place the muslin into the funnel to act as a strainer. I carry an additional clean cloth in a plastic bag and spread it on the ground to place the funnels, muslin, and accessories on. Pour the flower-petal water through the cloth and the funnel into the bottle that already contains brandy, grain alcohol, or apple cider vinegar. If you are making more than one flower essence, it's important to use a different funnel and a clean cloth for sanitation and to assure capturing each individual flower essence.

Label the filled bottle with the name of the flower, the date, and the location where you made the essence. Write "MT" for "mother tincture" indicating that this is a concentrated form of the essence straight from the flower's blossoms, or use the symbol "Ø." This will remind you to use the mother tincture as a reserve from which to make stock bottles — a diluted form of the mother tincture. The mother tincture can have an indefinite shelf life if properly stored in a cool, dark place.

When you are done, place the mother tincture bottles, the funnel, cloth, and your other tools in a basket, bag, or backpack, packing them carefully for their ride home.

---

step seven: flower essence features and returning the essence to the earth

Once you've filled, marked, and packed the bottles, you can sit and drink the remaining flower essence from the bowl. This is truly a highlight of the process for me and a time to reap the rewards. It's an opportunity to make a toast to the flower, thank it for its gifts, and receive its blessings by taking in the essence. It's especially rewarding to share the flower essence water — and the whole experience — with a friend.

Before tasting it, I notice the color of the flower essence water. Usually the water is clear, but in some cases it has been various shades of yellow, milky white, or even lavender. Then I smell the flower essence water and allow myself to absorb its odor. I record the water color and the odor; these tell me more about the essence of the plant and the sensations of the flowers.

Next I close my eyes, say another prayer of thanks, and take a sip or two, noticing the taste of the water and any sensations I experience from drinking it. I usually feel something energetically, sometimes very subtly and sometimes more obviously. Often I feel a definite tingling sensation in certain areas or chakras of my body. Sometimes I feel certain temperatures when drinking an essence, such as an intense heat in my solar plexus or a cooling sensation in my throat and lungs. I may also feel an energetic vitality like a pick-me-up, while with other flowers I may feel very quiet and mellow inside. Each flower essence water is different in some way and adds to my understanding of the personality and presence of the flowering plant. I write down my experience with drinking the flower essence water in the Flower Essence Features section. I almost always experience a connection between the Flower Essence Features, the Plant Journey, and the Doctrine of Signatures.

When you are through sipping the water, leave enough to return some to the earth and the remaining plant. Gently pour the water and the flowers that are still in the bowl onto the ground at the base of the plant. I say a prayer of thanks to all the elements — the earth, air, sun, and water — and to the nature spirit of the plant for sharing its gifts with me. I thank my own spirit for receiving these blessed gifts, and I ask that I will carry them with me as I return to my other world. I pack the rest of my items, leaving the place as clear as possible, and return with a refreshed and energized sense of self.

step eight: preparation of the mother tincture to make elixirs

When you return home with the mother tincture (MT) bottle, you can make the MT into a "stock bottle." Place two to four drops of the MT into a sterilized 1-ounce amber or cobalt bottle filled one-third with brandy, grain alcohol, or apple cider vinegar and two-thirds with purified water. (I prefer brandy to grain alcohol because it's milder, tastier, and easier on the stomach.) Then secure the MT bottle with a regular cap, rather than a rubber dropper (to avoid a rubbery taste and possible contamination), and place it in a cool, dark place for indefinite shelf-life. It must not be exposed to sunlight. If a slight sediment appears at the bottom of the MT bottle, the contents may be refiltered into another sterilized bottle and relabeled.

Seal the stock bottle with a dropper

cap, label it and date it, then succuss it three times by holding the bottle in one hand and striking it on the palm of your other hand. Succussion energizes the essence; it creates a noticeable change in the quality of the essence, releasing its power to heal and influencing its vital force. Due to the minimal succussion of flower essences (3 to 6x, as compared to 100x and more in homeopathy), I do not consider flower essences to be potentized remedies in the same way that homeopathic remedies are. The essences are naturally potentized by the elements and again in brief succussions, but the method is not the same as the one used in making homeopathic remedies. This is another way in which flower essences differ from homeopathic remedies.

From the essence in the stock bottle, some people create a "dosage bottle" or "treatment bottle," which is used for daily consumption. The dosage bottle is prepared by putting two to four drops from the stock bottle into a sterilized 1-ounce amber or cobalt bottle filled one-third with brandy or apple cider vinegar and two-thirds with purified water.

I prefer to use stock bottles for my customers because I appreciate the powerful effect and energetic vibration of the stock essence. I seldom bottle essences into a dosage bottle unless I am working with an alcoholic or an alcohol-sensitive person. If a recipient needs to avoid consuming alcohol, you can also dissolve the flower essence in hot water to volatilize the alcohol.

You can also add vegetable glycerin to a treatment bottle as a preservative and to give a sweeter taste. I generally put one-eighth to one-fourth of a bottle of vegetable glycerin and one-fourth of a bottle of brandy or apple cider vinegar in the dosage bottle, fill the bottle with purified water, then add the two to four drops from the stock bottle.

Taking a Flower Remedy

After selecting the appropriate flower remedy for a given situation (see chapter 7), the recipient should take three or four drops of flower essence from the dosage bottle under the tongue or in a cup of water about four times per day for at least a week and up to several months. The frequency and duration depend on the recipient's needs and level of sensitivity. The essence should be taken at least fifteen to thirty minutes before or after consuming food or liquids other than water. It's good to take the essence upon first getting up in the morning, twice during the day, and at bedtime, taking time to focus on one's intention, enter one's inner silence, and connect with the essence. The impact of flower essences is strongest between sleeping and waking due to the changes in our consciousness at this time. It's also helpful to create special times in the day, even if only for five minutes, to honor what one is working on with the essence and to help one stay connected with oneself and one's intention. It helps to take time to feel the effects of the essence, be with the effects, monitor internal dialogue, and observe moods and energy shifts.

The frequency of the dosage creates a devotion to the process and allows time for inner growth and outward manifestations to occur. A person may decide to take the flower essence more frequently (such as six to eight times a day) for the first several days to heighten sensitivity to the flower. The frequency should then gradually be reduced each day according to personal needs. In the case of a crisis or trauma, a person may want to take the essence more often until a sense of calm returns.

When taking a flower essence to treat a chronic condition (such as deep depression, a deep-seated unresolved trauma, an unresolved childhood issue, cancer, arthritis, obesity, AIDS, etc.), a person may want to take the essence for a month or longer until there is an inner release and movement. After that time, a different remedy may be appropriate.

If one is taking a flower essence to treat an acute condition, such as a sudden onset of fear, anger, agitation, or sadness, one may only need to take the essence once or a few times to cause an energy shift. If one needs a higher dosage, it is more effective to increase the frequency of doses than the quantity of each dose. Most flower essence practitioners have adopted the homeopathic principle of "less is more." It isn't always important to take more drops, but it is important to take them consistently.

Some people, such as children or the elderly, are highly sensitive to flower essences; they may only need to take the essences one to three times per day. Observe their responses and choose the frequency accordingly.

When the flower essence has helped a person make the desired energetic shift, and that shift feels stable, it is probably time to stop taking the essence. It's a good idea to go four days to a week or more without taking any flower essences before beginning to take another one. This will allow any residual effects from the previous essence to diminish and prevent carry-over into the next cycle.

Usually, the stronger one's intention is for taking a flower essence, the more noticeable the results will be. The flower essence acts as catalyst in the awareness of Self, and its vibration or frequency creates an inner shift. It's best to take time to feel the effects of the essence, be with the effects, monitor one's thoughts, and observe moods and energy shifts. Keeping a journal can be helpful.

Flower essences can be used concurrently with other treatments, such as chemotherapy for cancer, and those treatments should not be discontinued without a physician's approval. Flower essences are used as a treatment to help a person deal emotionally with a condition; they are not a cure. Please see your healthcare professional for any medical concerns.

Flower essences can also be added to bath water to relax or invigorate the body/mind/spirit, or added to spray bottles to freshen the air and promote the vibration you want. Flower essences can also be added to the family water pitcher to give a group uplift or even to a pet's water bowl.

Expectations of flower essences

Flower essences can work subtly or dramatically. Sometimes it may take only seconds or a few minutes to feel an energy shift after taking a flower essence. In other cases, it may take several days or longer to observe and feel the effects of flower essences and how they influence our lives. I have found flower essences to be most helpful for people who take personal responsibility for their physical, emotional, mental, and spiritual well-being.

Flower essences are one tool among many that help us find greater understanding and guidance into the depths of our innermost natures. If you choose to take a flower essence seriously, you will realize that you are working with your whole person in many ways. You will become more aware of your emotions, mental activity, dreams, inner voice, intuition, psychic abilities, and reflections of your life patterns, including diet and health.

Flower essences offer an awakening into a deeper perspective on who we are and who we are becoming. The plants and their flowers are guides, teachers, and companions to the human and animal kingdoms.

CHAPTER 9
How Do We Know Flower Essences Work?

As with the practices of herbalism and homeopathy, flower essence practitioners have collected case studies, personal anecdotes and testimonials, and more recently, flower essence research provings.

The use of flower essences involves a kind of truth that isn't based on hard scientific data. Instead, it is a truth based on witness, experience, and testimony. Dr. Bach, for example, collected case studies of his patients when he worked with his flower remedies. I, too, have collected case studies, personal testimonials, and stories over the years. But I also felt a need to explore the effects that flower essences have on people when they don't know which remedy they are taking.

The flower essence provers' project

My business, Living Flower Essences (LFE), conducted a flower essence provers' project that included about forty-five people over a six-month period. The results of this study validated for me how well flower essences work. In the project, provers (or testers) completed a seven-page diary for each flower essence they took; the testers did not know what flower essence they were taking. In general, six people took each essence. This is a small group, so the results may still be viewed as a bit subjective. However, I am sharing the results of this project as a way of demonstrating how flower essences worked for the testers.

How a flower essence proving differs from a homeopathic proving

I would like to clarify the difference between the flower essence proving I conducted and Hahnemann's method of homeopathic proving. These two methods are different, yet both collect important information about the prover (or tester) and the remedy itself.

Homeopathic provings first involve

healthy people, sometimes using toxic remedies of either low or high potency. In the flower essence provings conducted by Living Flower Essences, a stock bottle was consistently used for the remedy being tested, and each stock bottle was succussed three times. There were no different potencies or toxic substances involved.

The symptoms recorded in the flower essence proving included documentation of the physical/emotional/mental/spiritual levels of the person. This is similar to a homeopathic proving, in which the symptoms documented are based on the three levels of the organism: physical, emotional, and mental.

In a homeopathic proving, after a remedy is given to various "healthy" people, it is then given to a sick person, and its success is demonstrated by a "cure" of the whole organism. In Living Flower Essences' Research Provers' Project, remedies were given to people who were not necessarily "sick." They were given to people who wanted to take flower essences for their personal growth and awareness. Documentation regarding the follow-up of such remedies is not exact, as it is fairly subjective.

The proving process

The criteria for the testers who participated in Living Flower Essences' Research Provers' Project were

- Testers were aware of and open to the use of flower essences, but did not have to have prior experience with taking them; most testers

showed definite results from taking the flower essences, regardless of level of prior experience.

- Testers were between the ages of eighteen and fifty, and in fairly good overall health.
- Testers wanted to participate in the proving.
- Testers could live anywhere geographically; the majority lived in the United States.

The provers' diary included thorough documentation:

- Medical information, such as whether the tester was taking vitamins, herbs, or a homeopathic remedy
- Whether symptoms experienced were familiar or unfamiliar
- Dreams and sleep patterns
- Energy impact in relation to the chakras
- Physical sensations (tingling, energy boost, tiredness, sexual feelings) and what part of the body was affected, food cravings, fluid cravings and fluid intake, urination and bowel movements
- Emotional symptoms (any emotional experiences), the nature of the emotion, a change in emotions, and any particular activity that triggered an emotional state
- Mental activity — whether it stayed the same or changed and, if it changed, in what way it changed (mental confusion vs. mental clarity, groundedness vs. spaciness,

memory patterns, left-brained vs. right-brained, more or less creativity, more or less intuition, more or less understanding, etc.)

- Spiritual reflections, such as spiritual guidance or influences while taking the remedy, any significant awareness or spiritual understandings, and in what way spiritual practices such as meditation, prayer, or consciousness exercises changed or did not change while taking the essence;
- Positive healing patterns
- Patterns of imbalance
- Affirmations
- The overall effect of the flower essence
- Rubrics or keynotes for each flower essence
- Insights and recommendations about what the tester believed the flower essence could be used for

There were approximately six testers for each flower essence, although some flower essences had eight or ten testers. The flower essence was never identified to the testers before or during the time when it was taken. No testers shared information with each other that could have influenced the results.

The length of time during which the flower essence was taken varied from tester to tester, but the average was four to five days, with three to four days between different flower essences. Some testers took certain essences for longer periods of time, up to two weeks. Most testers experienced effects on the day they began taking the essence, and sometimes within hours or even minutes.

A placebo essence was also given, to which two out of ten people responded. The other eight testers showed no effects from taking the placebo.

testing results

In chapter 11, which gives detailed information on each of the essences in Living Flower Essences' repertory, you will find a section entitled "LFE's Research Provers' Project Findings" toward the end of each flower essence description. Summaries of the provers' diaries are recorded there.

The Provers' Project certainly validated the characteristics and personality types of the flower essences. For example, in nearly every proving, two testers experienced the pattern of imbalance, while the remaining testers experienced the positive patterns of balance. In the Calendula proving two female testers physically demonstrated the patterns of imbalance; they experienced dry scaly skin, skin rash, stomachache, nausea, hot flashes, physical exhaustion, anxiety, and distress. One of these testers later informed me that she was allergic to marigolds and experienced similar symptoms when around them; calendula and marigold have similar compositions and characteristics, and another name for calendula is "pot marigold." The other testers had a more calm, relaxed, soothing experience with the Calendula flower essence. It's important to note here that Calendula skin salves or creams are made to treat dry scaly skin and skin rash.

Calendula is also used to treat anxiety and distress. Much like Hahnemann's proving of cinchona, the Calendula flower essence caused the very conditions that it is intended to cure. This is a good example of applying "like treats like" with flower essences.

Another example involves the Indian Paintbrush flower essence. Indian Paintbrush is a root-chakra, survival-issue remedy. For one tester, it brought up deep fear and survival issues — "Where will I live? Can I take care of myself?" Patterns of imbalance among other testers included concerns about relationships, lack of confidence, fear of the future, living arrangement problems, and a sense of indifference. Patterns of balance among testers included increased levels of creativity, dream images, positive attitudes about family and job, and prayer and creative spiritual reflections. Again, these patterns are typical of Indian Paintbrush.

In response to taking the Mexican Hat flower essence, which is about surrendering emotions we have no control over, one tester wrote, "I felt that the out-of-control experience served to bring me ultimately to a much more clear and peaceful state by letting go of the clutter of dammed-up emotions inside," and later, "This essence showed me how deeply I can be gripped by the drama of life's emotions." Another tester wrote, "I realized how much emotional tension I was holding onto, and I felt all these emotions surfacing; this essence helped me release these emotions."

The Ox-Eye Daisy is a flower essence that provides deep relaxation, peacefulness, inner knowing, and a deeper spiritual wisdom leading to inner joy and happiness. It highlights a playful, optimistic, positive, fun-loving, nurturing nature, especially in relation to our inner child or to children in our lives. It also teaches us balance between intellect and intuition, providing greater wisdom in understanding, vision, and clarity in seeing the whole picture. Here are some comments made by testers while taking the Ox-Eye Daisy flower essence: "I felt playful and child-like," "I felt joyful and in harmony," "It stimulated my imagination," "It gave me positive mothering images," "It helped me have the wisdom to see ways to heal my wounded inner child in order to help my own children heal themselves," "It helped me tap into my inner happiness and be more optimistic about life," "It enhanced my imagination and trust in a higher power," "Abandonment issues in relation to my inner child came up."

The strengths of LFE's Provers' Project findings are as follows:

1. It utilized an open-ended questionnaire that allowed categorization of results and personal anecdotes.

2. It offers a point of reference for future studies.

3. It demonstrated consistent results in relation to the forty-eight flower essences described in this book.

4. It was a low-cost study with quick turnaround.

5. It was thorough.

6. The testers' enthusiasm, understanding, and relationships with both flower essences and themselves were enhanced despite the fact that the process was somewhat tedious and time-consuming.

The Blessing of Flower Essences

My own adventure in discovering the energetic alchemy of flower essences, my personal stories and the stories of others, and the research I have done all demonstrate the powerful impact of flower essences and plant studies on people's lives. Over and over, the transformational impact of flower essences has been verified by my personal contacts with others, including horses, dogs, cats, birds, men, women, teenagers, children, the elderly, and the dying. I have experienced the pro-found effects of flower essences through making flower essences, using them in ceremonies (solstice and equinox gatherings, weddings, rites of passage), telling stories about plants, plant journeys, plant and flower essence diaries, and art, as they all interrelate with the plant kingdom and the path to self-discovery, self-empowerment, and in all my relationships.

Flower essences are an important healing modality that provides a catalyst for growth, a source of nurturing and insight, and a vehicle for shaping a person's identity, self-awareness, self-esteem, and self-confidence. I feel blessed to have witnessed these effects in so many people's lives, in the lives of my animal friends, and especially in my own life and with the people who know me well. Please visit my website at www.livingfloweressences.com to read more stories and comments from people who have shared their personal experiences with flower essences.

PART IV

The Flower Essences

as one

You arise from beneath,
bringing beauty with your wake.
Within that beauty,
your free spirit holds the mystery
of its fading powers.

When I take your spirit into me,
as One I understand its presence.
No longer hiding in my shadows,
I see the Light
and break on through.

By Jenny Dawn Downey

completely free

Sitting in a green Pinyon tree
Listening to the gentle hum of the breeze
I feel as if I am completely free
Watching the sun go down,
No sight of any town.
Climb down the tree,
I'm happy and I'm free.

By Sarah Marie PallasDowney

CHAPTER 10
An Introduction to the Materia Medica

The detailed documentation of Living Flower Essences' Materia Medica in chapter 11 is intended to be easy to use. However, an introduction to the format and content will increase your understanding of how to apply the information in selecting and using the flower essences. My approach to flowers and their essences is similar to Dr. Bach's, but it also has unique aspects. Unlike Dr. Bach, I believe in an in-depth understanding of the "whole plant" concept, meaning that the appearance and physical characteristics of the whole plant and the flower, not just the flower's essence, are important components of its power and character. I also believe that the colors of the plants and flower blossoms relate directly to the chakras.

outline of the Materia Medica

In chapter 11, you will find the following basic categories of information for each flower essence:

- The plant's common, botanical, and other names
- The primary quality associated with the flower essence
- Where the plant grows naturally
- The energy impact of each flower essence and its relationship to the chakras — especially useful when you are consciously working with a particular chakra or chakras
- Whether the essence is an original Bach flower essence
- Rubrics: key words that describe the flower essence; obtained from my own studies and explorations, case studies, and the Research Provers' Project
- The plant's traditional use as an herb, as a homeopathic remedy, and as a flower essence
- Positive Healing Patterns: the positive qualities of the flower; what the recipient wishes to gain by taking the flower essence
- Symptoms and Patterns of Imbalance: the present symptoms the

recipient may be experiencing or that may be exaggerated when taking the essence (especially if this is an area one needs to work through)

- The qualities of the original flower-essence water, including odor, taste, sensations, and water color (Many people find these features not only interesting but helpful in developing a more intimate relationship with the plant and its flower.)
- Physical Makeup: a description of the plant and its flower; provides a clearer sense of the plant's physical qualities and how it grows
- Doctrine of Signatures: an additional guide to selecting a flower essence; offers more detailed information about a given plant
- Helpful Suggestions for Taking Each Remedy: tips, meditations, and exercises to deepen personal growth and the relationship with the plant
- Affirmations: positive phrases to plant in your body/mind/spirit as seeds of Divine consciousness that build hope, optimism, and guidance (Saying the affirmations daily, both when actually taking the flower essence and throughout the day, develops the power of your intention, intuition, and trust.)
- A case history to convey how the flower essence has affected another person
- LFE's Research Provers' Project Findings: a reference and a guide to help you understand how others were affected by taking the unidentified essence; this information may give you deeper insight into your own relationship with the flower essence

Reference charts

The following tables will also introduce you to LFE's flower essences. They provide an overview of some of the essences' basic features. The first table lists the forty-eight essences profiled in this book and their primary qualities.

Repertory of LFEs' forty-eight flower essences	
Name	**Quality**
1. Aster	Illumination
2. Bells-of-Ireland	Inner-Child Transformation
3. Black-Eyed Susan	Inner Peace
4. Blanketflower	Fire Dance
5. Blue Flag (Iris)	Stamina
6. Bouncing Bet	Mystic Union
7. Calendula	Calm
8. California Poppy	Purifier
9. Century Plant	Breakthrough
10. Chamomile	Serenity
11. Chicory	Interrelatedness
12. Cliff Rose	Positive Self-Image
13. Columbine	Divine Beauty
14. Comfrey	Service
15. Crimson Monkeyflower	Personal Power
16. Desert Larkspur	Graceful Passage
17. Desert Marigold	Flexibility
18. Desert Willow	The Empress
19. Echinacea	Rejuvenation
20. Evening Primrose (White)	Inner Strength
21. Honeysuckle	Harmony
22. Indian Paintbrush	Creativity
23. Lupine	Pathfinder
24. Mexican Hat	Release
25. Morning Glory	Liberator
26. Mullein	Security
27. Onion	Membership
28. Ox-Eye Daisy	Inner Knowing
29. Palmer's Penstemon	Self-Expression
30. Paloverde	Earth Wisdom
31. Peace Rose	Gift of the Angels
32. Pinyon	Patience
33. Pomegranate	Fruit of Life
34. Purple Robe	Plenty

Repertory of LFEs' forty-eight flower essences (continued)	
Name	**Quality**
35. Sage	Whole-Life Integration
36. Saguaro	The Guardian
37. Scarlet Penstemon	Courage
38. Strawberry Hedgehog	Passion
39. Sunflower	Fountain of Youth
40. Sweet Pea	Growing Child
41. Thistle	Balance
42. Vervain	Reach for the Stars
43. Wild Rose	Love
44. Willow	Forgiveness
45. Yarrow	Protection
46. Yellow Monkeyflower	Overcoming Fear
47. Yerba Santa	The Sacred Within
48. Yucca	Spear of Destiny

Quick Reference Chart for Chakras and Flower Essences

The purpose of this chart is to help you decide which chakra category best describes the condition or conditions you want to work with. Use this chart as a quick reference guide to help pinpoint the flower essences associated with the chakras. For example, if a person has a predomi-nantly emotional issue, begin by checking the second-chakra flower essences. If a person wants to explore spiritually, check the sixth- or seventh-chakra flower essences. Read the complete description of each flower essence in chapter 11 to help you choose the proper remedy or remedies. For more information about the chakras, refer to part II of this book, Chakras and Flower Essences.

quick reference chart for chakras and flower essences

	first chakra	second chakra	third chakra	
Also Known as	Physical, Root, or Base Chakra	Emotional, Spleen, or Regenerative Chakra	Mental, Personal Power, or Solar Plexus Chakra	
Element	Earth	Water	Fire	
Focus	Survival; Physical Security	Sexuality; Procreation; Emotions	Will; Purpose; Power; Self-Empowerment; Self-Honor	
Color	Red	Orange	Yellow	
Endocrine Gland	Adrenals	Gonad	Pancreas	
Function	Rectum; Circulatory System; Reproductive System; Kidneys; Lower Extremities	Reproductive System; Lower Back; Adrenal Gland; Lymph Gland; Spleen; Bladder; Pancreas; Kidneys	Adrenal; Stomach; Digestive System; Assimilation Process; Liver; Gall Bladder	
Flower Essences	Black-Eyed Susan Blanketflower Bouncing Bet Century Plant Crimson Monkeyflower Desert Willow Echinacea Indian Paintbrush Mexican Hat Paloverde Peace Rose Pomegranate Pinyon Saguro Scarlet Penstemon Strawberry Hedgehog Yellow Monkeyflower	Black-Eyed Susan Blanketflower Calendula California Poppy Century Plant Crimson Monkeyflower Echinacea Indian Paintbrush Mexican Hat Mullein Paloverde Pomegranate Scarlet Penstemon Yellow Monkeyflower	Aster Black-Eyed Susan Blanketflower Blue Flag Calendula Century Plant Chamomile Cliff Rose Columbine Comfrey Desert Marigold Desert Willow Honeysuckle Mexican Hat Mullein Ox-Eye Daisy Palmer's Penstemon Paloverde Pomegranate Purple Robe Saguro Scarlet Penstemon Strawberry Hedgehog Sunflower Wild Rose Yellow Monkeyflower	

fourth chakra	fifth chakra	sixth chakra	seventh chakra
Heart Chakra	*Throat Chakra*	*Third Eye, Eye of Wisdom, or Brow Chakra*	*Crown Chakra*
Air	*Ether*	*Radium*	*Magentum*
Love; Compassion; Forgiveness	*Communication; Sound; Vibration*	*Seeing; Visualization; Clairvoyance; Light; Psychic Perception; Intuition; Imagination*	*"The Thousand-Petaled Lotus"; Bliss; Understanding; Oneness with the Infinite; Peace; Expanded Consciousness; Communication with the Divine*
Pink/Green	*Blue*	*Violet/Purple*	*White/Gold*
Thymus	*Thyroid*	*Pituitary*	*Pineal*
Thymus Gland; Immune System; Circulatory System	*Larynx; Tongue; Mouth; Esophagus; Thyroid Gland Parathyroid Gland*	*Pineal Gland; Endocrine System; Immune System*	*Cerebral Cortex; Central Nervous System; Pituitary Gland; Electrical Synapses*
Bells-of-Ireland Bouncing Bet Comfrey Desert Willow Evening Primrose Indian Paintbrush Morning Glory Onion Palmer's Penstemon Peace Rose Pinyon Strawberry Hedgehog Sweet Pea Thistle Wild Rose Willow	Blue Flag Chicory Comfrey Crimson Monkeyflower* Desert Larkspur Desert Willow Palmer's Penstemon* Sage Scarlet Penstemon* Yellow Monkeyflower* Yerba Santa*	Aster Blue Flag Chicory Comfrey Desert Larkspur Echinacea Indian Paintbrush* Lupine Morning Glory Palmer's Penstemon Pinyon Purple Robe Sage Thistle Vervain	Aster Bells-of-Ireland Black-Eyed Susan Blue Flag Bouncing Bet Chamomile Cliff Rose Columbine Comfrey Desert Willow Evening Primrose Honeysuckle Lupine Morning Glory Onion Ox-Eye Daisy Peace Rose Sage Saguro Thistle Vervain Willow Yarrow Yerba Santa Yucca

* Refers to signature rather than color

living flower essences key rubrics guide			
flower	primary quality	key rubrics for positive healing patterns	key rubrics for symptoms and patterns of imbalance
aster	Illumination	insight, spiritual inspiration, wisdom	spirituality closed down, lack of direction, tendency not to be "down to earth"
bells-of-ireland	Inner-Child Transformation	trusting intuition, healing inner-child issues, union with self	insecurity, lack of trust, lack of protection, extreme vulnerability
black-eyed susan	Inner Peace	healing abusive/addictive relationships, strength	avoidance, resisting pain, emotional conflict within self
blanketflower	Fire Dance	joy, love of life, creative expression	inhibition, depression, low vitality, sadness
blue flag	Stamina	artistic creativity, inspiration, positive stress management	feeling "stuck," suppressed creativity, lack of discernment, attraction to superficial beauty
bouncing bet	Mystic Union	balance, harmony, intimacy, love, sexuality	closed down, dissociation from self and others, lack of feeling love and loved
calendula	Calm	soothing, peaceful, sensitive, radiant	anxiety, fear, impatience, nervousness
california poppy	Purifier	receptivity to emotional cleansing, sensitivity, sensuality, wisdom	emotional insensitivity, lack of care for self, closed down
century plant	Breakthrough	confidence, empowerment, strength, ability to survive, rebirth	lack of willpower, letting others dominate, holding on and not letting go
chamomile	Serenity	relaxation, emotional balance, peacefulness, comfort	anxiety, impatience, irritability, moodiness

living flower essences key rubrics guide (continued)			
flower	primary quality	key rubrics for positive healing patterns	key rubrics for symptoms and patterns of imbalance
chicory	Interrelatedness	respect and caring for others, unconditional love	demanding, insensitivity, lack of concern about others, self-centeredness
cliff rose	Positive Self-Image	self-acceptance, self-value, love of self, self-image	lack of self-acceptance and self-value, fear of expressing love
columbine	Divine Beauty	appreciation, love, inner beauty, cheerfulness, inner worth	egoic personal beauty, lack of self-worth, overemphasis on the material world
comfrey	Service	nurturing others to serve the best interests of all, compassion, protection, personal service	resistance to making personal sacrifices, lack of discernment, limited spiritual vision
crimson monkeyflower	Personal Power	communicating emotional bitterness in a positive way, male sexuality, confidence, courage	aggressiveness, anger, "sticky" relationships, verbal abuse
desert larkspur	Graceful Passage	ease in communication, positive attitude toward life changes, imagination, clarity	difficulty expressing self, resistance to change, lack of awareness
desert marigold	Flexibility	willingness to flow with life's circumstances, balance of wisdom and intellect	controlling, overstructured, rigidity, overly intellectual, lack of intuition
desert willow	The Empress	abundance, appreciation, beauty, communication, feminine sexuality, nourishing, nurturing	closed down sensually or sexually with self or partner, lack of love and nurturing

living flower essences key rubrics guide (continued)			
flower	primary quality	key rubrics for positive healing patterns	key rubrics for symptoms and patterns of imbalance
echinacea	Rejuvenation	vitality, cleansing and elimination of old patterns, understanding	confusion, exhaustion, rejection, repression, blocked emotions, thoughts, and insights
evening primrose	Inner Strength	awakening, purity, self-identity, healing issues related to mother, nurturing, bonding	depression, rejection, unclear identity, unclear values, issues with mother
honeysuckle	Harmony	balance, concentration, intimacy, integration, optimism	attachment, mental tension, nostalgia, lack of harmony with self and others
indian paintbrush	Creativity	creative expression, family values, passion, resourcefulness	abandonment, anger, codependence, insufficient family system, lack of resourcefulness
lupine	Pathfinder	appreciation of the moment, uplift, spiritual guidance	struggle in the past or future, inability to access a higher purpose in life
mexican hat	Release	self-empowerment, letting go of undesirable situations and people	abandonment, abuse, anger, addiction, fear, grief, hopelessness, suppressed emotions, holding on to the above
morning glory	Liberator	clarity, freedom, inspiration, love, new beginnings, vitality	closed down, not in touch with natural body rhythms, resistance to waking up
mullein	Security	intimacy, listening, purpose, positive masculine energy, protection, security, sensitivity	lack of intimacy, lack of direction and purpose in life, insensitivity

living flower essences key rubrics guide (continued)

flower	primary quality	key rubrics for positive healing patterns	key rubrics for symptoms and patterns of imbalance
onion	Membership	belonging to a group, bonding, releasing grief and suppressed emotions	confusion, disinterest, grief, lack of belonging, sadness, withdrawal, difficulty crying
ox-eye daisy	Inner Knowing	aloneness without feeling lonely, intuition, insight, optimism, understanding, wisdom	lack of trust in intuitive guidance, loneliness, misunderstanding, being overanalytical, worry
palmer's penstemon	Self-Expression	speaking one's truth from a higher perspective, sensitivity, clairvoyance	anger, misuse of communication, verbally abusive, lack of confidence in speaking
paloverde	Earth Wisdom	amend-making, groundedness, self-awareness, strength, survival	avoidance, blame, emotional miseries, being judgmental, lack of inner strength
peace rose	Gift of the Angels	compassion, forgiveness, inspiration, joy, love	burdens, depression, despair, facing death, grief, loss of a loved one
pinyon	Patience	appreciation, gentleness, introspection, purification, honoring death and dying	burdens, guilt, impatience, lack of perseverance, regrets, restlessness, shame, struggles with death/dying
pomegranate	Fruit of Life	abundance, creativity, loving, nurturing, passion, resourcefulness, self-empowerment, sexuality	hidden talents, lack of creativity, lack of passion and joy in life, inability to locate resources
purple robe	Plenty	abundance, clairvoyance, expansiveness, insight, vision, wisdom	dwelling on lack and being without, inability to see a broader perspective, lack of inspiration and insight

living flower essences key rubrics guide (continued)

flower	primary quality	key rubrics for positive healing patterns	key rubrics for symptoms and patterns of imbalance
sage	Whole-Life Integration	conscientiousness, insight, purification, spiritual inspiration, whole-life balance	bitterness, insensitivity, resistance to embracing spirituality in all realms of life
saguaro	The Guardian	endurance, honoring sacred space, perseverance, protection, purpose, stamina, wisdom	disrespect, lack of dignity, impatience, restlessness, feeling a lack of protection or vulnerability, lack of purpose in life
scarlet penstemon	Courage	creativity, confidence, self-expression, masculine sexuality, passion, intimacy	agitation, anger, depression, lack of courage and faith, lack of confidence
strawberry hedgehog	Passion	compassion, love, intimacy, sexuality, self-worth	aggression, insecurity, insensitivity, inhibition, shut-down sexuality
sunflower	Fountain of Youth	cheerfulness, determination, direction, expansion, playfulness, vision, warmth, wisdom	anger, despair, exhaustion, fear, guilt, hopelessness, panic, pessimism, lack of goals or direction, unworthiness
sweet pea	Growing Child	belonging, compassion, confidence, love, protection, social integration	desertion, fear, insecurity, lack of confidence, loneliness, feeling unloved and unprotected
thistle	Balance	calm, centeredness, confidence, clarity, inspiration, union, vision	anxiety, fear, lack of confidence, nervousness, tension, lack of inspiration and vision

living flower essences key rubrics guide (continued)			
flower	primary quality	key rubrics for positive healing patterns	key rubrics for symptoms and patterns of imbalance
vervain	Reach for the Stars	accomplishment, direction, insight, inspiration, leadership, motivation, purpose, uplift	complicated thoughts, being judgmental, lack of motivation, nervous exhaustion, being opinionated, rigidity, tending to be overstressed
wild rose	Love	beauty, compassion, devotion, freedom, protection, vitality	apathy, avoidance, depression, dissociation, disinterest, grief, weariness
willow	Forgiveness	clarity, compassion, flexibility, letting go, patience, understanding	blame, confusion, criticism, emotional bitterness, impatience, injust acts, resentment, resistance, rigidity, vengefulness
yarrow	Protection	cleansing, energy, insight, prevention, shield, inspiration	anxiety, exhaustion, over-responsibility, run down, "wounded warrior, wounded healer"
yellow monkeyflower	Overcoming Fear	cleansing, confidence, courage to communicate, self-expression, self-assertiveness, self-respect	abandonment, doubt, fear, restlessness, timidity, unworthiness, lack of confidence to communicate needs
yerba santa	The Sacred Within	cleansing, inner loving, receptivity, renewal, reverence for all of life, self-discovery, spiritual guidance	anxiety, impurities, inferiority, out of touch with self, psychic toxins
yucca	Spear of Destiny	higher consciousness, focus, perseverance, ability to act toward and stay focused on life's goals	emptiness, feeling lost in the darkness, lacking spiritual direction, purpose, and guidance

CHAPTER 11
Materia Medica

This chapter is a summary of my clinical endorsement of the *materia medica* as best as it can be at this time. This constitutes a reference work; it is not intended to diagnose, treat, or prescribe, and the information found here should be used with that understanding. The Research Provers' Project Findings are accurate for the provers who participated and are a source of information for future collections of research and documentation.

The compilation of this material provides a foundation for what is yet to come; it fulfills the purpose of being useful to students, practitioners, and the general public. You will need to discover for yourself the value of flower essences and the ways in which they benefit your relationship with all of life, thus creating your own experiences and your own foundation in the world of plants and nature.

Blessings to you on your journey.

ASTER (desert aster)

(Machaeranthera tephrodes)
PRIMARY QUALITY: ILLUMINATION

FAMILY: Sunflower (Compositae)

OTHER NAMES: Tansyleaf Aster, Tansy-aster. *Aster* is an ancient Greek word meaning "star."

WHERE FOUND: Dry hillsides, washes, desert flats, along roadsides, and on abandoned ground in the Western states. There are many species of asters throughout the United States.

ELEVATION: 1,000' to 3,500'

ENERGY IMPACT (CHAKRA CORRESPONDENCE): third, sixth, and seventh chakras

KEY RUBRICS FOR POSITIVE HEALING PATTERNS: insight, spiritual inspiration, wisdom

KEY RUBRICS FOR SYMPTOMS AND PATTERNS OF IMBALANCE: spiritually closed down, lack of direction, tendency not to be down-to-earth

OTHER RUBRICS: acceptance, aloneness, ambition, anxiety, awareness, beauty, brow, calm, chakra, clarity, cleansing, community, confident, crown chakra, depression, flexible, focus, gentleness, grace, grounded, happiness, higher knowing, illumination, images, insecurity, integration, intellect, intuition, irritability, joyfulness, loneliness, meditation, mellow, nurturing, organized, positive, quieting, radiance, sadness, security, sensitive, simplicity, solar plexus chakra, spirituality, strength, understanding, vibrant, vision, world, worry

traditional use

There are numerous species of wild asters varying in colors, including purple, white, and yellow. The various species of aster have been used as purgatives, to treat eruptive skin diseases, and as aromatic nervines. The entire plant of the smooth aster has been used in Native American traditions to furnish smoke in sweats and is also used as a smudge to uplift consciousness.

homeopathic use

Unknown to author.

positive healing patterns

- Offers spiritual balance and inspiration through vision and wisdom, opening our ability to see more deeply. If you're closed, it will open you; if you're too open, it will bring you deeper inside.
- Gives us illumination and insight, like a shining star, and helps us accept our path of spiritual evolution; offers a light, joyful disposition that helps lift depression.
- Gracefully gives us the focus to allow Spirit to move through us, and helps

us take the less complicated routes that avoid unnecessary downsides.

- Embraces higher community awareness and follow-through on higher spiritual principles of living and being in the world; teaches us to share our spiritual truths with our children and to hold our children in light and love.

symptoms and patterns of imbalance

Aster may be an appropriate flower essence for those who

- Lack a spiritual foundation or direction and are in need of spiritual inspiration
- Feel irritable, in disharmony, depressed, and spiritually closed down
- Demonstrate spiritual immaturity and lack of insight
- Tend to be overly spiritual and are in need of a spiritual framework that is grounding and integrative into the world.

features of the original flower-essence water

ODOR: subtly sweet
TASTE: sweet, strong, earthy "green" taste
SENSATIONS: tingling in the mouth and throat; a pulling sensation in the third eye to the crown chakra and slight tension in the forehead; an opening feeling in the pituitary
WATER COLOR: clear

physical makeup

ROOT, STEM, LEAVES/LEAFLETS, HEIGHT: Aster is a perennial that grows about 6 inches to 3 feet tall and reproduces by seeds. The root is hardy and doesn't pull easily. The stem is round, smooth, and spindly. The stem is firmer toward the bottom and more flexible toward the top of the plant; it branches out, forming clusters of flowers at the ends of its many stems. The leaves are pale, grayish green, and linear-lanceolate shaped. They vary from sparsely to densely hairy, and alternate along the branches. The leaves are larger at the bottom of the stem and shorter and smaller at the top. There is one slight center vein in the leaves. There are many species and varieties of asters.

FLOWER COLOR: Purple (violet) with a golden-yellow center

FLOWERS: The purple (or violet) ray flowers cluster at the ends of branches. They are about 1 inch to $1\,^1/_2$ inches in diameter and have a golden yellow disk in the center. There are approximately fifteen to thirty rays per flower head. The underside of the rays is pale and faded, while the topside has a deeper purple color. The flower has a slightly musty odor.

BLOOMING PERIOD: May to October

doctrine of signatures

- The plant has a strong foundation, yet its many branches are flexible, light, and uplifting.
- The flower's starlike shape represents simplicity, light, grace, and

illumination. Its rays reach out as if to embark upon the path of the flower's spiritual truth in joy. The flower also resembles a crown on top of a head, symbolic of the seventh chakra. This unique signature and energy center is a reflection of our ability to be drawn to a higher consciousness, to live in the here and now, and to plant and nurture the seeds of our thoughts with Divine Intelligence.

- The taste of the flower itself is somewhat bitter, especially in the center. The flower-essence water, however, is subtly sweet and pleasant. This represents the challenging aspects of disharmony, irritability, and bitterness, and also some of the flower's healing patterns such as inspiration, illumination, and brightness.

- The purple (violet) color of the flower is representative of the sixth (or brow) chakra or third eye, which embraces higher spiritual principles of being in the world. The yellow disk in the center of the flower is symbolic of our mind's eye, which is linked with the rational mind and to psychic energies and intuition, offering guidance, vision, wisdom, and insight. The energy center of the sixth chakra works with the mental aspects of the third chakra, allowing spiritual direction to guide our mental thought-forms.

- Asters grow in communities near

each other, showing support and the need for community.

Helpful suggestions

I once journeyed with the desert aster while sitting directly across from the doorway to the Great Kiva at Chetro Ketl in Chaco Canyon, New Mexico. Chetro Ketl is an Anasazi Indian ruin that dates from about A.D. 850 through 1100. Chetro Ketl is characterized by skilled masonry, good design, large scale, and geometry. Two beautiful desert asters were growing near "my spot" at this Great Kiva. The incredible architectural designs of the ruins were all around me. I held Sarah, my eleven-month-old baby, nursing in my lap as I studied and journeyed with this plant. The desert aster took me back in time. I felt invisible as I sat there watching the Anasazi Indians build their homes. The people seemed to know their duties and were skilled at what they did. They worked in silence and were very focused. I had a feeling of the peace and union they felt deep inside themselves, with the land, and with each other. I felt their joys and I felt their sorrows. They seemed to have a great vision for themselves, and they patiently held their vision with deep devotion.

Like the Anasazi people, the desert aster's petals reach out as if to embark upon a path of spiritual truth. The plant holds its character of strength and radiance despite life's pitfalls and challenges. It seemed so "right" for this plant to grow here — for its roots to grow from the sandy, rocky, barren earth and to evolve into a plant with many flowers that face the sky. I felt a great sadness for these people, for their hope, for all their hard work, and for whatever caused their departure. Yet I also felt the tremendous strength and vision that guided them.

As I opened my eyes, I felt drops of rain on my bare arms and legs. Sarah and I were the only people at the Great Kiva. In the silence, I could hear the soft tones of my husband Curt's flute in the distance. Sarah lay asleep in my arms as we sat in the gentle rain, washing away the passage of time and cleansing our souls.

Take several drops of the Aster flower essence, close your eyes, and enter the silence. Imagine your own eye as the center of the aster flower. With the flower as your mirror, take a look at the eye looking back at you. What do you see? Imagine the purple ray flowers of the aster flower circling around your third eye and extending outward in all directions. Feel the flower's grace. Look at its simple beauty. Let yourself be guided by the light and the higher vision this flower has to offer. Staying in your inner silence, allow yourself to see and stretch beyond time and space. Notice any lights, colors, or images that enter through your third eye. Notice your awareness. Allow yourself to experience your journey with the aster flower, and ask for its guidance to help you tap into the collective unconscious. Stay with your experience until you feel it is complete. Slowly open your eyes and remain in a relaxed state until you feel ready to do something else.

Affirmations

- "I see the deeper meaning behind all life situations and act from a place of wisdom and insight."
- "May Light flow within and around me and guide me to my highest good."
- "I accept all that is and will be. My future is bright before me and the path is easy to find. I trust my intuition; I am my own shining star."

Case History

Tanya, age nineteen, took the Aster flower essence. This is what she has to say about her experience:

"Each time I took the essence, I felt a physical rush of energy beginning at the back of my head, spreading through my solar plexus and then my calves and lower legs. Mentally, I became more aware that patience is a big factor in my life; it is the key that will help me reach my goals. I feel a greater understanding of how and why things are in the moment, and of how the present relates to my goals in life. I feel more accepting of what is and what will be. My emotions have been more stable. I feel less depressed. I can think about how I'm feeling before reacting to my emotions. I have more emotional control. I also have a better memory because I'm beginning to sort things out from the past as well as in the present. I'm more trusting of my feelings and have more insight into who I am and the direction I want to take. I am meditating more and experiencing a natural healing of my fears and confusion. The Aster essence has also helped me to focus on getting rid of things in my life that are hindering my path. My relationship with my boyfriend is more positive, and I'm more at ease in communicating my needs to him."

Lfe's Research provers' project findings

Physical Symptoms

Cravings: Salads, fruits, wanting to improve my diet

Sensations: Increased body warmth

Pain: None

Modalities:
  Worse: None
  Better: Improved sleep and more energy during the day

Head: None

Eyes: Increased depth perception, imagery

Face: None

Ears: None

Stomach: None

Abdomen: None

Bowel condition: None

Urine: None

Female: None

Male: None

Extremities: None

Back: None

Skin: None

Other: "I had more energy and was able to catch up on everything, like my laundry, shopping, and eating well. I also enjoyed exercising, which usually is a drag."

Emotional Symptoms

Patterns of Balance: "very mellowing and quieting; good in stressful periods," "very gentle," "settling," "relaxing," "generally made me feel better," "took the edge off stress," "I felt the need to spend time alone and focus on doing things for myself; I liked this essence because it gave me courage to be on my own again," "gave me a sense of security," "took time to nurture myself," "I felt happy, confident, and good," "I felt sensitive to others' loneliness," "calm," "aware of emotional dynamics," "I feel the strength to move on"

Patterns of Imbalance: "irritability," "loneliness," "inability to relate to the world," "anxiety related to cruelty — man's inhumanity to man," "feeling alone in a hostile world"

Mental Symptoms

Patterns of Balance: "softening of tension," "my mind was focused and I felt grounded and organized," "I was more organized and able to get things done," "I had the attitude of 'take it or leave it' and was also more flexible," "my mind was centered," "visions and images," "a seeing awareness and clarity"

Patterns of Imbalance: "anxiety," "worrying about other people," "more intense awareness of lonely feelings and sad thoughts"

Spiritual Reflections

"Made meditation easier and influenced a quiet reflection," "took time for myself to meditate more," "I felt this essence helped to prepare me spiritually for my next step," "I keep thanking Great Spirit"

DREAMS/NIGHTMARES

Most provers had increased dreams and many dream images: "I experienced more dream images while falling asleep. Once I saw two dark doorways, black as a night sky, with suffering faces: men, women, and children."

"I repeated the same dream twice. I was searching an industrial area for an airplane. I found the plane and, as I was setting up to take off, the plane was partly on the grass and partly on the water. Then I was flying around a city and power lines were a problem and I landed in the snow."

BELLS-OF-IRELAND

(Moluccella laevis)
PRIMARY QUALITY: Inner-Child Transformation

FAMILY: Mint (Lamiaceae, Labiatae)
OTHER NAMES: Shell Flower
WHERE FOUND: a garden flower able to grow in most areas throughout the U.S.
ELEVATION: most U.S. climate zones
ENERGY IMPACT (CHAKRA CORRESPONDENCE): fourth and seventh chakras
KEY RUBRICS FOR POSITIVE HEALING PATTERNS: trusting intuition, healing inner-child issues, union with self
KEY RUBRICS FOR SYMPTOMS AND PATTERNS OF IMBALANCE: insecurity, lack of trust, lack of protection, extreme vulnerability
OTHER RUBRICS: childhood, children, cleanse, communion, complain, crown chakra, feminine, frustration, gentleness, guidance, heart chakra, higher consciousness, impatience, irritability, light, love, masculine, nature, nurture, out of sorts, personal responsibility, security, spirituality, strength, wisdom

---

traditional use

Green bells-of-Ireland is a showy, attractive addition to the garden. No medicinal or other uses are known to the author.

homeopathic use

Unknown to author.

positive healing patterns

- Offers security, nurturing, and protection to our inner child.
- Helps us to communicate, commune, and connect with nature's kingdoms.
- Enhances our ability to transform inner-child issues and take personal responsibility for ourselves.
- Helps cleanse emotional wounds of the heart and provides a gentle strength necessary to trust again.
- Allows us to open, yield, and commune with our female receptive self and be guided by intuition and higher knowledge.
- Allows us to open, yield, and commune with our positive male self and demonstrate strength and determination though gentleness.
- Aligns us with our spiritual presence and an intrinsic knowing that is linked to our higher consciousness. As children (and at all ages), we intuitively know how we feel yet our intuitions are not trusted or respected by adults or those who seem to have power over us. This

essence helps us trust our intuition and realize the need to connect with our higher selves for guidance.

- Opens our awareness to the situations we find ourselves in, holding the Light and heart energy as our power.

symptoms and patterns of imbalance

Bells-of-Ireland may be an appropriate flower essence for those who

- Feel insecure, vulnerable, and unprotected (i.e., children who feel insecure at school, with certain family members, or in general; women who feel unprotected by men; men who feel unprotected by others; or people who have been abused); insecurities may be acted out through impatience, irritability, complaining, and generally feeling out of sorts
- Have difficulty setting boundaries
- Are overly trusting or who lack trust
- Are overly protective of their children or spouse
- Need to connect with nature and are out of touch with the natural world

features of the original flower-essence water

ODOR: sweeter and more flavorful than the flower itself
TASTE: very full, aromatic, and pleasant
SENSATIONS: a cool, smooth sensation in the mouth; felt pain and hurt deep inside heart chakra (slight tingling). The energy released and moved upward, stayed at the crown, then moved out the top of the head.
WATER COLOR: remained clear

physical makeup

ROOT, STEM, LEAVES/LEAFLETS, HEIGHT: The root is sturdy and hard to pull. The stem is square with rounded corners and is light, hollow-feeling, and fibrous. There is a hint of purple toward the base of the stem.

The leaves grow in opposite pairs with each cluster of flowers, and they alternate in opposite directions as they grow up the spike-like plant. Leaves have edges that are jagged yet smooth. The showy bell- or shell-shaped apple-green calyces carry the flowers from near the base and up the spike-like plant. Flowers are in whorls of three clusters with three calyces per cluster, alternating with two clusters with four calyces per cluster growing around the stem. Each calyx is very veiny (with a cup-like spider-web effect), with five primary veins each leading to a thornlike point — thus five points per calyx. A soft but prickly thorn grows at the base of each cluster. The spicy mint odor is both attractive and repulsive.

FLOWER COLOR: White and pale pink
FLOWERS: Each flower has two petals. The upper, pale-lavender petal emerges from a small, soft, phallus-shaped cap with white spindly stamens and two anthers that resemble testicles. The lower, whitish petal has two vagina-like lips that unfold and appear to have a clitoris in the center. The petals are soft, fuzzy, and velvety. The flowers smell slightly sweet.

BLOOMING PERIOD: Early spring to early fall, depending on the climate zone

Doctrine of signatures

- The flower is seated inside, and appears protected by, the outer shell. If you look closely at the flower, it resembles a small person wearing a hood sitting inside the shell facing out toward the opening. It is as if a small, vulnerable child is sitting inside the soft, protective, bell-shaped cup and feeling nurtured and protected by the nature spirits. This signature resembles a closeness and communion with nature.
- Looked at differently, the flower resembles male and female genitals, both protected by the outer shell. This signature demonstrates openness and communion between the feminine receptive and the positive male expressive in a cove of protection and security.
- The lightness, delicateness, and soft colors of the flower suggest the presence of radiant Light. The color of the flower is symbolic of the seventh chakra, aligning us with our spiritual nature and an intrinsic knowing that is linked to our higher consciousness. This signature is about trusting our intuition and realizing the need to connect with our higher selves to help and guide us.
- The pinkish color of the flower represents the fourth chakra, which is the heart chakra, and is a signature of opening our awareness and desire to bond between the heart and the upper chakras. It is about seeing ourselves as a system of energy, being aware of the kinds of situations we find ourselves in, and to hold the Light and heart energy as our power.

Helpful suggestions

Find a nice, quiet spot and give yourself some time to be with the bells-of-Ireland plant. Look closely at the bells-of-Ireland photo. Study the flower. What do you see? How does it make you feel? Then close your eyes. See yourself inside the cup or shell of the bells-of-Ireland. Imagine a soft, green color all around you, embracing you with a warm, fuzzy blanket of velvet. Lean against the inside of the shell. Feel its love and protection. Talk to yourself inside the shell, knowing that you are safe and protected. Talk to anyone else you feel you have something to say to, and know that you are safe and protected. If you have an unresolved childhood incident (or any incident) that needs healing and protection, embrace yourself inside the shell. Tell yourself that you are now safe and secure. Embrace the union of your inner male and female; feel their trust and guidance. Put your left hand on your heart chakra and ask for a healing vibration to come through you. Pray that your heart chakra will give you guidance in awakening compassion, love, and healing energies. Ask for guidance in awakening your sight into the deeper forces in the nature kingdom.

Pay attention to any images that come to you. Then imagine yourself being filled with white crystalline light pouring through every cell in your body. Feel the warmth, brightness, and power of the light. Ask Spirit for healing to occur. Stay with your experience until it is complete. Thank the plant for the gifts it gave you and make a choice, according to your own needs, about whether to remain in the shell or to step away from it.

Affirmations

- "I give myself the freedom to express vulnerability and trust in a safe, nurturing environment."
- "I am drawn to those of like mind who nurture, love, and protect my friendship with them."
- "I let love pour through my heart and heal my inner child."

Case History

Crystal, age forty-one, was drawn to flower essence therapy to heal her unresolved parental abuse and bad childhood memories. She also had a history of smoking and drinking, which she felt were related to the way she dealt with her childhood issues. She still felt unsafe, unprotected, and very "stressed" when childhood memories arose. This stress carried over to her relationship with her husband and affected her in many ways. She felt a need for spiritual guidance in resolving these issues, and she described herself as having a "hurting heart." Crystal felt that she had dealt with her anger, but hadn't resolved the tremendous wounds, loss of trust, and vulnerability she experienced as a child. Due to the childhood issues and the need for transforming these issues, the first essence given to her was Bells-of-Ireland.

Crystal said that, in taking this essence, "it helped me find my 'center.' It didn't make me feel so far down. It made me feel safe. My husband and the essence helped me work through some of these issues and release them. I felt peace within myself."

LFE's Research Provers' Project Findings

PHYSICAL SYMPTOMS

CRAVINGS: Good food, rice, vegetables, and fruits

SENSATIONS: None

PAIN: Pain in hip

MODALITIES: Inconsistent

HEAD: None

EYES: None

FACE: None

EARS: None

STOMACH: None

ABDOMEN: None

BOWEL CONDITION: None

URINE: None

FEMALE: Felt like she was having PMS

MALE: None

EXTREMITIES: Hip pain

BACK: None

SKIN: None

NOTE: Two provers reported no symptoms.

EMOTIONAL SYMPTOMS

PATTERNS OF BALANCE: "helped me get more real in how I was feeling"

PATTERNS OF IMBALANCE: "irritable, frustrated, impatient, complaining, and generally out of sorts," "I had mood swings and bottled-up feelings, not wanting to get up and face the day," "lack of self-worth, unsure of abilities, mood swings," "felt unsure of myself"

MENTAL SYMPTOMS

PATTERNS OF BALANCE: "helped me have more clarity and be more aware of my frustrations," "helped me face life's dilemmas with equanimity"

PATTERNS OF IMBALANCE: "worrying about assorted problems," "mentally sluggish," "experienced negative vs. positive thoughts"

SPIRITUAL REFLECTIONS

"Angels are messengers as protectors and guides," "children may be longing for the past, a childhood lost, or perhaps what I need is to get in touch with my inner child," "I feel I am being helped and protected and that new growth will come in spite of obstacles or lost longings"

DREAMS/NIGHTMARES

"A beautiful woman was supporting and helping me. I woke up feeling happy about this. I had many other dream images that included angels, many angels."

BLACK-EYED SUSAN

(Rudbeckia hirta)

PRIMARY QUALITY: INNER PEACE

FAMILY: Sunflower (Compositae)

OTHER NAMES: Golden Glow, Lance-Leafed Coneflower, Dormilon, Rudbeckia

WHERE FOUND: Grows on hillsides and in prairies, fields, and open woods in southern Canada and most of the United States from June until October.

ELEVATION: 5,000' to 8,000'

ENERGY IMPACT (CHAKRA CORRESPONDENCE): first, third, and seventh chakras

KEY RUBRICS FOR POSITIVE HEALING PATTERNS: healing abusive/addictive relationships, strength

KEY RUBRICS FOR SYMPTOMS AND PATTERNS OF IMBALANCE: avoidance, resisting pain, emotional conflict within self

OTHER RUBRICS: abuse, addiction, anger, breakthrough, brokenheartedness, calm, centeredness, challenge, change, clarity, cleansing, communication, confidence, courage, creativity, crown chakra, denial, depression, dreams, emotional bondage, faith, fear, feminine, freedom, healing, heart, hopelessness, inner peace, insight, isolation, judgmental, meditation, memory, mental bondage, pain, panic, patience, peace, prayer, prejudice, repression, root chakra, self-esteem, self-empowerment, sexuality, solar plexus chakra, trauma, uncertainty, understanding, unworthiness, victim, wisdom, worry

Traditional use

Diuretic with possible side effect of mild cardiac stimulation. It can be used to stimulate the water volume in urine, but not the solids. In New Mexico, the root has historically been used to relieve menstrual pains. Native Americans used the root to make a tea to treat colds and chest congestion. Some herbalists believe that black-eyed Susan was also used to treat boils, referring to the dark disk in the center of the flower.

Homeopathic use

Unknown to author.

positive Healing patterns

- Helps us embrace what we are resisting and to fill ourselves with a deep sense of inner peace.
- Teaches us to release emotional bondage through creativity and freedom of thinking.
- Helps us identify deep issues when we can't determine what we need to heal.
- Helps us heal past abusive and/or addictive experiences through understanding who we are now and that we can change our responses to those experiences that no longer serve us.

- Helps us connect with our higher self and integrate feelings, experiences, and thoughts with spiritual wisdom and understanding.
- Helps us find purpose and desire in life, and to empower ourselves.

symptoms and patterns of imbalance

Black-Eyed Susan may be an appropriate flower essence for those who

- Resist facing painful or undesirable parts of their personality
- Tend to suppress, avoid, or fear facing emotions
- Avoid looking at experiences that were traumatic and painful
- Tend to overanalyze situations, let emotions cloud their judgment, lack mental clarity and the ability to focus, and lack mind power in relation to fear, worry, anger, hatred, prejudice, unworthiness, etc.
- Feel stuck in "hairy" situations
- Misuse their personal power.

features of the original flower-essence water

Odor: a mild musty smell, similar to that of a sunflower

Taste: light and sweet, with a gentle sweet aftertaste

Sensations: a strong feeling of calm; a tingling sensation moved from the root chakra up to the crown chakra, releasing tension along the way

Water Color: clear

physical makeup

Root, Stem, Leaves/Leaflets, Height: The dull olive-green leaves are very hairy, dry, sticky and coarse, sometimes bearing tiny glandular purple dots. The lower leaves can be 2 to 4 inches long and vary in shape; they may be lance-shaped, oval, or egg-shaped, with or without teeth. The leaves become smaller and more tapered as they get closer to the flower. The strong, bendable yet rigid stems are also coarse, fuzzy, hairy, and bristly. They stand 1 to 4 feet tall.

Flower Color: Golden yellow with a dark brown center

Flowers: The flower heads are 2 to 3 inches in diameter. Seeds grow around and up toward the dark chocolate-colored center disk, which is surrounded by up to twenty golden-yellow daisy-like ray petals. Tiny florets encircle the disk in successive bloom (not all at once) and create a yellow halo when the pollen is ripe. Two creases in each petal create three symmetrical sections. The petals have several layers, creating an alternating effect. As the outer layer dies, a younger layer takes its place. The golden-yellow ray petals are without stamens or pistils. Several flowers branch out from one stem.

Blooming Period: June to October

doctrine of signatures

- The dark core spreading out into light petals is symbolic of this plant's ability to bring release and of the shadow-self embracing the light. The dark core also represents the darkness of the earth and our connection with our first chakra, or root chakra; this is the energy center that connects us with the earth and helps us build a foundation for understanding who we are and what direction we will choose in our lives.

- The yellow halo or crown is symbolic of our conscious awareness and our ability to embrace the light and higher power, giving a feeling of connection and freedom. The yellow petals also represent the third chakra, or solar plexus chakra, which gives us our ability to think and reason, to find our purpose in life, and to empower ourselves. This center strengthens our mind to pursue a state of peacefulness, stableness, courage, faith, humor, and joy, bringing about a balanced mental state. By working with this flower and chakra center, we can dissolve criticisms, learn to deal more effectively with our anger, understand what we avoid facing within ourselves, and unplug from our fears. Black-eyed Susan is a powerful flower that helps us understand and embrace our pains so that we can release them. It also teaches us the powerful influence our thoughts have on our lives.
- The coarse, hairy stem and leaves represent our rough, "hairy," potentially dangerous risks, losses, and injuries.
- The energy impact of the flower-essence water gives a strong feeling

of calm tingling energy from the root chakra all the way up to the seventh chakra, releasing tension along the way and creating a sense of peace from deep within.

Helpful suggestions

Take three to four drops of Black-Eyed Susan flower essence and find a quiet place to be alone. Take several deep, long breaths. Imagine yourself breathing out the bad and breathing in the good. Tune in to your body. How does it feel? Does it hurt anywhere?

Tune in to your feelings. How are you feeling? Is there something in your past that continues to bother you? Tune in to your thoughts. What is your inner voice saying? What kind of thoughts have you had recently? Is there something about yourself that bothers you, that you don't like? Do you intuitively feel that there is something hidden that you need to explore? Is there something in particular that you know you need to explore to help you heal? Find out what it is and try to stay with it. Explore your thoughts and feelings about it. Look at this part of your life and how it affects who you are.

Next, face whatever you need to look at and try to connect with it. Relive an experience through your imagination if need be. Take a close look and get in touch with all the levels involved: mental, emotional, physical, and spiritual. You may need to consult a friend, partner, therapist, counselor, or healer to help you. Depending on the intensity of your issue, it could take days, months, or longer to work through your healing process.

Ask for guidance in working through this issue. Keep your intention clear and focused. Pray for understanding about this situation or part of yourself that gives you great pain. Pray for letting go and for inner peace.

CAUTION: If you aren't able to confront the issue within four or five days, I suggest that you stop taking this essence and try another essence. On the other hand, if you feel you are becoming emotionally drained by taking this essence, I also encourage you to discontinue using it and to try another essence.

affirmations

- "I give myself permission to embrace my pains and to release all pain to God so that I may feel inner peace."
- "I am willing to be transformed, restored, and rejuvenated and to claim all parts of who I am."
- "I am free and whole. I have the power to believe in myself and to feel at peace with who I am."
- "May I stir the power within me to create loving and peaceful thoughts."

case History

Roby, age forty-one, sought flower essence therapy to help her confront the emotional and physical disharmony she was experiencing. She had tightness in her chest, which she associated with sup-

pressed emotions, especially fear issues. Roby felt she needed to face and release some core issues before she could make needed changes in her life. I immediately felt that Black-Eyed Susan flower essence and its release properties would serve her.

When she began taking the Black-Eyed Susan essence, Roby found herself crying easily as she experienced a series of healing crises that went back to her childhood. She discovered that parts of her melted away as she recognized them, confronted them, and let them go. "Black-Eyed Susan seemed to intensify my emotions," Roby says. "I felt moved with the first few doses. Its ability to bring up deep-seated feelings is dramatic and powerful. As I continue to take the essence, I find myself getting in touch with my true thoughts and emotions. I am able to settle unresolved issues, move beyond the pain, and — finally — heal. I feel a deep inner peace and love for myself that I have not experienced before."

Lfe's Research provers' project findings

PHYSICAL SYMPTOMS

CRAVINGS: Sugar, chocolate

SENSATIONS: Tingling, pressure on top of head, tiredness, hurried feeling, warm sensation in throat and stomach

PAIN: Tightness of head

MODALITIES:

  WORSE: Late at night

  BETTER: Early morning

HEAD: Top of head tight and pressured, headaches, cloudiness in head

EYES: Vivid images

FACE: Cold sore on lip

EARS: None

STOMACH: Digestive problems, tension in stomach lessened temporarily, warm sensation

ABDOMEN: None

BOWEL CONDITION: More frequent bowel movements

URINE: None

FEMALE: Sexual issues

MALE: Inappropriate sexual thoughts, hemorrhoid cleared up

EXTREMITIES: "Pin pricks" and tingling of hands

BACK: None

SKIN: None

OTHER: Weight gain, lack of sleep, staying up late

EMOTIONAL SYMPTOMS

PATTERNS OF BALANCE: "urge to create and change," "felt more powerful and confident in knowing what is right for myself," "strong emotional strength to stand up for myself," "courage and belief in myself," "felt more relaxed and calm in present crisis"

PATTERNS OF IMBALANCE: "depression," "feeling distant from myself," "irritable," "moody," "discouraged," "disharmony," "tired," "nervous anxiety," "emotions like a roller coaster"

MENTAL SYMPTOMS

PATTERNS OF BALANCE: "I first felt depressed, then I experienced relief and release," "mental clarity," "improved memory," "more creative," "increased mental analysis in regard to relationship problems," "negative, then positive, mental activity," "internal dialogue more quiet"

PATTERNS OF IMBALANCE: "depressed thoughts," "fuzzy thinking," "thoughts are out of balance," "dull," "anxiety," "brought back memories of previous crises (death of a close friend, divorce, breakup, abusive relationship)"

SPIRITUAL REFLECTIONS

"The crown chakra is about integration, and my thoughts are drawn to this theme," "I had more spiritual creativity and freedom, higher awareness of the 'cosmic perspective,'" "more firm 'knowing' of universal energy and a desire for more quiet time and stillness"

DREAMS/NIGHTMARES

"I found myself with a white bag over my head and tape over my eyes, nose, and mouth. There was also tape around my throat and I was panicking or suffocating. I managed to break free, and I experienced immediate relief from panic and a sense of freedom that was more than just physical."

"My ex-husband (who was a mean, abusive bully) was demanding that I do something he wanted. I was able to tell him that I refused to do it. He started yelling at me, but again I held my ground and ignored him. Once again, I felt my power!"

Some provers had more nightmares than usual, but with positive endings.

BLANKETFLOWER

(Gaillardia pulchella)
PRIMARY QUALITY: FIRE DANCE

FAMILY: Sunflower (Compositae)
OTHER NAMES: Firewheel, Indian Blanket, Gaillardia
WHERE FOUND: along roadsides, on plains, in fields and clearings in pinyon-juniper woodlands and ponderosa forests, and on dry, sandy, or rocky slopes, from Colorado and Utah to Texas, Arizona, and New Mexico
ELEVATION: 3,500' to 5,500'
ENERGY IMPACT (CHAKRA CORRESPONDENCE): first, second, and third chakras
KEY RUBRICS FOR POSITIVE HEALING PATTERNS: joy, love of life, creative expression
KEY RUBRICS FOR SYMPTOMS AND PATTERNS OF IMBALANCE: inhibition, depression, low vitality, sadness
OTHER RUBRICS: abandonment, abdomen, aggressiveness, anger, anxiety, breakthrough, carefree, centered, cheerful, colorful, confidence, energetic, expressive, fears, fire, free, grounded, impatience, inspiration, intimacy, intuitive, light, liveliness, passion, patience, radiance, root chakra, self-empowerment, sexuality, solar plexus chakra, spleen chakra, strength, sun, warmth, will, wisdom, vigilance, vitality, worry

Traditional use

Hopi Indians use the *Gaillardia pinnatifida* species as a diuretic. Other uses are unknown by the author. There are five species of gaillardia in Arizona.

Homeopathic use

Unknown to author.

positive Healing patterns

- Serves as "the fire that melts the ice," instilling warmth and exuberance for life when feeling inhibited or shut down.
- Offers a fun-loving attitude and the willingness to take the brighter side, helping us embrace radiance, compassion (warmth), and Light.
- Teaches us the power of our emotions and the energetic impact they have in our lives.
- Gives us the freedom to express our sexuality and our world of sensation. As we come into our identities, a freedom that we have not experienced before is felt. Blanketflower helps us to feel that freedom and to take new steps in the dance of life that stirs passion and excitement for living.
- Represents a joyful, creative expression of our vital life-force nature,

offering a grounding energy that connects us with the earth and her colors and with the sun and his colors.

- Strengthens our minds and our vision to feel self-empowered with a purpose in life that is guided by our Higher Will.

symptoms and patterns of imbalance

Blanketflower may be an appropriate flower essence for those who

- Feel inhibited or shut down
- Need an energy boost and want to look and feel brighter
- Experience depression, sadness, low energy and vitality, feeling down and unempowered
- Lack creativity, joy, and love of life.

features of the original flower-essence water

ODOR: musty sunflower-like smell
TASTE: strong and full, musty-like only sweeter than smell
SENSATIONS: cooler at the throat; warm, tingling sensation into the belly, abdomen, spleen, and solar plexus that is strengthening, yet calm
WATER COLOR: slightly golden-yellow

physical makeup

ROOT, STEM, LEAVES/LEAFLETS, HEIGHT: Roots are hardy, with a stiff yet flexible slightly fuzzy stem. The tall, slender stems are green with a reddish purple tint. The fuzzy, slightly prickly, hairy leaves alternate. The upper leaves are oblong and the lower leaves are lobed and average 2 to 3 inches long. The plant grows up to 2 feet high.
FLOWER COLOR: Bright yellow and reddish orange
FLOWERS: The bright, showy flowers have a strong musty smell, and each flower looks like a fiery pinwheel. They are reddish orange ray flowers with bright yellow tips. The outside rays are divided into lobes of three, and within each divided petal of the lobe are three symmetrical wedge-shaped creases. There are usually eight lobes per flower head. The disk is reddish orange with a golden-yellow dome-shaped center; reddish stamens with golden-yellow anthers grow in and around the disk. The anther heads appear to split into pairs. The center dome is tightly packed with many individual flowers.
BLOOMING PERIOD: April to September

doctrine of signatures

- The bright yellow and reddish orange colors of the plant resemble the fiery, colorful elements of the sun; this correlates with the third or solar plexus chakra, the first or root chakra, and the second or spleen chakra. The fiery presence of the blanketflower represents a joyful, creative expression of life, with warmth and exuberance. The flower is a positive expression of feeling the warm fire glowing from within to without, giving the signature of a strong, healthy vital life-force.

- The golden-yellow dome-shaped center represents the brightness within the core and the sunlike ability to embrace radiance, compassion (warmth), and light. This center also symbolizes the solar plexus, or third chakra. This signature indicates our ability to strengthen our minds and our vision, to be self-empowered with a purpose in life that is guided by our Higher Will.

- Another signature representative of the blanketflower's fiery colors and sun features is the warm sensation felt in the solar plexus, spleen, and abdomen when drinking the flower essence. The water color is also slightly golden-yellow, and the flower's odor is musty, like the sunflower.

Helpful suggestions

Take three to four drops of the Blanketflower essence. Find a comfortable position and close your eyes. Imagine yourself sitting in a field blanketed with vibrant colors of red, orange, and yellow. Take a deep breath and breathe the color red into your root chakra. Feel the red expand through the base of your spine and your pubic bone. Take several more deep breaths, continuing to see and feel the red in this area.

Now move your awareness up into the reproductive system and the spleen area (bladder, pancreas, kidneys). Continue breathing deeply, and visualize the color orange in these areas. You may want to concentrate on any areas of weakness or emotional blocks that you are aware of.

See the warmth of the orange dissolving the blockage and energizing that area. Visualize the orange expanding in this area as you continue to breathe.

Now move your awareness up to the solar plexus area, which includes the stomach, adrenals, digestive system, liver, and gall bladder. Breathe yellow light into these areas and again focus on any inner dialogues that may be preventing you from experiencing your power or your Higher Will. Fill this area with the yellow light and the warmth of the sun, and imagine this area expanding as you continue to breathe. Get in touch with how you would like to feel more passion, creativity, self-empowerment, and vitality in your life. See these vibrant colors surrounding you and swirling within you as flames of warmth and exuberance.

Depending on how you feel in the moment, either visualize yourself or actually participate in the following movement. Standing up, take a deep breath in. Raise your arms with open hands, with the intention of gathering the energy from the colorful swirling flames. As you exhale, send that energy out with your hands, arms, breath, belly, hips, legs, feet — your entire body — and dance in celebration of your inner flame! Continue this movement and/or visualization until you feel you have dissolved your blockages and you feel the juices of your passionate life-force energy moving!

Affirmations

- "I am a sacred flame of the Divine, dancing with joy and celebrating life."

- "Passionate consuming flames burn away all my fears."
- "May I arouse the fire within me to move forth in life with warmth and exuberance."

case History

The following is a case history as documented by Selina, age forty-seven:

"My intention in taking the Blanketflower essence is to merge with this sacred golden-red gift of nature to melt any denial that may prevent warmth, joy, abundance, and vitality in my creative expressions. I also have the intention to vibrantly bring this exuberance deeply into my marriage.

"The first morning after the initial full day of taking the Blanketflower essence, I woke up laughing and continued to laugh all day long. It was wonderful, and I noted a feeling of lightness opening me up again to a broader vision. The next day, I experienced an old, familiar symptom of pain and constriction in my heart, which was stimulated by taking the essence. An associated feeling of fear and a thought of abandonment and loss followed. I increased the frequency of taking the essence from two to four times that day, and the symptoms disappeared to be replaced by lightness and joy. There has been no discernible pattern or cycle to this symptom. I do believe its appearance was related to retracing an old pattern, for this was the first time the pain and fear had no lingering effect as long as I continued to take the essence.

"I have noticed a deeper softness (akin to compassion for myself and others), one that doesn't seem to even need protection. I have experienced a new level of joy and carefreeness. The major physical symptom has been a deep pain in my heart, accompanied by feelings of loss; this triggered a thought that led to an affirmation that countered the symptom. This led me to a spiritual lightness. I have had a deepening and changing energetic and sexual appetite. Blanketflower essence seems to be allowing me to process changes in a gracious, graceful, joyous manner without the heaviness of fear, and with resolve and strength of will.

"I definitely feel more grounded when I take the Blanketflower essence. There has been a renewed energy around my lower chakras and my heart, triggering creative expression with a deep level of trust and joy. I am less fearful of others, and I don't seem to be getting caught in old emotional patterns."

Lfe's Research provers' project findings

PHYSICAL SYMPTOMS

CRAVINGS: Cold water
SENSATIONS: Sneezing
PAIN: None
MODALITIES: Inconsistent
HEAD: None
EYES: None
FACE: None
EARS: None
STOMACH: None
ABDOMEN: None

BOWEL CONDITION: None
URINE: None
FEMALE: None
MALE: Hemorrhoids returned
EXTREMITIES: "I felt a numbness in my right hand; sometimes three fingers would go numb, and sometimes the whole hand would be numb."
BACK: None
SKIN: None

EMOTIONAL SYMPTOMS

PATTERNS OF BALANCE: "I felt anxiety coupled with gratitude," "I was able to help others more this week, and I had more patience," "I felt more creative," "strength," "I felt peaceful and relaxed," "I feel more balanced"
PATTERNS OF IMBALANCE: "anxiety," "fear," "impatience"

MENTAL SYMPTOMS

PATTERNS OF BALANCE: "felt more creative, more intuitive, felt a desire to make artwork," "this flower essence made me reflect on the good things in life"
PATTERNS OF IMBALANCE: "worry," "anxiety"

SPIRITUAL REFLECTIONS

"In spite of adversity, fear, and worry, we are able to smile again, to grow and to help others. It is like death and resurrection." "I'm grateful for my life, my energy, my gifts, friends, and family."

DREAMS/NIGHTMARES

"In my dream, I saw an Indian face steadily gazing at me. I can't figure out why I am dreaming of Indian people."

"I saw images of a mountain, a rose, and a cross with a jewel in the center."

BLUE FLAG (IRIS)
(Iris missouriensis)
PRIMARY QUALITY: STAMINA

FAMILY: Iris (Iridaceae)

OTHER NAMES: Snake Lily, Wild Iris, Western Blue Flag, Water Flag, Rocky Mountain Iris, Lirio (New Mexico), Fleur-de-Lis (France), and "many-leafed broad plant" (Navajo). The Latin name *Iris* comes from the Rainbow Goddess, referring to the colorful flowers.

WHERE FOUND: wet areas, moist meadows, marshes, shores of ponds, wet mountain areas in California, higher mountains of Arizona and New Mexico, and from North Dakota to British Columbia

ELEVATION: 5,500' to 9,500'

ENERGY IMPACT (CHAKRA CORRESPONDENCE): third, fifth, sixth, and seventh chakras

KEY RUBRICS FOR POSITIVE HEALING PATTERNS: artistic creativity, inspiration, positive stress management

KEY RUBRICS FOR SYMPTOMS AND PATTERNS OF IMBALANCE: feeling "stuck," suppressed creativity, lack of discernment, attraction to superficial beauty

OTHER RUBRICS: accomplishment, addictions, aspirations, beauty, bogged down, bridge, brow chakra, calm, centered, cheerful, clarity, confidence, crisis, crown chakra, elegance, feminine, focus, gentle, grounded, harmony, healing, idealism, insight, intuitive, love, perseverance, positive, relaxed, self-empowerment, simplicity, solar plexus chakra, stamina, strength, sweetness, throat chakra, uplifting

Traditional Use

The principal component of blue flag is a toxic substance called "irisin" or "iridin." An extraction of the roots is used as an emetic and cathartic, activating the production of pancreatic enzymes and bile. Blue flag has also been used to treat jaundice, but is not recommended for treatment of chronic or acute liver malfunctions. Frequent minimal doses of blue flag can also be used to treat hypoglycemia and as a diuretic, stimulating both saliva and sweat.

Due to its powerful properties, it is recommended that blue flag be used in combination with other herbs.

Some Spanish New Mexicans have used sliced iris roots as a necklace around their throats to treat smallpox. The Navajo Indians reportedly use a wild iris to make green dye. Iris is also used by the Navajo as an emetic in the Holy Way and Lightning Way ceremonies. The silky leaf fibers of the iris plant were used by Native Americans to make twine and rope for fishing and hunting.

Iris, affiliated with the Greek Goddess of the rainbow, represents hope and the eternal spirit; it was used as an herb to celebrate the passing of death and the incarnation of a new life. In Egypt, iris was a sacred symbol of the Pharaoh.

Rootstalks and leaves of iris are poisonous to eat, but are known to be used in potpourri, powders, soaps, and cosmetics. The orris-root powder used in toilet formulas comes from a European species of iris.

Homeopathic use

Mother tincture is prepared from the fresh root in early spring or autumn. The primary use of Iris versicolor (the homeopathic term for blue flag) is to treat migraine headaches with blurred vision, especially occurring before the headache, following with marked nausea and vomiting. It is also used to treat problems of the thyroid, pancreas, salivary glands, stomach, abdomen, sexual organs, and gastrointestinal mucous membrane. It is also used in cases of headache, colic, diarrhea and dysentery, impetigo, eczema, liver, neuralgia, morning sickness, shingles on the right side of the abdomen, skin disorders with headaches (such as psoriasis or herpes), internal burning from the mouth to the rectum with burning diarrhea, rheumatism, and vomiting. It also increases the flow of bile.

positive Healing patterns

- Teaches skillful pacing in order to prevent burnout and builds stamina

when it is necessary to experience and go through the crisis — "The Law of Healing Crises."
- Draws us upward, directing us to rise above the material, mundane, and self-centered aspects of self, addictions, and the world's inflictions.
- Offers an innate understanding, appreciation, and experience of beauty that comes from within, founded in spirituality.
- Helps us attract the rainbow colors by expressing our creativity and making a bridge between what enters and leaves us.
- Inspires creativity and artistic imaginative talents; helpful for writers, artists, speakers, and anyone interested in fulfilling their creative desires.

symptoms and patterns of imbalance

Blue Flag may be an appropriate flower essence for those who

- Have difficulty managing stress and dealing with crises
- Get "stuck in the bog," can't seem to rise above themselves or their situation, and eventually fall back into addictions and old habits
- Are fascinated by external and superficial beauty, giving no credit to the beauty that lies within
- Experience suppressed creativity and are unable to discern or guard between the light and the dark forces.

features of the original flower-essence water

ODOR: very sweet
TASTE: strong and sweet
SENSATIONS: tingling and stimulation in the crown chakra and pituitary; feels like a band of energy connecting all the way around the head
WATER COLOR: slightly yellow

physical makeup

ROOT, STEM, LEAVES/LEAFLETS, HEIGHT: Blue flag is similar to, but smaller than, the common garden iris. The creeping reddish brown rootstalk (or "rhizome") grows in clumps and is protected by a covering of leaf scales from former growth. Several tall stems often grow from one thick, horizontal stem and can reach a height of up to 3 feet. The smooth, slender, pale green leaves are sword-shaped and up to 20 inches long and $3/4$ inch wide. The leaves have a tendency to overlap and either arch or stand up.
FLOWER COLOR: Pale blue to lavender-violet veined with white; yellow center/base
FLOWERS: Three-parted, nearly regular perfect flowers bloom one by one and form a green bract or leaflet at the tip of a somewhat irregular leafless stem, followed by a slender oblong capsule with six ribs, up to $1\,1/2$ inches long and $3/4$ inch wide. The significance of the flower is the number three. There are three layers of three petals each, with three stamens that are hidden and inserted at the base of the three larger and more showy divisions of the flower.

Three petal-like drooping and wider sepals stand out or curve downward. Each division is a soft blue or violet and beautifully veined with a deep violet or purple, over a whitish ground tinted with a yellow center base. Three lighter blue or violet narrow petals stand up. The inferior ovary is three-celled. The flowers are up to 4 inches wide and have a sweet fragrance. Flowers are succeeded by a three-celled leathery seed pod.
BLOOMING PERIOD: May to September

doctrine of signatures

- The three layers of the flower correspond to the three levels of the psyche, commonly known as the "higher self," the "conscious self," and the "lower self." Iris represents our choice to be stuck in the "lower self" of addictions and unawareness, which provokes the "Law of Healing Crises." Going through the crisis builds stamina and teaches us to protect who we are, rise above the mundane, and reach toward a higher way of living and being. "The Law of Healing Crises" is a further unfoldment of our evolution and can occur at any layer or level.

- Indigenous of the "murky bog where dead and decaying matters lie," iris lives several years creeping along the outer layer of the bog, collecting enough nutrients to nurture her roots and shoot up a long, slender stem with an elegant flower of beauty and simplicity. Matthew Wood observes, "This 'hibernation' is her period of testing. Will she get stuck and return to the bog from which she is attempting to rise, or will she shoot up and show that it is toward heaven that she looks?"[1]

- The simplicity, beauty, and grace of the flower is indicative of its inherent nature and its ability to rise from the bog, reach toward the sky, and honor its beauty.
- The rootstalks have the ability to store water and feed it to the plant as needed. This is indicative of learning to pace ourselves, building stamina and not burning all our energy up at once.
- The rainbow colors build a bridge that connects our physical, emotional, mental, and spiritual aspects. It brings together any splits, inspiring us to reach toward our aspirations and to freely express our true creative selves. These colors specifically indicate the third, fifth, sixth, and seventh chakras.

Helpful suggestions

Are you feeling stuck in a bog? Do you lack inspiration or creativity to help you find your way out? Are you ready and willing to move out from under the bog? What one specific thing can you do for yourself that would help you turn around in your muck and reach toward a higher way of living and being?

If you feel really caught in the muck, you might ask for a healing crisis to help you go through the experience and elevate your conscious awareness, giving you the needed lessons and insight. Ask for guidance in helping you to recover your inner beauty and creativity. Ask or pray for the stamina needed to go through the crisis, for ways to pace yourself and prevent any unnecessary whirlwinds. Give thanks for the stamina that you are building and for your inner strength and awareness. State out loud to yourself three aspects of your inner beauty that you appreciate about yourself.

Affirmations

- "I face life's setbacks with creativity and inspiration to spiral upward."
- "I trust that my perseverance and stamina will help me get through any healing crisis that I need to encounter."
- "I fully embrace my inner beauty and integrity in the perfect image of my Divine being."

Case History

Michael, age forty-two, had a history of alcoholism, including participation in a recovery program. He was reaching a point of awareness in which he realized he needed to go further within himself. He had been feeling bogged down from his past and wanted to have the perseverance to look upward on his path. He felt a new door was opening, and he was ready for a life change. He also was an artist and felt that he wanted more inspiration to write, so he began taking a creative writing class. When he used the words "bogged down" to describe how he had been feeling, I immediately thought of Blue Flag. Then he added "perseverance" and the need for inspiration, and again Blue Flag seemed to be the appropriate remedy.

Michael describes the flower essence as a "positive place to focus, giving me inspiration and helping me to center myself." It helped him to persevere and stay focused on his goals, directing him toward his aspirations. It also helped him express his inner creativity through writing, which in turn, built stamina in his discipline to focus and to "stay on the path."

LFE's Research provers' project findings

PHYSICAL SYMPTOMS

CRAVINGS: Drank more water, fewer cravings for soda pop

SENSATIONS: A slight floating feeling as if "walking on air"

PAIN: None

MODALITIES: All times of day stabilized

HEAD: None

EYES: None

FACE: Acne and oily skin on face

EARS: None

STOMACH: More relaxed

ABDOMEN: None

BOWEL CONDITION: None

URINE: More frequent urination

FEMALE: None

MALE: None

EXTREMITIES: None

BACK: One prover had kinks in back, which caused less sleep.

SKIN: One prover had more oily skin and acne on face.

EMOTIONAL SYMPTOMS

PATTERNS OF BALANCE: "emotionally uplifted during trying situations," "felt a softer, sweeter, gentler aspect," "had been irritable but felt stronger," "calmer," felt more control over my emotions," "felt energetic with a positive attitude," "more confidence," "felt able to accomplish tasks," "more relaxed," "felt like things will get better," "less emotional"

PATTERNS OF IMBALANCE: "irritable," "feelings of desperation"

MENTAL SYMPTOMS

PATTERNS OF BALANCE: "more creative," "more right-brained and intuitive," "better understanding," "lightening of negative or frustrating thoughts," "helped me stay focus without analyzing," "helped me follow through mentally with tasks"

PATTERNS OF IMBALANCE: No comments from provers.

SPIRITUAL REFLECTIONS

"I prayed a lot more than usual; I 'let go and let God' take care of my problems for me," "I felt God helped carry me through the rough times," "helped me feel spiritually uplifted from circumstances that are trying, difficult, or chaotic," "helped me find a gentler approach to circumstances," "increased awareness and acknowledgment of the importance of spiritual growth," "I am one with the universe," "I am in the right place at the right time"

DREAMS/NIGHTMARES

A prover woke up one morning internally hearing the song "When Irish Eyes Are Smiling." Another day while taking this essence, the same prover woke up with the song "You Are So Beautiful To Me" "You're everything I hoped for, Everything I need..." She feels that these songs are referring to herself: "I'm the Irish eyes hearing the angels sing and knowing that I'm everything I need!"

Other provers seemed to have normal dreaming with no increase or decrease in dreams.

OTHER COMMENTS

One prover had a strong urge to dig up her irises, which she did (she didn't know that she was taking the Blue Flag flower essence). She dug up one bed of irises that were twelve years old and threw them away. She said that this particular bed "repulsed, annoyed, and offended" her because they were brown-tipped and not in bloom. She also said how much she loves irises, and that it was unlike her to dig them up, but that they were on her mind. She added that her tendency is to not finish a project, and that this essence helped her stay focused on completing the task. She later told me that digging up the irises felt like getting rid of part of her past and that she was ready for an upward change in her life.

BOUNCING BET

(Saponaria officinalis)
PRIMARY QUALITY: MYSTIC UNION

FAMILY: Pink (Caryophyllaceae)

OTHER NAMES: Soapwort, Soaproot, Fuller's Herb, Sheep Weed, Saponaire, Bruise-wort, Latherwort, Wild Sweet William, and Herba Fullonis

WHERE FOUND: Native to western Asia and locally naturalized in temperate North America and Europe. Grows in average to poor, well-drained soil in full sun to light shade along wooded areas or hedgerows. Also common on roadsides, railway embankments, fence rows, ditch banks, and waste places. In natural settings, the plant shows a preference for stream banks, damp woods, and moist conditions with partial shade.

ELEVATION: 4,800' to 7,500'

ENERGY IMPACT (CHAKRA CORRESPONDENCE): first, fourth, and seventh chakras

KEY RUBRICS FOR POSITIVE HEALING PATTERNS: balance, harmony, intimacy, love, sexuality

KEY RUBRICS FOR SYMPTOMS AND PATTERNS OF IMBALANCE: closed down, dissociation from self and others, lack of feeling love and loved

OTHER RUBRICS: abandonment, abdomen, acceptance, appreciation, blissful, calm, centered, clarity, communication, compassion, confidence, crown chakra, erogenous, expression, feminine, healing, heart chakra, kundalini, leadership, masculine, meditation, misunderstanding, passion, radiance, receptivity, repression, root chakra, self-empowerment, sensuality, softness, strength, tenderness, transition, understanding, union, wholeness

Traditional Use

The active ingredients of bouncing bet are saponins found in the leaves and roots of the plant. By boiling the leaves and roots, you produce a sudsy solution that creates a cleansing lather to be used for laundering, to revitalize old delicate fabrics, and as a water softener. Medicinally, bouncing bet is an effective expectorant for use in treating bronchitis and dry coughs. It is also used as a dynamic laxative, although it can cause stomach upsets, and as a mild diuretic. A lotion can be made for soothing sore, irritated skin caused by eczema, acne, or poison ivy rashes.

In the Middle East, bouncing bet has also been used for its ability to eliminate toxins, especially from the liver, and to relieve problems caused by venereal disease. Bouncing bet has also been used in the United States to treat venereal disease. In medieval times, Arab physicians used the plant to treat leprosy, to promote sweating, to treat rheumatism, and to purify the blood. In India, treated rhizomes of the plant are used to increase the milk flow of nursing mothers.

The flowers of bouncing bet can be added to salads and have been used to increase the "head" in beer. They also can be dried and used in potpourri.

homeopathic use

Unknown to author.

positive healing patterns

- Offers receptivity, balance, openness, union, and harmony, both in relation to one's self (the "inner marriage") and with a partner.
- Awakens sexual energy; is a wonderful essence for partners in love and who consciously work with the kundalini force in their lovemaking.
- Opens the desire realms for passion, channeling and circulating erogenous energies of ecstasy.
- Opens the heart, helping us to love and be in harmony with ourselves.
- Helps us consciously experience the vibrant energy impact of all the chakras working harmoniously together.

symptoms and patterns of imbalance

Bouncing Bet may be an appropriate flower essence for those who

- Feel out of balance and disharmony with self or with their partner
- Feel closed down sexually and lack passion with their partner
- Have difficulty loving themselves
- Feel disassociated from others, withdrawn, hopeless, or depressed.

features of the original flower-essence water

ODOR: bittersweet and spicy
TASTE: full, sweet, and spicy
SENSATIONS: a centering and feeling of balance along with a blissful wave of ecstasy passing through the desire realms of passion
WATER COLOR: clear

physical makeup

ROOT, STEM, LEAVES/LEAFLETS, HEIGHT: The fibrous rootlets grow on pinkish brown runners $1/4$ inch to $1/2$ inch thick, are white inside, and contain a high concentration of lathering saponin. The stem base has a lower concentration of saponin than the roots and has a sturdy, stout, erect, slightly thick, cylindrical, light-green stem. The stem grows up to 3 feet tall. Leaves are oval-lanceolate, pointed, smooth, soft, and pale green, marked with three distinctive parallel veins. They grow in opposites, with two offshoot leaves off each larger leaf that clasp the stem and narrow to a point. The leaves also contain saponin.
FLOWER COLOR: Subtle creamy lilac or pale pink and whitish

FLOWERS: The showy flowers are sweet, spicy, and aromatically intoxicating. They form dense terminal clusters and are about 1 inch across, with five pink, creamy lilac, or whitish petals and ten stamens. The clusters are said to appear as bouncing young girls. The petals are notched at the apex and spread. The flowers grow in single and double forms. Each flower petal has two identical, mirror-image parts. If you look closely, the two parts form a heart shape. The buds on the plant have a phallic shape, coated with whitish creamy liquid (saponin); some also resemble a soft spiraling candle flame. The flower heads are very feminine, resembling a flowering vulva; they are very sensually arousing. The phallic bud opens and becomes the feminine flower head. The oblong, toothed capsules are composed of many dull black, rough-surfaced, kidney-shaped seeds that are about 1 1/2 inches wide.

BLOOMING PERIOD: June through September

Doctrine of signatures

- The smooth leaves grow in pairs and the soft petals have two parts, representing balance, union, and harmony: left/right, yin/yang, male/female.
- The sensuality of the plant and its expression of male/female, penis/vulva, also represents balance and the awakening of sexual energy rising up the spine as the kundalini force and spiraling up to the heart.

This signature corresponds with the first chakra or root chakra with energy currents rising up to the crown chakra. The plant is an expression of wholeness and union with oneself as well as with a partner.

- The pale pink and creamy lavender colors represent the fourth or heart chakra, radiating compassion, oneness, bliss, and love. This energy center provides the union for the lower and the upper chakras, radiating creative life-force energy and power.

Helpful suggestions

Try this deep-breathing exercise:

1. Close your eyes and breathe in what you want to be open to in yourself. Think of feelings, thoughts, or truths that you want to experience more of. Take a deep breath and bring whatever that particular focus is into your entire being through your breath. Say the word, such as "love," "harmony," "union," or "balance," as you breathe in.

2. As you breathe out, breathe out the "bad stuff" — whatever you don't want for yourself. Be specific about what no longer serves you and what you need to get rid of so that you can receive the "good stuff." Again say what you're releasing as you breathe out; get into the feeling of letting it go.

3. Stand up with your feet at a comfortable distance apart. Take a step with your left foot as you breathe in, then take a step with your right foot as you breathe out. Walk comfortably in a circle, breathing in with your left step and out with your right step.

4. Once you are in the flow with your breath and the steps, put your hands in front of you. Move them toward your chest as you step with your left foot and breathe in, then move them away from your chest as you step with your right foot and breathe out.

This exercise stimulates balance and inner harmony. Try to do it for fifteen minutes a day while taking this essence (and longer, of course, if you so desire) — or make up your own exercise that promotes a feeling of balance and harmony.

Affirmations

- "I am the power of love singing deep into my heart."
- "I awaken the love in my heart to fulfill my most intimate passions."
- "Let the doorway of my heart open wide for love to flow freely through me."

case History

Joan, a woman in her late forties, felt out of balance with her inner masculine and feminine. She tended to feel uncomfortable with her femininity, causing her to externalize her masculinity. Joan was also aware that she lacked harmony and love for herself. All of these factors affected her relationship with her husband, especially in her desire to be sexually open with him.

Joan was given Bouncing Bet to help her in these areas. She discovered a new love of herself, which opened her heart toward a higher union with herself and her partner.

LFE's Research Provers' Project Findings

PHYSICAL SYMPTOMS

CRAVINGS: Water, salt, coffee

SENSATIONS: Tingling in head and abdominal areas, all around to buttocks

PAIN: None

MODALITIES:

  WORSE: None indicated

  BETTER: Longer and stable sleep

HEAD: None

EYES: None

FACE: None

EARS: None

STOMACH: None

ABDOMEN: Tingling sensation

BOWEL CONDITION: None

URINE: None

FEMALE: Increased sexual energy

MALE: Increased libido

EXTREMITIES: None

BACK: None

SKIN: Developed unusual skin sore on nose, rash under armpits

OTHER: Higher energy level

EMOTIONAL SYMPTOMS

PATTERNS OF BALANCE: "healing of heart pains have been noticed with this remedy," "felt more relaxed and at peace with self," "emotional highs," "had issues with love," "felt more confident, especially when dealing with relationship," "more control of emotions," "able to express myself and work out relationship problems," "ready for new beginnings," "more calm and ease with relationship situation," "felt more cheerful and happy with myself," "more self-acceptance"

PATTERNS OF IMBALANCE: "sour grumpy moods," "emotional lows"

MENTAL SYMPTOMS

PATTERNS OF BALANCE: "felt more reflective and less reactive in relationship with partner," "more understanding," "more intuitive," "more creative," "more clairvoyant"

PATTERNS OF IMBALANCE: None noted

SPIRITUAL REFLECTIONS

"Desire to pray more," "meditated more frequently," "coming to a deeper acceptance of myself and my influence," "I want to and am ready to follow my heart."

DREAMS/NIGHTMARES

Light dreaming.

CALENDULA

(Calendula officinalis)
PRIMARY QUALITY: CALM

FAMILY: Sunflower (Compositae)

OTHER NAMES: Marybud, Pot Marigold, Holigold, Golds. "Calendula" comes from the Latin *kalend* or *calends,* which refers to the long-flowering blooms and the fact that the plant blooms on the first day of every month.

WHERE FOUND: Well-drained, light, sandy soil in full sun. A native of the Canary Islands through southern and central Europe and North Africa to Iran. Grows in most regions in the United States.

ELEVATION: most U.S. climate zones

ENERGY IMPACT (CHAKRA CORRESPONDENCE): second and third chakras

KEY RUBRICS FOR POSITIVE HEALING PATTERNS: soothing, peaceful, sensitive, radiant

KEY RUBRICS FOR SYMPTOMS AND PATTERNS OF IMBALANCE: anxiety, fear, impatience, nervousness

OTHER RUBRICS: acceptance, aggression, anger, apathy, balance, calm, clarity, comfortable, communication, confidence, creativity, depression, exhaustion, grounded, healing, inner, insecurity, insight, irritability, lack, meditation, memory, mindfulness, misunderstanding, moody, paranoia, quiet, revealing, self-empowerment, sensitivity, smooth, solar plexus chakra, sorrow, spleen chakra, tension, understanding, uneasy, vulnerable, warmth

Traditional use

Calendula is a versatile herb with a wide array of uses. Ancient Egyptians found the herb to be rejuvenating. Europeans used the plant to treat skin problems such as varicose veins, skin cancer, frostbite, and athlete's foot; they also used it as a flavoring for soups and stews and to color butter and cheese. The leaves of the plant were used to treat open wounds on the battlefield in the American Civil War. Calendula is also known to treat cuts, inflammations, bruises, cracked and blemished skin, skin ulcers, chapped lips, and minor burns and scalds. It has been used to strengthen eyesight and the heart as well as to treat digestive inflammations, gastric and duodenal ulcers, liver and gall-bladder problems, jaundice, water retention, cramps, toothaches, fever, flu, stomachaches, and viral and bacterial invasion. It is a normalizer for menstruation and, as an emmenagogue, helps bring on delayed menses.

Persians and Greeks used the bright yellow and orange petals to garnish and flavor salads and foods, while Hindus used them to decorate temple altars. Calendula is also used as an ornament, dye, and cosmetic. It brings out highlights in blond, brunette, and red hair. Used as an herb in the bathtub, it will stimulate the body.

homeopathic use

Mother tincture is prepared from the flower and leaves. In the form of a cream or tincture, it is used homeopathically to promote healing. It also controls bleeding and is used for minor cuts and abrasions, burns, fissures, and after childbirth to treat perineal tears. A homeopathic tincture can also be used effectively as a mouthwash for mouth ulcers and sore throats, and to control bleeding after tooth extractions. Calendula is used internally to treat jaundice and fever in which irritability, nervousness, and acute hearing are affected. Calendula is also used to treat skin cancer, genital warts, fright, injury to the eye, deafness, heartburn, distention, and suppressed menses.

CAUTION: Calendula lotions or salves prepared with alcohol can irritate the skin or cause excessive drying.

positive healing patterns

- Deeply heals the emotions and mind in a soothing, calming way. Calms nervousness and brings a quiet centering to the abdomen and solar plexus, which also builds confidence.
- Helps those who have undergone emotional work with themselves and are already in touch with their feelings; helps us to relate to ourselves and others in a nonconfrontational, soothing way.
- Promotes sensitivity and understanding with others.

- Provides an inner warmth and radiance that extends outward.

symptoms and patterns of imbalance

Calendula may be an appropriate flower essence for those who

- Are nervous, anxious, distressed, or fearful
- Lack confidence
- Demonstrate insensitivity toward others and have difficulty relating to others with ease
- Have a confrontational or stressful personality type (stressful to be with, and/or tending to become stressed out easily).

features of the original flower-essence water

ODOR: distinct, somewhat pungent, strong
TASTE: strong; similar to odor
SENSATIONS: Feels peaceful and calm in the belly and in the temple regions above the ears. Head also feels at peace and balanced, with soothing tingling sensation.
WATER COLOR: clear

physical makeup

ROOT, STEM, LEAVES/LEAFLETS, HEIGHT: Calendula stands erect with many branching stems growing from the same root. The green, succulent, angular stems are thick and sturdy, yet flexible; they are covered with fine hairs that are slightly soft and fuzzy. The green lower leaves are paddle-shaped and the middle to upper leaves are oblong or lance-shaped with lemon-lime centered veins. They are hairy, soft, and fuzzy on both sides, and they are both basal and alternate on the stems. The leaf edge is smooth to finely toothed. The lower leaves are short-stemmed and grow to $2^3/_4$ inches long, and the middle to upper leaves clasp the stem. The plant averages 1 to 2 feet in height. Calendula bears fruit that ripens from green to brown, shaped like a boat with yellowish seeds of various winged to curled shapes.

FLOWER COLOR: Golden yellow-orange

FLOWERS: The golden yellow-orange ray flowers are layered and multi-petaled with single or double flower heads. The ray florets radiate from the pronounced center golden-yellow florets, have a feathery look, and are 2 to 3 inches across. Each petal has two folds with three triangular tips. The buds are round and fuzzy and form pointed tips. The base of the flower head is held by small green petals with pointed tips. The thinner outside florets die first, and then the inside florets die. As the petals die, they become stringlike. Calendula is known for its long flowering period.

BLOOMING PERIOD: Spring to fall

Doctrine of signatures

- The colors of the flower correspond with the orange color for the abdomen, or second chakra (spleen), and yellow for the third chakra, or solar plexus chakra; they also relate to sensations and emotions in regard to one's self and others. By working with these chakras we can release prejudice, judgments, criticism, and emotional patterns. We can also learn to take time out for ourselves by doing things that are nurturing, relaxing, and calming.

- The soft, fuzzy hairs on the leaves and stems represent soothing, calm, and nurturing.

- The golden glow at the center of the plant indicates warmth and radiance.

- The dry, dead petals, in their string-like appearance, look like nerve endings — another indication of the plant's relationship to the nerves and calming the nerves.

Helpful suggestions

Imagine yourself stepping inside the golden yellow-orange center florets of calendula. Look around you. Feel the softness of her color. Breathe in the color and imagine it filling your entire body. Place your hands on the velvety petals and bring to mind a healing that has taken place or needs to take place. Take the color into your root chakra and visualize it blending there with the color red. Fill your root chakra with the energetic vibration you are experiencing. Feel your root chakra filling with warmth and radiance.

Then take the color to your second chakra area and blend it with more orange. Fill your pelvic area with the energetic vibration you are experiencing. Feel your pelvis filling with warmth and radiance.

Next take the golden yellow-orange

color into your solar plexus and repeat the process with yellow. Then take the color to your heart chakra, and blend the colors golden yellow-orange with green and then with pink. Fill yourself with warmth and radiance in your heart. Take the golden yellow-orange color to your throat chakra and blend it with the color blue. Observe any changes that you feel inside. Feel warmth and radiance in your throat chakra. Take the golden yellow-orange to your brow or third-eye chakra and again blend the colors, allowing warmth and radiance to be felt in your third eye. Then take the golden yellow-orange color to your crown chakra and blend it with the color white. Feel warmth and radiance in your crown chakra. Observe how you feel.

Then put yourself inside the golden yellow-orange and feel its energy impact on your entire body. Stretch your arms and legs and allow the color to spread out of your extremities and into your auric field. Feel the calm yet stimulating, revitalizing effect this exercise and calendula have on you. Remember this feeling and this exercise when you take Calendula flower essence, and repeat the process as often as you can.

Affirmations

- "I fill myself with a gentle glow of orange and yellow light."
- "I allow peaceful, easy emotions to emerge and be felt."
- "I create positive, calm, thoughtful energy."

Case History

My sister, Linda, age forty-five, who was a prover in LFE's research project, took Calendula flower essence without knowing which one she was taking. (All essences were unknown to provers during the time they were taken.) Linda had some reactions to Calendula, which included nervousness, depression, tiredness, emotional distress, and general unhappiness. In a follow-up phone call, Linda asked me what she had been taking that provoked these symptoms. Before I could respond, she asked if it was related to the marigold family. I found her inquiry fascinating; how did she know? She went on to tell me that she was allergic to the marigold family and that the symptoms she experienced were typical of her allergic reactions! She had taken the essence for three days and had become so exhausted and depressed that she decided to stop. I wonder if she would have experienced a healing crisis had she continued! She didn't want to take the chance.

Linda experienced all the symptoms of patterns of imbalance for Calendula. The other provers, with the exception of one who experienced symptoms similar to Linda's, all shared the positive healing traits of Calendula and nearly unanimously reported that Calendula helped them feel calm and relaxed.

I have found the Calendula flower essence to be especially helpful for children to lessen irritability and induce calmness, somewhat like Chamomile. It's a great remedy to have on hand for your child during emotional times — and for your-self as well!

life's research provers' project findings

PHYSICAL SYMPTOMS

CRAVINGS: Water, yogurt, peanut-butter-and-jelly sandwiches

SENSATIONS: Hot sensation like a heat wave; lingering sensation in mouth and tongue

PAIN: None

MODALITIES: Inconsistent

HEAD: Felt physical release in head

EYES: Vision intensity and depth perception enhanced; eyesight improved

FACE: None

EARS: Increased sensory perception, more acute

STOMACH: Fullness in belly; stomach "queasy"

ABDOMEN: Fullness

BOWEL CONDITION: Good bowel movements, more frequent

URINE: Increased urination

FEMALE: Increased sex drive

MALE: None

EXTREMITIES: None

BACK: Lower back sensitive

SKIN: None

EMOTIONAL SYMPTOMS

PATTERNS OF BALANCE: "comfortable," "balanced," "calm," "quiet inner happiness," "balanced and smooth," "peaceful," "relaxed and grounded," "creative energy," "confident," "felt balanced," "deep calmness," "released anger," "felt uplifted," "helped to release a weight I've been carrying for a long time," "felt revitalized"

PATTERNS OF IMBALANCE: "insecure," "more sensitive to judgment from others," "nervous," "paranoid," "anxious," "moody," "uneasiness," "sadness," "tension," "vulnerable," "released anger"

MENTAL SYMPTOMS

PATTERNS OF BALANCE: "memory improved, more clarity, anxious; worried about what people think of me," "sharp, aware, peaceful thoughts; more relaxed mentally," "handled increased demands better," "more mindful," "release of mental struggles," "increased conscious awareness," "helped me activate resources and make better use of my time"

PATTERNS OF IMBALANCE: "mentally depressed and uneasy," "mental confusion"

SPIRITUAL REFLECTIONS

"I felt connected to an ancient race," "I experienced a broader range of emotions, including calm and trust; paranoia and anxiety are absorbed in a deeper knowing," "less meditation, more conscious activity"

DREAMS/NIGHTMARES

Dreams were inconsistent, from being very vivid to not being able to remember them.

CALIFORNIA POPPY

(Eschscholzia californica)
PRIMARY QUALITY: PURIFIER

FAMILY: Poppy (Papaveraceae)
OTHER NAMES: Gold Poppy. The plant was named for Dr. Eschscholzia, a Russian surgeon and naturalist.
WHERE FOUND: slopes, grasslands, lower mountain meadows, plains, foothills, mesas, and yards near moisture in the spring; New Mexico, Arizona, Colorado, Utah, Texas, Nevada, and west and south of the Sierra Nevada
ELEVATION: below 7,000'
ENERGY IMPACT (CHAKRA CORRESPONDENCE): second chakra
KEY RUBRICS FOR POSITIVE HEALING PATTERNS: receptivity to emotional cleansing, sensitivity, sensuality, wisdom
KEY RUBRICS FOR SYMPTOMS AND PATTERNS OF IMBALANCE: emotional insensitivity, lack of care for self, closed down
OTHER RUBRICS: abdomen, blame, bowels, breakthrough, brokenhearted, burden, calm, centered, cheerful, clarity, compassion, confidence, creativity, doubt, dreams, emotions, father, fear, grief, guilt, healing, heart, inner knowing, insight, intellectual, intuitive, love, meditation, memory, misunderstanding, mother, passion, patience, perception, protection, purification, reproductive, sexuality, shame, sorrow, spleen chakra, strength, toxins, transition, vulnerability

Traditional Use

American Indians used California poppy to treat colic pains. The infusion has been used as a mild sedative and analgesic to treat overexcitability and sleeplessness, especially in children. Similar to opium poppy, California poppy contains flavone glycosides, which are alkaloids. Unlike opium poppy, California poppy is nonaddictive although not as potent. It is known to relieve pain and is used to treat gall-bladder colic and as an antispasmodic.

Homeopathic Use

Animal research has shown that California poppy is more powerful than morphine, as it can cause a deep and unnatural sleep that is harmless. California poppy can also cause general weakness, lethargy, rapid breathing, paralysis of the limbs, and slowed circulation.

Positive Healing Patterns

- Offers a cleansing effect and purifies emotional toxins.

- Helps us take care of ourselves emotionally; gives an "inner knowing" of when to be receptive and open and when to protect our vulnerability.
- Heightens sensitivity and aids "inner insight" and wisdom.
- Opens ourselves to the spark of fire deep within our sensuality and sexuality, expanding our heart so that we can feel its radiant glow.

symptoms and patterns of imbalance

California Poppy may be an appropriate flower essence for those who

- Need to cleanse emotional toxins and "purify" their emotions
- Need to learn how to care for themselves emotionally
- Are emotionally insensitive and lack an inner connection with self
- Are emotionally closed down in their sensuality and sexuality.

features of the original flower-essence water

Odor: very subtle spicy, sensual smell
Taste: strong and refreshing
Sensations: Mouth, throat, and teeth feel refreshed with slight tingling. There is a sense of "stirring" from root to crown, giving a solid peaceful state throughout the body.
Water Color: clear

physical makeup

Root, Stem, Leaves/Leaflets, Height: Many stems cluster from one root, and the stems are smooth, juicy, and moist but not milky. There are green lines from bottom to top of each stem, and the stems are sturdy yet bendable. Clumps of well-dissected bluish green leaves grow at the base of the plant and are up to $2^{1}/_{2}$ inches long. The leaves are light, airy, feathery, and fernlike, resembling tiny fingers, hands, or soft parsley. The plant grows between 1 and 2 feet tall.
Flower Color: Deep, rich orange
Flowers: The showy orange flowers have four wide overlapping petals, with a reddish purple ring at the base and thin orange stamens in the center. They appear elegant in their simplicity. The petals are thin, delicate, soft, and velvety; they fall off easily requiring gentle care. They are highly sensitive, opening only in the sunlight, and staying closed on cloudy days and at night. Each flower ripens into a seed pod that is phallic in shape, with the reddish purple ring around its base.
Blooming Period: February to October

doctrine of signatures

- The clear juice from the plant's stems represents its cleansing or purifying nature.
- The color of the plant and its second-chakra relationship indicate the power of its ability to detoxify

and purify, especially at the emotional level. Its fiery color also allows for greater inner growth, warmth, and deep wisdom. The color also indicates the reproductive system and sexuality associated with the second chakra.

- The lightness and airiness of the leaves represent the plant's highly sensitive and emotional nature.
- The openness of the flower and its simplicity demonstrate receptivity, and the closed state of the flower in the night or in cloudy weather shows its ability to protect itself and its vulnerability.

Helpful suggestions

Take three drops of California Poppy flower essence and find a comfortable position. Identify any emotional toxins you feel you need to let go of; be specific about what they are. Close your eyes and imagine the deep rich orange flower petals of California Poppy wrapped snugly around you. Let the fiery glow of the petals warm the area of your second chakra. Breathe into the warmth and let it fill you. Hold each breath as long as comfortable. As you exhale, breathe out any emotional toxins you wish to release. Stay present with each breath in and out, keeping your body filled with the warm glow and the protection of California Poppy. Let yourself be in the moment with this experience. When ready, slowly open your eyes. If you wish, write your experience in your journal or simply be with it for a while longer. Make up your own affirmations in regard to the emotional toxins you want to release; use these affirmations as often as possible throughout the day. You can also use the affirmations given for California Poppy and replace any words as desired.

Affirmations

- "I release my emotional toxins and pray for emotional cleansing."
- "I am the power of purification. May my thoughts and feelings be purified."
- "I radiate light, wisdom, and love."
- "I stir my passion and excitement for life and living."

Case History

Irene, a woman in her forties, wanted to rid herself of old emotional toxins, especially those related to her boyfriend and her lack of self-esteem. She also had some doubts and fears about possibly having breast cancer, which aroused some old emotional patterning. She felt she needed to rid herself of these no-longer-needed emotions in order to purify and become strong. Irene realized that she wasn't taking care of her emotional needs and that she was also closed down in her sensuality and sexuality in her current relationship. She also felt a lack of connection with herself and wanted to tap into her "inner knowing."

Irene had several dreams while taking California Poppy flower essence. The first night, she dreamed of her old boyfriend and felt insecure. She felt that she had to prove to him that she was "good enough" to be his girlfriend. Several nights in a row, Irene had more dreams related to her old boyfriend that consistently brought up more insecurities and lack of self-worth. She also felt that California Poppy helped her look at some old emotional issues in a positive way and that she was able to cleanse and "purify" these issues. She found that she was able to connect with herself in a new way, tapping into innate knowing and inner truths.

LFE's Research Provers' Project Findings

PHYSICAL SYMPTOMS

CRAVINGS: Sweets, artichokes, vegetables, poultry, liquids

SENSATIONS: Tingling in the heart and chest, hot flashes, circulation in the heart

PAIN: None

MODALITIES:

  WORSE: None

  BETTER: Deep sleep

HEAD: None

EYES: None

FACE: None

EARS: None

STOMACH: Felt a "release"

ABDOMEN: None

BOWEL CONDITION: Some provers had bowel retention, while others had diarrhea and bowel cleansing.

URINE: One prover had urine retention, while another had more frequent urination.

FEMALE: "Sexually awesome"

MALE: None

EXTREMITIES: None

BACK: None

SKIN: None

EMOTIONAL SYMPTOMS

PATTERNS OF BALANCE: "a deep feeling of love, caring, and compassion," "a stronger connection to all involved on the earth," "more heart space," "more confident," "experienced a deep knowing," "I experienced an emotional cleansing," "awareness of relief"

PATTERNS OF IMBALANCE: "hurt feelings surfaced, which were succeeded by a deepening of these feelings," "slightly depressed state colored with an awareness of relief"

MENTAL SYMPTOMS

PATTERNS OF BALANCE: "sharp," "perceptive," "accurate," "clear," "improved memory," "more alert," "increased understanding," "more creative," "more intuitive," "mental cleansing," impulse to think back on old wounds," "had more focus and concentration," "deepening of perceptions," "awareness of the need for more personal time"

PATTERNS OF IMBALANCE: "experienced more mental exhaustion"

SPIRITUAL REFLECTIONS

"I experienced a profound connection to the miracle of life, of a new human arriving into the world; I felt compassion for the mother and her child."

"I just feel a deep knowing with no confusion; I feel like I'll always know and I always have known."

"I felt very connected to the earth; one day while taking this essence, a raven flew over me and dropped a feather."

"Spiritual cleansing," "felt connected with my guidance," "deepening reflection," "better unification of energies," "disciplined meditation"

DREAMS/NIGHTMARES

A prover shared the following dream:

"Sarah, my eighteen-year-old, was having a party. I didn't like it. I was going around telling everyone to leave and that it wasn't okay with me. She was ignoring me, but she got everyone to leave. Then she came back with another group of people to have another party, but this time they were my friends. I still didn't like it and I asked everyone to leave again."

Several provers had dreams related to trying to get rid of something or someone. Others had vague or no dreams.

CENTURY PLANT

(Agave parryi)

PRIMARY QUALITY: BREAKTHROUGH

FAMILY: Agave (Agavacae)

OTHER NAMES: Agave, Maguey, Parry's Century Plant, Mescal

WHERE FOUND: Grows in New Mexico, Arizona, Sonora, and throughout the West along mountainsides, mesa slides, and limestone slopes, and in high deserts and rough terrains

ELEVATION: 2,000' to 8,000'

ENERGY IMPACT (CHAKRA CORRESPONDENCE): first, second, and third chakras

KEY RUBRICS FOR POSITIVE HEALING PATTERNS: confidence, empowerment, strength, ability to survive, rebirth

KEY RUBRICS FOR SYMPTOMS AND PATTERNS OF IMBALANCE: lack of willpower, letting others dominate, holding on and not letting go

OTHER RUBRICS: abuse, abdomen, ambition, anxiety, apathy, appreciation, birth, boundaries, breakthrough, calm, celebration, challenge, clarity, clairvoyance, cleansing, codependence, compassion, courage, creativity, death, defensiveness, depression, denial, discernment, doubt, dreams, emotional balance, enthusiasm, envy, exhaustion, exuberance, faith, focus, freedom, groundedness, guilt, harmony, honoring self, impatience, insight, lack, nurture, paranoia, patience, power, purification, purpose, receptivity, release, repression, responsibility, rest, root chakra, self-empowerment, self-esteem, solar plexus chakra, spleen chakra, tension, transition, victim, warmth, will, wisdom

Traditional use

The stalk is known for its high alcohol content. It is collected and fermented to make alcoholic beverages, some of which are distilled commercially such as mescal, pulque, and tequila. The leaves and root contain soapy substances used in manufacturing steroids. Expressed leaf sap or dried leaf boiled in tea is used to treat indigestion, stomach fermentation, and chronic constipation. Burns, cuts, and skin abrasions can also be healed with the fresh sap. Either fresh or dried root of the century plant can be used to make a soap or to treat arthritis. Continuous use is not advised. The century plant has been used in Mexico to treat jaundice. More recently, the dried stalk of the century plant has been used in the Verde Valley of Arizona for making didgeridoos, an Australian musical instrument usually made from a hollow limb.

Homeopathic use

Another species, *Agave Americana,* is a home-opathic remedy used to treat swollen and bleeding gums, painful erections in cases of gonorrhea, and legs covered with dark purple blotches that are painful, hard, and swollen.

positive Healing patterns

- Teaches fortitude and the inner and outer strength necessary to survive in a harsh environment.
- Helps us take time to nurture our-selves in order to feel strong and empowered.
- Helps us to stay focused on life goals and feeds us with strength, praise, joy, harmony, confidence, and creative expression.
- Embraces a new cycle of birth and celebration. Helps us celebrate the departure of an old pattern and a renewal of energy in a new and positive direction.
- Reminds us of the need to surren-der, particularly when faced with death at any level. This could include the death of a loved one or even oneself, or the dying of an old emotional, mental, or soul pattern.

symptoms and patterns of imbalance

Century Plant may be an appropriate flower essence for those who

- Lack willpower and self-confidence, letting others dominate

- Tend toward pleasing another, even when it goes against one's own best interest
- Tire easily, become "victims," and feel stuck in that role
- Don't take time to nurture and love themselves.

features of the original flower-essence water

ODOR: a very strong, powerful, musky odor
TASTE: a strong, powerful taste, sweeter than the musky odor it produces
SENSATIONS: a feeling of strength and tingling in the belly, with this sensation moving upward through all the chakras and out the crown
WATER COLOR: golden-yellow

physical makeup

ROOT, STEM, LEAVES/LEAFLETS, HEIGHT: This century plant takes eight to twenty-five years to send up the only flower stalk it will ever produce. After blooming, the plant dies and new plants already growing on the root system replace the old one. The name "century" comes from the many years it takes for the plant to blossom. Its 12-to-18-foot stalk is sturdy and feels like a soft wood. It can be up to 3 or 4 inches in diameter. The base of the century plant is thick with grayish green, spatula-shaped leaves up to 20 inches long growing in a basal rosette. The fibrous leaves are con-cave on the upper surface, with hooked spines on their margins and pointed tips.

Flower Color: Reddish-purplish orange, which turns yellow after opening

Flowers: Flowers are grouped in large terminal clusters that face upward to the sun and the sky. There are six petal-like parts to each bud and the blooms are up to 3 inches long.

Blooming Period: June, July, August

Doctrine of signatures

- When holding the strong, sturdy stalk firmly, a feeling of strength, power, and endurance is experienced that empowers us to feel strong, powerful, and enduring and helps us make a breakthrough in our life's circumstances.

- The massive clusters of blooms reach toward the sun, which also give a feeling of strength and fortitude. It takes eight to twenty-five years for this plant to produce its only flowering stalk, which is another signature of the plant's strength and endurance. The birth/death process of this plant plays a significant role in understanding and experiencing the cycles of birth and death in our lives.

- The colors of golden-yellow and orange/red/purple are like the colors of the sun and represent the fire of life, the will. These colors relate to the first, second, and third chakras and to the expression of joy, creativity, warmth, exuberance, sensuality, and self-empowerment. The century plant helps us feel a new freedom, giving us the strength needed to break through our barriers. Its

clusters of blooms are symbolic of being guided by the light of the sun, and are associated with our own abilities to strengthen our minds and visions to empower us to find purpose and direction in our lives.

Helpful suggestions

Take three to four drops of Century Plant flower essence. If you are able, take time to sit in the sun and close your eyes. Feel the warmth of the sun against your face and body. Imagine that you are a small child standing on the earth and that your feet are protected by a circle of long, fibrous leaves that form a pointed tip. As you begin to grow, you feel guided by your own strength and a desire to continue along your journey. You feel nurtured by the earth below and led by the sky above. As you grow taller, you grow in strength, power, wisdom, and understanding to their fullest. Whenever you meet an obstruction or a setback, you listen to the breath within you and direct it upward. Finally, you produce groups of beautiful golden-yellow droplets with orange-red blossoms and you raise your blossoms toward the sky.

You have risen to your glory. You feel your strength from the top of your head to the soles of your feet, and you let light come through to every part of your being. You feel the magnitude of this strength and of the ability to break through life's barriers. Slowly open your eyes.

Here are a few exercises to do:

1. Think of something you would like to do that would give you strength

and confidence, and visualize yourself doing it.

2. When someone asks you to do
   something that doesn't feel "right,"
   stop and ask yourself how you feel;
   act according to what would serve
   you and the other person best.

3. Whenever you find yourself not
   meeting your needs, stop and ask
   yourself what you're doing, what
   you're thinking, and how you're
   feeling, and get in touch with what
   would serve your highest interests.

4. Participate in physical exercises and
   activities that help you feel strong.

Affirmations

- "I am willing to let go of the old and
  become who I see myself to be."
- "I take action for my own growth
  and changes."
- "I empower myself to be focused
  and creative, and to embrace my
  highest goals."
- "I am creating each moment."

Case History

Marie was a woman in her thirties who
divorced an abusive partner two years ago.
She described herself as having dug a hole
in a deep dark tunnel and now realized it
is time for her to come out of the tunnel
and face the light. Through her past abusive relationship, she lost her will to nurture herself and to regain her power. She
also lost the intention to pursue her life
goals and she felt weakened by her lack of
enthusiasm for life. Marie said that she

was in need of letting go of the old and
wanted to create a new expression for herself in the world.

The Century Plant helped Marie
regain her intention to follow her dreams
and lifetime goals. By accepting her old
situation as something that was and is no
longer, Marie felt empowered to regain her
strength and confidence by finding new
ways to express herself. She began daily
affirmations and focused on the messages
of the century plant. She visualized herself
as the century plant and journeyed with
the plant in her dreams. Marie continued
flower-essence therapy with the Century
Plant and eventually returned joyfully
back to the world with a new job that supported her creative expression. She began
participating in community activities,
made new friends, and found new
resources.

Marie experienced a new zest for life
and discovered a part of herself that was
able to celebrate her power and strength as
she gradually surrendered her past and let
go of the bondage she had felt. In her
words, "I finally accepted my past relationship by understanding the lesson of
what it is to give away my personal power
to another person. Now that I am regaining that power, I feel stronger to act in
ways that embrace a higher wisdom and
that keep me focused on my life goals."

Life's Research Provers' project Findings

PHYSICAL SYMPTOMS

CRAVINGS: Sweets
SENSATIONS: None

PAIN: None

MODALITIES:

  WORSE: Evening

  BETTER: Morning, sleep

HEAD: None

EYES: None

FACE: None

EARS: None

STOMACH: Cramps

ABDOMEN: Cramps

BOWEL CONDITION: Looser stools

URINE: Urination reduced in frequency

FEMALE: None

MALE: Improved prostate condition

EXTREMITIES: None

BACK: Lower back pain, backaches

SKIN: None

OTHER: Loss of appetite

EMOTIONAL SYMPTOMS

PATTERNS OF BALANCE: "sentimental feelings, wondering about old friends," "acceptance," "increased comfort in daily activities," "increased confidence," "eased tension and pressure," "more relaxed," "increased energy level and creativity," "experienced more emotional balance," "uplifting," "felt ready to meet the challenges of the day," "self-acceptance," "desire to nurture self," "felt empowered," "energy shifts of experiencing a 'breakthrough' after feeling depressed and directionless"

PATTERNS OF IMBALANCE: "low emotions," "conflicting anxiety," "depressed," "directionless," "feelings of depression and directionless," "lacking in confidence," "confusion," "insecurity," "challenged," "pushed," "tired," and "insecure"

MENTAL SYMPTOMS

PATTERNS OF BALANCE: "clairvoyant," "thoughts of old friends," "eased mental tension and pressure," "more calm," "quiet," "relaxed," "insightful," "intuitive awareness," "thoughts and dialogues with myself about wanting to take time to do things for myself and to be with myself," "improved memory," "more understanding," "more creative in general and having creative solutions to everyday concerns"

PATTERNS OF IMBALANCE: "feeling dull and spacy," "indecisive"

SPIRITUAL REFLECTIONS

"Influenced through integration of dreams and deeper insights," "increased conscious realms," "more conscious consideration of personal life," "this essence enabled me to take time to reflect with myself," "this essence worked as a transitional bridge over a difficult time"

DREAMS/NIGHTMARES

Several provers had dreams of old friends or characters from the past not seen in many years. Provers also experienced an increase in vividness and quantity of dreams, with a deepening of reflective thought patterns during the waking state.

"I am pregnant and ready to give birth. As the dream progresses, the pregnancy disappears. My body returns to normal before I can give birth."

"I am overhearing a group of people talking about me and saying that I am too singly focused and they need someone with a broad vision to do the job."

CHAMOMILE (German)

(Matricaria chamomilla)
PRIMARY QUALITY: SERENITY

FAMILY: Sunflower (Compositae)

OTHER NAMES: Ground Apple, Wild Chamomile, Manzanilla ("little apple"), Maythen (one of nine sacred herbs of the *Lacnunga,* an ancient Anglo-Saxon manuscript), Matricaria. *Mater* is the Latin word for "mother," and *matrix* refers to the womb. Germans call Chamomile *alles zutraut,* meaning "capable of anything."

WHERE FOUND: Meadows, roadsides, gardens, and abandoned areas, with preference for full sun and a light, moist soil. A native to Europe, Africa, and northern Asia, chamomile has become naturalized in the United States and is commonly cultivated.

ELEVATION: most U.S. climate zones

ENERGY IMPACT (CHAKRA CORRESPONDENCE): third and seventh chakras

KEY RUBRICS FOR POSITIVE HEALING PATTERNS: relaxation, emotional balance, peacefulness, comfort

KEY RUBRICS FOR SYMPTOMS AND PATTERNS OF IMBALANCE: anxiety, impatience, irritability, moodiness

OTHER RUBRICS: aches, addiction, anger, apathy, babies, breakthrough, calm, centered, change, cheerful, children, clarity, cleansing, colic, confidence, congestion, criticism, crown chakra, depression, digestion, doubt, dreams, exhaustion, fear, gentle, grief, grounded, guilt, healing, indigestion, inner peace, insight, insomnia, menses, mindful, nervous, nightmares, pain, paranoia, parenting, patience, personal awareness, protection, restful, restless, self-empowerment, sensitivity, serenity, soothing, shame, skin, sleep, solar plexus chakra, sorrow, stability, stress, surrender, tension, thirst, upset, wisdom

Traditional use

There are several plants in the Compositae family that use the name chamomile. The two chamomiles used in herbal medicine are "German" *(Chamomilla matricaria)* and "Roman" *(Anthemis nobilis);* throughout history their names have been interchanged. They both contain a blue volatile oil that is derived from the flowers.

Over the centuries, chamomile has been known for its sweet apple scent and its soothing qualities. In early Egypt, chamomile was used to treat malarial fever characterized by regularly returning chills or fevers. Baths and poultices of chamomile were used by herbalist leaders such as Dioscorides and Pliny to treat headaches and kidney, liver, and bladder dysfunctions. Even in the fairytale "The Tale of

Peter Rabbit," Peter's mother gave him chamomile tea to relieve his headache. In medieval England, chamo-mile was used as a fragrance to freshen the air, and in Spain chamomiles were used to flavor sherry. Chamomile was also used as an insect repellent and as a natural hair highlighter for blondes.

Today, chamomile is a favorite among the herbs. In addition to its traditional folk uses, it is known as the "baby remedy"; it is used to treat colic and as a sedative for whining, crying, impatient, irritated babies and children with earaches, teething, pains, and difficulty sleeping. Chamomile is also used as an anti-inflammatory for various ailments of the skin and mucous membranes; as an antispasmodic for the treatment of such conditions as indigestion, upset stomach, heartburn, flatulence, tension related to the liver, and menstrual cramps; and as an anti-infective for conditions such as fevers, asthma, bronchitis, and colds. The uses of chamomile are too numerous to mention, thus its name "capable of anything."

Homeopathic use

The homeopathic tincture is prepared from the whole plant. Dr. Samuel Hahnemann, originator of homeopathy, refers to Chamomilla as the "Children's Remedy." The keynotes of the homeopathic Chamomilla remedy are children's conditions, one cheek hot and flushed, the other cheek cold and pale, and green diarrhea during teething that smells like a rotten egg. Inconsolable children demand to

be carried, and they have the tendency to throw things away that are offered to them. Chamomilla is also commonly used to treat colic. Chamomilla is used to treat those who are hypersensitive, irritable, angry, impatient, thirsty, intolerant to pain, and oversensitive to coffee.

positive Healing patterns

- Releases tension and restores a serene, peaceful, calm, relaxed disposition, offering emotional balance and stability.
- Creates a peaceful, balanced emotional relationship with our illness through understanding and bonding with the underlying emotion that caused the illness.
- Induces sleep and relaxation.
- Can be used during pregnancy, premenstrual or menstrual cycles, and menopause, as well as for babies and children.

symptoms and patterns of imbalance

Chamomile may be an appropriate flower essence for those who

- Feel moody, upset, anxious, impatient, or irritable
- Need to bond emotionally with their illness or symptoms
- Have insomnia, restlessness at night, or nightmares
- Are women with PMS and irritability, especially related to menses or lack thereof, and for babies and

children who get easily upset and moody.

features of the original flower-essence water

ODOR: hint of honey-like lemon; sweet
TASTE: fruity, like watermelon
SENSATIONS: soothing, calming, relaxing, sleepy, light, and mindless
WATER COLOR: clear

physical makeup

ROOT, STEM, LEAVES/LEAFLETS, HEIGHT: Chamomile has a creeping rootstalk that spreads, creating a carpetlike surface. The roots are delicate and easy to pull. The smooth, round, tall, erect, branching stems grow up to 3 feet tall. The delicate bright-green leaves have a lacy fernlike appearance and have no stalk. They are light and airy, and may alternate or grow parallel on the stems.

FLOWER COLOR: White with yellow centers
FLOWERS: The scent of the flowers is a pleasant combination of honey and apple. Single, daisy-like, symmetrical flowers have marked conical, fuzzy, hollow yellow centers and grow on the long stems. The flowers have a bitter yet pleasant taste. The seeds are ribbed.

BLOOMING PERIOD: Early summer to mid-autumn

doctrine of signatures

- The flower's gentle appearance and sweet fragrance offer a sunny, peaceful, relaxed, light disposition with its white ray flowers open and its yellow center facing toward the sun. Chamomile's white ray flowers extend toward the light and are symbolic of the seventh or crown chakra. It is as if they are stretching toward higher consciousness and the simplicity of oneness.

- The yellow center refers to the third, or solar plexus, chakra, which links emotions with the digestive system, adrenals, stomach, liver, and gall bladder. The third chakra is the energy center that strengthens our mind toward positive faith, joy, and humor, bringing a balanced state of serenity, peace, clarity, and wisdom.

- The flower contains a blue volatile oil that offers a soothing, peaceful presence and is undoubtedly included in the flower's essence. The flower essence itself is light and fruity — very calming to taste and experience.

- The delicacy of the plant's root, stems, and leaves represents the plant's sensitive nature.

helpful suggestions

Take four or five drops of Chamomile flower essence whenever you feel nervous, tense, moody, impatient, or irritable. When you take the drops, take time to sit, relax, and center yourself. If it's possible to be outside, place your feet on the earth. Get in touch with the places in yourself that feel nervous and tense. Feel them flow out of you through the soles of your feet. With each intake of breath, breathe in calm, light, and relaxation.

If you're dealing with children, take time to hold and nurture them or engage in a low-key, soothing activity with them. Sing a soft song and rock the child (it's nice to do this with your inner child if you're alone). Tell your child to imagine the grumpiness as a disliked color and to let the color leave. Tell the child that the drops will make the grumpies happier.

Have Chamomile available in your first-aid kit to give to members of your household or friends as needed.

Affirmations

- "I choose thoughts, feelings, and activities that comfort me emotionally."
- "I take time out to relax and center myself."
- "I release my anger, irritability, and impatience and seek inner peace and inner guidance."

case History

Chamomile flower essence has been used successfully as a subtle approach in helping children attain inner peace and serenity. My daughter, Sarah, responds well to three or four drops of Chamomile in a vegetable glycerin base before going to sleep at night. I also frequently use Chamomile with Sarah during emotional upsets. I have found that a blend of Chamomile, Calendula, and Mon-

keyflower works well in treating restlessness, emotional upsets, fears, and nightmares. Generally, this essence takes effect quickly.

I have a personal story to share regarding Chamomile. One day, I was writing about this essence on my computer. After hours of work, I somehow managed to lose the file when I attempted to transfer it to a disk. I immediately began to panic and noticed that my back ached and that my throat was dry. I became very thirsty and drank two cups of water. My stomach ached, inner tension skyrocketed, nervousness accelerated, and I was really out of sorts. Then Sarah came in feeling upset herself! I had taken the Chamomile essence several hours before this incident, and the bottle was sitting right in front of me; it seemed to be screaming to me to take some. I gave both Sarah and myself some drops and was able to redirect her almost immediately. I also felt calmer and at peace within a few minutes. I then called my computer buddy and asked for help, and was able to relax as he helped me step by step to find my lost document.

LfE's Research provers' project findings

PHYSICAL SYMPTOMS
CRAVINGS: Sweets
SENSATIONS: Sore throat, throat and jaw feel tight
PAIN: Back and stomach aches
MODALITIES:
  WORSE: Night in sleep: tossing and turning
  BETTER: Felt better immediately after taking essence any time of day or night

HEAD: Headaches
EYES: Dry; eyesight improved
FACE: Dry and scaly
EARS: None
STOMACH: Stomachache, nausea
ABDOMEN: None
BOWEL CONDITION: Slight constipation, bowels "tighter"
URINE: Increased
FEMALE: Hot flashes
MALE: None
EXTREMITIES: "Restless limbs"
BACK: Backache
SKIN: Dry and scaly; skin rash
OTHER: Lack of hunger. "Ease in bronchi and opening in nasal passages. Gave to one-year-old with cold and allergies and noticed immediate improvement. Congestion cleared. Felt 'physically pacifying.'"

EMOTIONAL SYMPTOMS

PATTERNS OF BALANCE: "patient," "calm," "cool," "collected," "peaceful," "relaxed," "confident," "grounded," "inner peace," "emotionally balanced," "able to contact some long-held resentments and find a way to work with them," "experienced sadness by being more aware," "able to be more detached emotionally; gives quietude and openness without destroying personal boundaries"
PATTERNS OF IMBALANCE: "restless," "impatient," "emotional and physical intolerance," "irritable," "shakiness," "quietly screaming"

MENTAL SYMPTOMS

PATTERNS OF BALANCE: "personal awareness; objectively seeing myself as if outside of my body," "mentally balanced," "memory not as strong but felt more detached mentally," "helps me make decisions more easily," "quiets my mind," "simplifies things for me," "gave me clarity"
PATTERNS OF IMBALANCE: "restless," "impatient," "intolerant," "confused"

SPIRITUAL REFLECTIONS

"I took more time for myself and for centering," "the light is inside me and inner peace washes over me," "spiritual relaxation," "experienced a better understanding of my limitations and boundaries without trying to please everyone," "I have better contact with my guidance."

DREAMS/NIGHTMARES

A mother who is emotionally bonded with her son and who was worried and anxious about him shared this dream: "One night while on this essence, I was dreaming about my twenty-year-old son. In the dream I was wondering where he was. At that moment, he called me in reality and said 'Mom, I'm thinking about you so much right now.' What a trip!"

CHICORY

(Cichorium intybus)
PRIMARY QUALITY: INTERRELATEDNESS

FAMILY: Sunflower (Compositae)

OTHER NAMES: Succory, Coffeeweed, *Barbe de Capuchin*, Endive, Garden Chicory, Blueweed, Blue Dandelion, Blue Sailors, Ragged Sailors, Witloof. *Cichorium* derived from its Arabic name, *intypbus* derived from *tybi*, Latin and Egyptian name for the month of January when it was usually eaten.

WHERE FOUND: Fields, roadsides, old pastures, and waste areas on light, sandy soil in all of our states. Native to Europe.

ELEVATION: below 9,300'

ENERGY IMPACT (CHAKRA CORRESPONDENCE): fifth and sixth chakras

BACH FLOWER REMEDY: Bach Flower Remedy Chicory is for those who are possessive, selfish, and demanding — who want others to think and be like them. The positive trait for Chicory, according to Bach, is a genuine concern and care for others.

KEY RUBRICS FOR POSITIVE HEALING PATTERNS: respect and caring for others, unconditional love

KEY RUBRICS FOR SYMPTOMS AND PATTERNS OF IMBALANCE: demanding, insensitivity, lack of concern about others, self-centeredness

OTHER RUBRICS: aggressiveness, appreciation, arms, awareness, balance, bitterness, breathing, brow chakra, chest, cleansing, collective, compassion, concern, connection, consciousness, control, creativity, defensiveness, depression, devotion, dreams, energetic, exhaustion, eyes, fluids, groundedness, hands, harmony, healing, heart, holding on, impatience, insight, inspiration, legs, letting go, lungs, meditation, movement, patience, possessive, relations, release, responsibility, rigid, self-pity, selfless love, sensitive, sharing, sleep, spiritual, spiritual vision, surrender, tension, throat chakra, truth

traditional use

Chicory was cultivated in Egypt 5,000 years ago, and the ancient Egyptians and Arabs blanched and ate the leaves. Since the early nineteenth century, chicory roots have been roasted and ground to flavor and smooth out coffee. Queen Elizabeth I drank chicory broth for its nutrients.

Chicory contains two bitter substances, lactucin and lactucoprin, which act as a sedative on the central nervous system. It is said that mixing chicory with coffee soothes the central nervous system and the heart. Chicory can be used as an antiseptic or astringent like its relative, dandelion. Herbalists use a decoction of the root as a mild tonic, diuretic, carminative, digestive aid, or laxative, or to treat liver inefficiency. The bruised leaves can be used as a dressing for swellings, and the milky sap in the stems can be used to treat poison ivy and sunburns. Chicory tea releases phlegm from the stomach, cleansing the liver, spleen, and gall bladder, and aids conditions of gout, rheumatism, and joint stiffness.

Herbalists have also recommended chicory flower water for sore and inflamed eyes, however, excessive use of any form of chicory can impair the retina. Chicory has also been used as a food item; the leaves can be eaten fresh or cooked like spinach. The young root can also be steamed as a vegetable, and the fresh flowers can be used to garnish salads. The boiled leaves make a blue dye.

Homeopathic use

The Mother tincture is prepared from the dry root and is used to treat dimness of vision, constipation, and headache.

positive Healing patterns

- Helps us to respect, honor, and see all life forms as an expression of our Creator, teaching us to live in harmony with one another.
- Opens our consciousness toward understanding natural laws (such as "what goes around comes around"), which opens us to experiencing "selfless love," heartfelt concern for others, and genuine sharing.
- Expands our spiritual awareness,

opening a doorway for genuine caring and unconditional love without the need to control.
- Teaches us that we are all interrelated and come from the same Source.

symptoms and patterns of imbalance

Chicory may be an appropriate flower essence for those who

- Are self-centered, unconcerned, and insensitive toward others
- Have bitter personalities that feed off of negative attention, are possessive and demanding, have a tendency toward self-pity, refuse to be responsible for their actions and thoughts, and want others to be like themselves
- Are rigid and hold on so tight that they lose sight of what they're doing and how they impact others through their need for control and continual correction of others
- Are lacking in spiritual direction, creativity, and willpower
- Are suppressed and who may have pent-up emotions, anxiety, or nervousness, and who tend to feel unappreciated
- Have a strong need to care for others and to want people they care for to be near to them without true consideration of the others' needs
- Seek attention from others and withdraw in self-pity when not responded to in the way they want.

original flower-essence water features

ODOR: very subtle

TASTE: slightly bitter

SENSATIONS: restlessness and stirring in solar plexus; impatient, bitter mood immediately changing to a very peaceful, spiritually inspiring state

WATER COLOR: translucent

physical makeup

ROOT, STEM, LEAVES/LEAFLETS, HEIGHT: Chicory's long brownish-whitish taproot grows quite deep and contains a bitter, milky, saplike substance. Its erect dark-green stem can grow from 1 to 6 feet tall, and it is rigid, sturdy, hollow, and furrowed with many branches growing at obtuse angles. The stem, like the root, is covered with tiny hairs and contains a bitter milky substance. The lower grayish green leaves are quite large (up to 8 inches long) and raggedy, petioled, and coarsely toothed. There is a large vein on the underside of each leaf, with many tiny veins branching and subbranching off it. The large leaves form a rosette at the base of the plant, similar to dandelion, and they ooze a bitter milky substance when broken. The upper leaves are small, sessile, clasping, and less divided than the lower ones; arrow-shaped leaves diminishing in size toward the top of the stem, which appears nearly naked. When the roots are forced in warmth and darkness, blanched heads called "chicons" (also known as Belgian endives), grow midway up the stem. The plant produces tiny, hard oval brown seeds.

FLOWER COLOR: Iridescent lavender-blue

FLOWERS: The musty-smelling flower heads grow in clusters or pairs at each leaf joint, looking similar to dandelions. Each flower head has square-tipped ray flowers with five square-edged teeth or straps on its outer rim. Five tiny pale lines extend from the teeth to the center of the flower, where they form a small tube on which dark lavender stamens with faded anthers protrude from a small stalk. In overcast weather the flowers bloom all day long, but in sunny weather they close in the noonday sun approximately five hours after they open. Chicory's starlike petals and its iridescent color create a heavenly experience.

BLOOMING PERIOD: June to October

doctrine of signatures

- The heavenly lavender-bluish color of the flowers opens our devotion to seeking spiritual vision and understanding of collective consciousness and of all relations. This allows us to act unconditionally and to speak our spiritual truths. The colors of the flower are symbolic of the fifth chakra of communication and the sixth chakra of spiritual insight and vision.

- The bitterness of the milky, saplike substance represents the patterns of imbalance that produce possessiveness, demands, emotional blackmail, and bitterness when things don't go the "right" way. Even the flower essence is slightly bitter, yet it offers a very peaceful and spiritually inspiring state.

- The many-branched stems and veins represent our connections with each other and with all our relations.
- The flowers growing at the joint demonstrate their need to "hold on," teaching us about our own need to hold on and about when to let go. This signature also refers to joint stiffness.
- The deep taproot, along with the heavenly and inspirational flower, represents spiritual groundedness.
- Chicory plants grow abundantly in communities, and each plant has multiple flower heads, symbolizing new opportunities and growth.

Helpful suggestions

Most people tend to get tired and have less energy around midday. When we're tired, we tend to express our negative impulses more freely. Observe yourself around this time of day. Instead of feeding on the tiredness or anxiety, take time to be silent with yourself and go within to be with the Source. Be like chicory; take the time to close down and revitalize yourself. If you can, prepare a special place for yourself. Perhaps that means removing the clutter in a certain area, lighting a candle, burning your favorite incense, breathing in a favorite aromatherapy oil, or sitting in your back yard. Get comfortable, then take three to four drops of Chicory flower essence. Let the drops slowly move down your throat. Close your eyes and follow the energy of the flower essence. Stay in each moment and let the moment take you on your journey. Enter the silence from within and let yourself relax. When you open your eyes again, observe how you feel. Ask yourself to hold the energy of this feeling and to share this feeling with others in the way you communicate and express yourself.

Affirmations

- "We are all connected. We are all one family."
- "I honor and respect all life forms as an expression of our Creator."
- "May I listen to the wind within my voice, and sing and speak in beauty."

Case History

By taking the Chicory flower essence and being devoted to seeking higher truths, Clara found herself more relaxed with others, less demanding, less possessive, and more energetic in serving her own needs as well as the needs of others. By being more connected, open, and loving with herself, she felt more connected, open, and loving with others. She also learned to pace herself in her work and to take time to be alone and nurture herself as needed. Clara felt that her experience with Chicory helped her to respect and honor herself, and for this she is grateful.

LFE's Research Provers' Project Findings

PHYSICAL SYMPTOMS

CRAVINGS: Pizza, beer, fluids, water, fresh fruit, raw vegetables; general increased appetite

SENSATIONS: Tingling in arms and hands
PAIN: Tension in back
MODALITIES:
  WORSE: Tired mid-afternoon
  BETTER: Nighttime sleep, more energy in early morning
HEAD: None
EYES: None
FACE: None
EARS: None
STOMACH: None
ABDOMEN: None
BOWEL CONDITION: Moist bowel movements
URINE: More frequent
FEMALE: Increased libido/creativity
MALE: None
EXTREMITIES: Tingling in hands; energy moving through the heart center and out the arms
BACK: Increased tension near one vertebra
SKIN: None
OTHER: Increased (even exaggerated) creative physical energy

EMOTIONAL SYMPTOMS

PATTERNS OF BALANCE: "tears and emotions were close to the surface, cried easily and it felt good," "the tears were in response to the beauty of the way someone would express their truth," "releasing was more spontaneous than usual," "mellow," "even-tempered in the face of difficult situations," "grounded"
PATTERNS OF IMBALANCE: "sadness," "tension," "irritability"

MENTAL SYMPTOMS

PATTERNS OF BALANCE: "realization of holding onto old baggage; able to let go of being so mental," "helped me put things in perspective," "more mellow," "less analytical," "in places of turmoil in my mind, I kept getting the message to just love and listen"
PATTERNS OF IMBALANCE: No responses from provers

SPIRITUAL REFLECTIONS

"Increased meditation," "I realized I was lacking in my spiritual self," "I had a beautiful time with my higher state and it rooted a good spiritual connection," "I wanted to work on being more spiritually healed and balanced," "I felt the connection through all things; the feeling of unity was uplifting and joyful — feeling my connections to the collective consciousness," "more prayer," "felt more open spiritually in general"

DREAMS/NIGHTMARES

"I was physically younger but still emotionally/mentally/spiritually the same. I felt that what my elder family members were telling me was untrue and rather ignorant. I was looking at them dubiously and wondering, 'Do they really think this is how it works?'"

In general, dreams were vivid and clear.

CLIff ROSE

(Cowania mexicana)

Primary Quality: Positive Self-Image

Family: Rose (Rosaceae)

Other Names: Stansbury Cliffrose, *C. stansburiana,* Quinine Bush, Buckbrush, and *'awééts' áál,* or "baby cradle" (Navajo).

Where Found: in oak/pinyon/juniper woodland openings, on dry open rocky slopes and mesas, and on hillsides, cliffsides, canyon rims, and plateaus in upper desert and grasslands, from southeastern California through Nevada, Utah, Arizona, western New Mexico, southwestern Colorado, and south to central Mexico

Elevation: 3,500' to 8,000'

Energy Impact (Chakra Correspondence): third and seventh chakras

Key Rubrics for Positive Healing Patterns: self-acceptance, self-value, love of self, self-image

Key Rubrics for Symptoms and Patterns of Imbalance: lack of self-acceptance and self-value, fear of expressing love

Other Rubrics: acceptance, agitation, anxiety, appetite, awaken, back, bowels, brain, change, child, clarity, cleansing, confidence, confusion, crown chakra, detachment, doubts, emotional bitterness, empowerment, faith, fear, gentleness, healing, heart, impatience, inner child, insight, love, personal growth, perspective, positive, purifier, quiet, release, restless, revitalizes, sadness, self-confidence, self-empowerment, sexuality, solar plexus chakra, spiritual, strength, transition, trust, uplifting

Traditional Use

Indians of the Southwest have used cliff rose for a variety of applications. The tea is used as an emetic for traditional singers during sweats and in various ceremonies. The Navajo shredded the bark for padding cradleboards and making "baseballs." Navajo women used the wood to make prayer sticks, and the leaves and stems were ground along with juniper branches to make a yellowish golden dye. Ceremonial arrows were made from the straight branches. The leaves and twigs were made into a tea by the Hopi to cause vomiting and as a cleansing agent for sores and wounds. The Hopi also used the wood to make arrows. Basket makers of various tribes made clothing, sandals, mats, and rope from the shredded bark.

Chopped stems and leaves can be boiled and made into a tea to treat the early stages of a chest cold and as a gargle for sore throat. It also increases perspiration and loosens mucus, and the same tea can be used to treat diarrhea, liver ailments, and backaches. Cattle, sheep, and deer depend on the bitter-tasting foliage during the winter.

homeopathic use

Unknown to author.

positive healing patterns

- Increases self-acceptance and self-value while removing doubts and fears.
- Heightens spiritual sensitivity and the feeling and expression of love.
- Awakens us to empower and love ourselves and to be guided by our "higher good," thus creating a positive self-image.
- Cleanses and purifies inner emotional barriers that no longer serve us.

symptoms and patterns of imbalance

Cliff Rose may be an appropriate flower essence for those who

- Aren't accepting themselves or their life situation
- Are doubtful and afraid to express love
- Lack self-confidence and are afraid to be themselves
- Need a gentle, uplifting spiritual boost.

features of the original flower-essence water

Odor: a subtle fruity, rose-like smell
Taste: tastes like it smells

Sensations: soothing and relaxing in the throat; gives a peaceful feeling of knowing who you are
Water Color: slightly yellow, with a creamy tint

physical makeup

Root, Stem, Leaves/Leaflets, Height: Cliff rose is a medium to large shrub, ranging from 5 to 10 feet tall, or a small tree growing up to 20 feet tall with gnarled, open branches. The older, thicker branches have soft, shreddy, gray bark, while the younger branches are shiny and reddish brown. Branches and twigs are covered with glandular-dotted, pinnately lobed, somewhat sticky dark-green leaves that are white and woolly underneath. The leaves are divided into three or five narrow lobes, have a leathery wrinkled appearance, and can be quite juicy. Cliff rose foliage contains resinous compounds that are bitter and unpleasant in taste, giving rise to the name "quinine bush." When in full bloom, the entire shrub or tree is covered with flowers and is quite picturesque.
Flower Color: Cream to pale yellow
Flowers: The sweetly fragrant orange blossom and rose-like scent of the abundant flowers is an attraction to the hiker or the passerby. You can smell the sweet aroma even if you don't see the shrub at first. The flowers first bloom a pale yellow but then become a soft cream color. Each flower is about 1 inch wide and has five petals with a bunch of short golden stamens in the center. While collecting pollen from the stamens, insects casually

brush against the pistils and transfer the pollen from flower to flower. A single-seeded fruit called an achene emerges from the fertilized pistil. Each achene has a long, fuzzy, stringlike, feathery tail called a "plume," which grows about 2 inches long. Up to ten plumed achenes can grow from one flower head; as the wind catches them, their seeds are scattered. A plant called "Apache plume" also has plumed achenes, but the flowers are larger and usually more white or pinkish, and the Apache plume's leaves have no dots.

Blooming Period: April to September

Doctrine of signatures

- The subtle creamy color of the flower corresponds to the seventh chakra; it is cleansing and purifying, and heightens us toward spiritual sensitivity. The golden center, like a golden halo, relates to both the seventh chakra and the third chakra, which strengthens, revitalizes, and awakens the sense of self. The golden color also helps us love and empower ourselves and come to terms with who we are and what we desire. As a member of the rose family, cliff rose is also a symbol of expressing love.

- The long, fuzzy, feathery tail represents the subtle softness and gentleness of this flower and its ability to flow with the wind and plant its seeds (representing our seeds) for new growth.

- The bitter, unpleasant taste of the leaves is like our own emotional bitterness that causes doubts, fears, and nonacceptance. Yet the flower and the flower-essence water smell fragrantly sweet and have a soft, gentle taste. This signature speaks of our ability to rise above our doubts and fears, empowering who and what we are.

Helpful suggestions

Make a commitment to yourself to take Cliff Rose flower essence for at least three to four weeks with the intention to work on one or two specific issues that relate to your self-image, self-confidence, self-esteem, and ability to love yourself.

Begin in silence or meditation. "Tune into" yourself and try to tap into what would help you feel more focused and positive about yourself. What is your relationship with yourself like? Do you do loving things for yourself? Do you take care of yourself? What could you do differently that would help you feel better about yourself? List your doubts and fears. What gets in the way? Write the responses to these questions in a journal and allow yourself to go with your own writing flow as you plant new seeds for further personal growth.

Read and write in your journal every day. Record any dreams you have. Try to detach from your emotions and look at yourself from a deeper perspective. Observe your emotions and thoughts. Decide on one or two actions that would help you move toward your intention — and most of all, value yourself!

Affirmations

- "I think well of myself and respect who I am and where I came from. I see myself in the eyes of others."
- "I release self-doubts and fears, and allow myself to be who I am."
- "I allow the body of Light to embrace me."

Case History

Amber, age eleven, had a history of working with flower essences and responded well to them. Her parents were getting a divorce and she was having a difficult time. In addition to that, she was being pressured by her peers to have a boyfriend, and her regular school teacher (whom she liked) was absent from school due to a death in the family. Amber was lacking in self-confidence, self-esteem, self-acceptance, and positive self-image; was riddled with self-doubt and fear; and feeling heart torn between her parents.

Cliff Rose was the first flower essence given to Amber to help her rebuild a positive self-image and deal more effectively with her emotions. Therapeutic counseling and body work was also advised. Amber liked Cliff Rose and said that it helped her feel "quiet inside." She was better able to let go of what others thought of her and be herself — and to love both parents despite the tendency to want to take sides.

LFE's Research Provers' Project Findings

Physical Symptoms

Cravings: Fresh food
Sensations: Felt a vibrational shifting
Pain: None
Modalities:
    Worse: Noon to mid-afternoon, night during sleep
    Better: Evening
Head: None
Eyes: None
Face: None
Ears: None
Stomach: None
Abdomen: None
Bowel condition: Looser stools
Urine: More frequent urination
Female: Increases libido
Male: None
Extremities: None
Back: Back pain close to my heart; I felt blocked emotionally
Skin: None
Other: Increased appetite

Emotional Symptoms

Patterns of Balance: "emotionally stable," "learning to trust myself emotionally," "needing more personal time with self," "I had the ability to detach myself from feelings and thoughts and accept things that have bothered me or confused me," "experienced emotional release," "was able to detach myself from my emotions and feel them but also observe them more clearly," "melancholy"

PATTERNS OF IMBALANCE: "slight agitation and nervousness," "a feeling of 'slowing down' slightly," "delayed reaction influence," "slightly stressed," "weak and irritated," "impatient with self," "anxiousness," "frustration," "sadness"

MENTAL SYMPTOMS

PATTERNS OF BALANCE: "feeling in touch with self," "I had a deepening of experience of the way my mind works," "a clearer seeing of patterns and blockages despite my confusion," "I felt the need to understand and explain," "I experienced a deepening of seeing," "detachment of my thoughts gives me clarity, which cleared emotional and mental confusion," "able to see myself more clearly"

PATTERNS OF IMBALANCE: "worried and restless energy"

SPIRITUAL REFLECTIONS

"Felt quiet spiritually," "I lost a lot of faith without noticing it until now . . . I've had a lot of people reject my spiritual self simply because we were at different levels in our growth," "I am saying good-bye to this bad habit," "I need to have more faith in my spiritual self," "increased prayer and meditation," "understanding the meaning of taking care of and being myself in the moment," "realizing how much I hold onto my mental activity as to who I am — and how much I identify with and cling to the patterns of my mind in reality," "seeing deeper into fears and limitations"

DREAMS/NIGHTMARES

A prover shared the following dream: "There is a wild horse in my bedroom. The door is open a crack and I shut it for fear of him escaping and I wouldn't be able to catch him. I am taking care of three children and they are also in the room. I am afraid for their safety. The horse is running in circles around the room, up and over the bed at full speed. The horse then becomes a greyhound dog and runs so fast that it turns into a blur. One of the children, a boy, gets up on the bed and puts his legs out into the blur. This stops the dog, and the dog comes at the boy viciously biting. The boy continues to kick and provoke the dog. I am very afraid for his safety and also am unable to speak."

COLUMBINE (yellow)

(Aquilegia chrysantha)
PRIMARY QUALITY: DIVINE BEAUTY

FAMILY: Buttercup (Ranunculaceae)

OTHER NAMES: Yellow Columbine, Golden Columbine; the Latin word *aquila* means "eagle," and the Italian word *columbina* means "dove."

WHERE FOUND: beside streams, springs, and waterfalls, and in rich, damp, fertile soil in shaded forests and alpine meadows from southern Colorado to New Mexico, Arizona, and northern Mexico

ELEVATION: 3,000' to 11,000'

ENERGY IMPACT (CHAKRA CORRESPONDENCE): third and seventh chakras

KEY RUBRICS FOR POSITIVE HEALING PATTERNS: appreciation, love, inner beauty, cheerfulness, inner worth

KEY RUBRICS FOR SYMPTOMS AND PATTERNS OF IMBALANCE: egoic personal beauty, lack of self-worth, overemphasis on the material world

OTHER RUBRICS: acceptance, alertness, anxiety, breakthrough, burden, clarity, cleansing, crown chakra, depression, divinity, eyes, feet, goodness, hands, happiness, head, healing, heart, hidden, inner gifts, insight, joy, meditation, menses, nurture, quietness, receptivity, release, relief, sadness, self-empowerment, sexuality, solar plexus chakra, spontaneity, tingling, understanding, union, uplifting, wisdom, worry

traditional use

Columbine flower has been known for its traditional use as a love potion; sweethearts mashed the seeds and rubbed them on their bodies. Before meeting their woman, Native American men would blend columbine seeds with tobacco and have a smoke for good luck. In traditional folklore, columbine was referred to as "folly" or an " abandoned lover."

Contrary to the previous reference, columbine represented the "Holy Spirit" in religious circles due to the Italian word for "dove" in its name. Columbine root, with medical direction, has been used to treat external skin diseases. Fresh roots were mashed and rubbed on swollen, aching joints. The boiled leaves and root have been used to treat scurvy, plague, fever, dizziness, diarrhea, and bladder problems. The leaves, eaten raw, have been used to treat swollen glands or adenoid problems. The leaves were commonly used in potions to treat sore mouths and throats. The entire plant, boiled, is said to stop venereal diseases. According to Parkinson in 1640, "A dram of seeds taken in wine with saffron opens obstructions of the liver, and is good for jaundice, causing profuse sweating."

homeopathic use

Treats problems of the nervous system, hysteria, menopausal women who vomit a green substance, especially in the morning, and dysmenorrhea in young girls.

CAUTION: The seeds contain hydrocyanic acid, a poison that can be fatal for children. It is now considered poisonous to use the leaves and flowers as diuretics.

positive healing patterns

- Allows us to appreciate, nurture, love, and accept ourselves and to receive the goodness of life.
- Helps us to capture the beauty of life and the beauty within and without, allowing us to feel and express our Divine beauty.
- Offers healing energy right where it is needed.
- Teaches us to treasure our inner gifts.
- Transforms negativity by offering a higher insight and the ability to focus visually.
- Offers wisdom, joy, and positive life-energy.

symptoms and patterns of imbalance

Columbine may be an appropriate flower essence for those who

- Are closed down and burdened, and don't see their own inner worth and beauty

- Have difficulty loving and accepting themselves, and who deny the good things in life
- Need a loving guide to find their hidden treasures and to share their treasures with others
- Thrive on an egoic personal inner and outer beauty, and who are ready to discover and express their Divine beauty.

features of the original flower-essence water

ODOR: full-bodied and fragrantly sweet
TASTE: powerful, fragrant, and full
SENSATIONS: Feel more bright, senses are heightened, hearing the smallest sounds, "seeing" at a higher level, face is more relaxed.
WATER COLOR: clear

physical makeup

ROOT, STEM, LEAVES/LEAFLETS, HEIGHT: Columbine has a brownish orange rootstalk that is erect and short. Its erect, woody, sticky, fuzzy, round, slender stem can grow up to 4 feet tall. The green stem has a hint of purplish-bluish coloring. This species is the largest of the columbines. The bluish green leaves grow mostly at the base of the plant, in clusters of three. The leaflets are rounded and toothed and are $1\frac{1}{2}$ inches wide and long. The veins on the leaflets look like tiny hands, sometimes with five points.
FLOWER COLOR: Canary yellow
FLOWERS: Columbine flowers have a

strong honey-sweet scent with five yellow, soft, fuzzy, cuplike yet nodding petals that are prolonged into a narrow funnel-like tube of spurs 2 to 3 inches long that project backward. The spurs give the plant a unique appearance, resembling an eagle's talons or a "dove drinking at a fountain or spring." A clump of golden stamens emerges from the center.

BLOOMING PERIOD: April to September

Doctrine of signatures

- The cuplike petals appear open and receptive, receiving light and the goodness of life.
- The long, tubular ends of the spurs hold a sweet nectar — like having a treasure and goodness deep inside.
- The whole expression of the flower captures the beauty of life, within and without. The flower is like a fairy who comes and sprinkles cheerful fairy dust in your face and changes how you perceive yourself and how you feel about things.
- The yellow color of this flower is like a halo of the seventh chakra, giving healing where it is needed and offering a deep wisdom and understanding of one's inner and outer beauty. It is also symbolic of the third chakra, offering wisdom, joy, and positive energy, and linking our rational mind to our psychic energies and intuition.
- The eagle and the dove both represent powerful healing qualities and the illumination of Spirit.

Helpful suggestions

Take three or four drops of Columbine flower essence. Sit or lie very still. Imagine yourself stepping into an open petal of the flower. Sit down inside the petal while leaning up against the petal wall. Gently scoot your bottom toward the edge of the tubular spur, then close your eyes and take a giant leap. You have landed in a sweet, juicy nectar at the base of the spur! Breathe in its sweet fragrance. Swim in the nectar. Allow yourself to laugh and play. Capture your own essence of pure enjoyment and beauty. Stay with your feeling. Drink and breathe in your Divine beauty. Hold onto it. Feel it and embrace it. Give yourself permission to keep it, to treasure it, and to share it when appropriate. Climb back out of the petal; you may slip and slide some. Brace yourself against the petal wall again and scoot on up toward the opening. Feel and see the light shining down on you. Take in all the treasures and goodness you experienced as you climb back out of the open petal and as you embrace the world again.

Affirmations

- "I treasure my inner gifts and willingly share these gifts with others."
- "I capture the beauty of life, opening myself to my own Divine beauty within and without."
- "I embrace myself in golden yellow light."

Case history

Columbine flower essence usually gives an immediate feeling of joy when taken.

There have been several comments from people about the receptivity, beauty, cheerfulness, and appreciation of self that this flower gives to them. My friend Veronica Vida says, "It's like being hugged by a teddy bear or an angel. It gives me hope and optimism."

LFE's Research provers' project findings

PHYSICAL SYMPTOMS

CRAVINGS: None

SENSATIONS: Tingling in feet and hands

PAIN: None

MODALITIES:

WORSE: No response

　BETTER: Sleep, early mornings

　HEAD: Heaviness at back of head just above the neck, became foggy, then experienced relief of these symptoms

EYES: Slightly blurry, temporarily out of focus

FACE: None

EARS: None

STOMACH: Physical release, lightness

ABDOMEN: None

BOWEL CONDITION: None

URINE: None

FEMALE: Menstrual flow lighter, great sex

MALE: None

EXTREMITIES: Tingling in feet and hands

BACK: None

SKIN: None

OTHER: Physical boost energetically, heart pain on left side of heart

EMOTIONAL SYMPTOMS

PATTERNS OF BALANCE: "spontaneity," "joy," "love," "heart opening," "emotional uplift," "release," "happiness," "feeling higher than normal," "helps me feel relief in a worrisome time," "felt hopeful," "needed more quiet time and personal space"

PATTERNS OF IMBALANCE: "fear," "anxiety"

MENTAL SYMPTOMS

PATTERNS OF BALANCE: "increased awareness," "releasing worries and anxieties," "mentally uplifted," "more mental clarity," "more understanding and knowing," "more alert"

　PATTERNS OF IMBALANCE: "slightly foggy and less clear," "worried," "anxious"

SPIRITUAL REFLECTIONS

"I feel grateful for this remedy and for the relief it gave me; the gratefulness I experienced was a spiritual reflection," "I experienced an increased awareness of the balance concerning male/female union and in relationships."

DREAMS/NIGHTMARES

No significant dreams to share. Minimal dream activity with this flower essence.

COMFREY

(Symphytum officinale)
PRIMARY QUALITY: SERVICE

FAMILY: Borage (Boraginaceae)

OTHER NAMES: Boneknit, Gum Plant, Healing Herb, Nipbone, Blackwort, Bruise-wort, Sumplant, Slippery Root, and Wallwort; Greek word *symphytum* means "to join or unite; mend or knit together (as in broken bones)."

WHERE FOUND: Grows naturally in moist fertile soil and along ditches, streams, and river banks. A native of Europe and temperate regions of Asia, comfrey has become naturalized and is commonly found throughout the United States where there is water or when watered well.

ELEVATION: most U.S. climate zones

ENERGY IMPACT (CHAKRA CORRESPONDENCE): third, fourth, fifth, sixth, and seventh chakras

KEY RUBRICS FOR POSITIVE HEALING PATTERNS: nurturing others to serve the best interest of all, compassion, protection, personal service

KEY RUBRICS FOR SYMPTOMS AND PATTERNS OF IMBALANCE: resistance to making personal sacrifices, lack of discernment, limited spiritual vision

OTHER RUBRICS: anxiety, balance, bowels, bridge, brow chakra, centeredness, clairvoyance, clarity, cleansing, confidence, connection, courage, creativity, crown chakra, depression, discernment, division, doubt, dreams, fear, groundedness, harmony, healing, heart chakra, imbalance, insight, inspiration, integration, love, lungs, meditation, opening, paranoia, perspective, perseverance, release, separation, silence, skin, solar plexus chakra, sorrow, spiritual vision, strength, surrender, throat chakra, transition, understanding, whole, wisdom

traditional use

Comfrey has been known as an invaluable remedy for centuries and is claimed to be a "miracle worker." The leaves contain many useful substances, such as calcium, potassium, phosphorus, copper, zinc, and vitamins A, C, and B12; they are also a good source of amino acids, and the leaves contain more protein than any other herb or plant. Both the leaves and the root contain allantoin, a chemical that stimulates cell division and promotes healing, both inside and out. The roots contain the highest amounts of allontoin in the spring and autumn. Comfrey has demonstrated success as a wound healer and bone knitter, healing stubborn leg ulcers, wounds, fractures, sores, broken bones, athlete's foot, bedsores, burns, insect bites, bruises, sprains, and skin problems such as eczema and psoriasis. Comfrey also feeds the pituitary, strengthens the body skeleton, promotes the secretion of pepsin, and aids digestion. Comfrey can be used as a general healing tonic to treat respiratory ailments such as bronchitis and irritable cough, gastric and duodenal ulcers, hiatal hernia, ulcerative colitis, and hemorrhages, and is effective in destroying harmful bacteria.

Poultices, oils, and teas can be made from the roots and leaves. Fresh leaves can also be cooked or eaten fresh like spinach. Comfrey can be added to baths and lotions to soften the skin, and can be used to make a brownish yellow dye.

Caution: There is some opinion in the medical field that comfrey should not be taken internally in herbal form and especially not on a daily basis.

Homeopathic use

Mother tincture is prepared from fresh root-stalk. It is used primarily for injuries of the bone, sensitive or painful periosteum, fractures, sprains, and phantom limb pain following amputation. It is also used to treat trauma to the eye, abscess, backaches caused by sexual indulgence, cancer, sore breasts, enlarged glands, gunshot wounds, hernia, stopped menses, psoas abscess, and general wounds.

Caution: Because this remedy is also known as "boneknit," do not give this remedy before the bones have been set in proper position.

Positive Healing patterns

- Teaches us to put things in perspective while staying connected to and in harmony with the whole.
- Offers protection and compassion when making personal sacrifices in order to serve the highest good of all concerned.
- Opens us toward spiritual vision, wisdom, and higher clairvoyance, especially during times of service that is for the best and highest interests of the whole.
- Builds a bridge of healing from within to without while providing nurturing and solitude, prayer and meditation.
- Gives us the ability to speak our truths from a spiritual knowing that come from within and to express harmony and balance in times of personal service.

Symptoms and patterns of imbalance

Comfrey may be an appropriate flower essence for those who

- Have difficulty putting life's circumstances in their place and integrating with the whole
- Resist making personal sacrifices even when they know it is for the highest good of all involved
- Feel closed down spiritually and limited in their spiritual vision and wisdom
- Are in need of coming together

within themselves to build their own bridge that connects from within to without.

features of the original flower-essence water

ODOR: slightly like sweet clover; fruity, earthy, "green"

TASTE: tastes like it smells, only stronger

SENSATIONS: warmth in the back of the throat, deeply penetrating from throat to solar plexus and back up through all the chakras

WATER COLOR: clear

physical makeup

ROOT, STEM, LEAVES/LEAFLETS, HEIGHT: Comfrey's brownish black, thick, hearty, tapering, penetrating taproot can be up to 1 foot long, carrying moisture and valuable nutrients to the upper soil levels. Its stem is winged and three-sided, liquid and fibroid inside, rough, hairy, and strong on the outside. The stem branches near the top and is about 2 to 3 feet tall. The dark-green, hairy leaves are thick-ribbed and alternate on the stem until they reach the flowers. Near the base of each flower cluster appear two smaller leaves that grow in opposites and are shaped like wings. Leaves are oval and lance-shaped on a nearly sessile stalk, with the underside rough and prickly and the top side soft and fuzzy. They have pronounced veins that are more prominent on the leaf's underside, and the veins look like skin.

FLOWER COLOR: Lavender to mauve and yellowish white

FLOWERS: The flowers taste and smell like a sweet, earthy green. The buds taste like squash or a raw potato. Flowers grow in clusters on a short, drooping raceme and are somewhat incurved toward the top and turn toward the same side. The purplish green, fuzzy sepal is divided into five lanceolate sections, and each tiny, drooping, tubular flower also has five segments with curved yellowish white edges. Each segment has a darker lavender stripe vertically in the center, and a yellowish white horizontal stripe around the middle. There are five short stamens shaped somewhat like a bear claw, with short, erect, yellowish white anthers. The pistil has a long yellowish white "tongue" emerging from the center. The fruit consists of four angular, shiny brown-to-black nutlets. The flower fades quickly after being picked.

BLOOMING PERIOD: May and June

doctrine of signatures

- The division of the sepal, the striking division of the flower's unique segments (along with the plant's physical ability to stimulate cell division), and the structure of the leaves' veins represents a proficiency for putting things into perspective while acknowledging integration and harmony of the whole.

- The tubular, clustered flowers droop toward the ground and are protected by the plant's leaves, making a statement of protection, surrender, and service for the highest good.

- The lavender color of the flowers represents the sixth chakra and comfrey's spiritual vision, wisdom, and clairvoyant perceptions that are especially needed during times of sacrifice for the greater good. The yellowish white colors represent the third and seventh chakras and our ability to transcend thoughts to arrive at our higher consciousness, empowering ourselves to seek Divine intervention and to act in the best interests of the highest good for all.
- The rough, prickly underside and the soft, fuzzy topside of the leaves symbolize the coming together of opposites, building a bridge of healing from within to without, transcending emotional barriers with spiritual guidance.
- The protruding tongue-like center of the pistil emerging from the core of the flower symbolizes our inner voice and the taste and expression of our sweet essence that comes from deep within; this signature guides us to access prayer and meditation to help us speak our spiritual truths, and to communicate sensitively with others.

Helpful suggestions

Comfrey flower essence is especially recommended for those times when one must make a personal sacrifice in order to serve the whole. This could refer to a personal sacrifice within yourself that doesn't include other people, or it could refer to a personal sacrifice that includes other people, be it your family, work colleagues, or friends. Take three to four drops of the flower essence when you have time to be alone during the daytime or at night before bed. Visualize the inside of the drooping, tubular flower. It may be difficult to sit inside it because you will probably slide out as it droops to the ground. Just take a peek and look inside from below. Notice the flower's ability to seclude itself and its sense of protection. Look at the colors inside the flower's walls as they shine from the outside light. Notice the bright lavender/mauve colors and all the concise lines and divisions that the petals have, yet how they are all connected in a circle with each other. Feel the humbleness and the strength of this flower. Get in touch with the service you will need to make that will benefit the whole of your situation. Pray for spiritual guidance and insight that will help you offer this service and that will guide you to your highest needs.

Affirmations

- "I seek spiritual guidance within and pray for vision and truth that will help me see the highest good for my situation."
- "I am developing the capacity to help myself so that I can help others."
- "I acknowledge that this is a cycle in my life in which personal service is needed and that I will continue to love, protect, and nurture myself and seek spiritual guidance during this time."

case History

Joan, a woman in her early forties and a doctor of Oriental medicine, experienced the Comfrey flower essence as a birthing plant that helped her "build bridges" that came together and supported her while making a sacrifice to the best good of a situation. Joan felt caught between her own career needs and those of her husband, in addition to her clients' personal and medical needs. She was torn between the security of her career practice and relocating with her husband on his "mission."

With Comfrey, Joan felt that she was able to find inner words that helped her reach out in her communication and speak her spiritual truths to her husband from deep within. She was able to let go by seeing the greater connection, including her role in the community. Joan felt sad while letting go, and she experienced a release with help from her own spiritual guidance, clarity, and wisdom. She realized that by offering service to her husband through offering to relocate, she created a greater understanding of this cycle in her life, and that the service she gave was a cycle in time that would change when the next cycle took its course. Joan also felt balanced and whole in the decision she made to serve a higher purpose.

Now, several years later, Joan is reaping the rewards of her choice. Her husband has fulfilled his career needs as a pastor, and she not only has a lucrative practice, but also works with her husband on their shared mission in the church.

LfE's Research provers' project findings

PHYSICAL SYMPTOMS

CRAVINGS: None

SENSATIONS: Sighing, constriction in the throat that then opened up from throat to the top of the head, increased intensity of heartbeat — stronger, not faster, for about fifteen minutes

PAIN: None

MODALITIES:

    WORSE: None indicated

    BETTER: Evening and early A.M.

HEAD: Cloudy

EYES: None

FACE: None

EARS: None

STOMACH: None

ABDOMEN: None

BOWEL CONDITION: Diarrhea

URINE: None

FEMALE: None

MALE: More sexual energy

EXTREMITIES: None

BACK: None

SKIN: Rash on chest that went away when remedy no longer taken

EMOTIONAL SYMPTOMS

PATTERNS OF BALANCE: "more grounded yet spiritually connected," "anticipation of big opening and breakthrough," "fewer fears," "emotional cleansing," "hope," "optimism," "love," "creative expression," "fear lifted," "depression lifted as essence was taken longer"

PATTERNS OF IMBALANCE: "emotional ambivalence," "slightly depressed," "teary,"

"vulnerable," "anxiety," "depressed," "sadness," "felt growth through 'painful' emotions," "felt fear"

MENTAL SYMPTOMS
PATTERNS OF BALANCE: "higher mental
clarity," "more intuitive," "felt my depression
lift as I continued to take the essence longer"
PATTERNS OF IMBALANCE: "depressed and
weighted down"

SPIRITUAL REFLECTIONS
"Cosmic awareness," "opened a channel of
insight," "new sense of spiritual discipline
with conscious concentration," "feels more
open," "experienced a connection with
being guided spiritually," "more prayer and
awareness of prayer being answered"

DREAMS/NIGHTMARES
Dreams in general were more frequent and
more powerful in the moment, but not
always remembered.

One prover commented that she
experienced strange images as she fell
asleep, with small lizard-like animals peer-
ing out of the dark undergrowth: an eye
with a star, a comet, and a rising sun. She
also had an image of a male Native American staring intently at her from a dark
doorway, as if in an adobe shelter of some
sort, which left her wondering who he
was and why he appeared. She felt that
he might be a spiritual guide or a spiritual seer.

CRIMSON MONKEYFLOWER

(Mimulus cardinalis)
PRIMARY QUALITY: PERSONAL POWER

FAMILY: Snapdragon or Figwort (Scrophulariaceae)
OTHER NAMES: Scarlet Monkeyflower, Mimulus
WHERE FOUND: In clumps and groups along cliffs and hillsides near and in wet places; along flowing mountain brooks, streams, springs, and seeps in shady places from Montana to Alaska and throughout the West; native to North America
ELEVATION: 1,800' to 8,000'
ENERGY IMPACT (CHAKRA CORRESPONDENCE): first, second, and fifth chakras
KEY RUBRICS FOR POSITIVE HEALING PATTERNS: communicating emotional bitterness in a positive way, male sexuality, confidence, courage
KEY RUBRICS FOR SYMPTOMS AND PATTERNS OF IMBALANCE: aggressiveness, anger, "sticky" relationships, verbal abuse
OTHER RUBRICS: abandonment, addiction, bullying, calm, challenge, cleansing, communication, community, compassion, conscious, family, fears, flow, frustrated emotions, expression, highest good, impulsiveness, menses, moodiness, overcome emotions, passion, personal power, possessiveness, powerlessness, purification, release, restless, root chakra, self-confidence, self-respect, solar plexus, spleen chakra, strength, support, throat chakra, unworthiness, voice, water, worthiness

Traditional use

Historical medicinal use is unknown by the author. The fresh plants, though slightly bitter, may be eaten raw for salad and greens.

Homeopathic use

Unknown to author.

positive Healing patterns

- Takes us back to our roots or past to heal emotional bitterness such as anger, addictions, impulsiveness, sexual obsessions, bullying, possessiveness, inability to get along with others, an overall feeling of powerlessness, and fears at the core level.

- Helps us let go of sticky relationships or situations that we find ourselves in.

- Helps us tap into our own sweet nectar to gain or regain personal power by exploring, identifying, releasing, and working with our core emotions.

- Allows us to become compassionate, strong, courageous, and full of passion for life by claiming our personal power.

- Teaches us to express ourselves from our highest nature as we nurture and feed ourselves from our own sweet nectar.

symptoms and patterns of imbalance

Crimson Monkeyflower may be an appropriate flower essence for those who

- Are stuck in core emotions such as anger, resentment, and overall emotional bitterness
- Tend to keep their emotions bottled up inside, yet one slight emotional trigger will cause them to "blast out" their emotions and anger
- Feel stuck in "sticky" relationships or situations, and want help getting out
- Have lost the taste of the sweetness of life.

features of the original flower-essence water

Odor: very fragrant, with a bittersweet tinge
Taste: fruity, fragrant, and light
Sensations: uplifting, gentle, soothing, warm tingling from throat to genitals
Water Color: clear

physical makeup

Root, Stem, Leaves/Leaflets, Height: The roots of crimson monkeyflower are stronger than those of yellow mon-

keyflower, and the stems tend to be tall, slender, and erect, growing up to 3 feet high. The stems are fuzzy, resinous, round, and bright green. Crimson monkeyflower's dark-green, long, oval-shaped leaves (up to $4\frac{1}{4}$ inches long) grow in opposites and are sticky, hairy, and coarsely toothed, with clasping stems. The leaves have several noticeable parallel veins that appear indented.
Flower Color: Crimson red to reddish orange
Flowers: The flowers have a spicy smell although they taste sweet, especially at the center. The irregular, two-lipped, sticky flower is about 2 inches wide and 1 inch long with five petals or lobes; it is a little larger than the yellow monkeyflower. The petals join in a long tube or funnel, with the upper lip's two broad lobes pointing upward and the lower lip's three notched broad lobes pointing downward. Two sets of fuzzy yellow stamens line the throat of the flower, and the sepals are also hairy and sticky.
Blooming Period: March to October

doctrine of signatures

- Like yellow monkeyflower, the most prominent signature of crimson monkeyflower is that it grows in or near flowing water. Water represents emotions, moods, and feelings. The fact that the plant prefers flowing waters demonstrates movement and cleansing of feelings and emotions.
- The hairiness and stickiness of this plant represent the kinds of sticky

situations or relationships that we find ourselves in, yet with help from flowing waters or by letting our emotions flow with our feelings we have the capability to let go of whatever it is we feel stuck in.

- The crimson red and reddish orange colors of crimson monkeyflower represent the root and spleen chakras, or first and second chakras, which relate to emotions such as reactivity, moodiness, aggression, anger, impulsiveness, sexual obsession, bullying, inability to get along with others, possessiveness, worrying, and powerlessness. These emotions are powerfully linked to our creative consciousness and can be overcome. The fuzzy yellow stamens represent the solar plexus and include emotions or attitudes such as fear, uncertainty, judgment, mental bullying, worrying, and moodiness.

- The lobes of the flower taste bitter, yet at the deep end of the tube that joins the flower's petals is a sweet nectar. The bitterness represents our own emotional bitterness, which can be overcome when we go back into our past to heal what was lost or stuck. Through the healing process, we are able to tap into our own sweet nectar, regaining personal power, compassion, strength, courage, and a passion for life.

- Like the yellow monkeyflower, and as a member of the snapdragon family, the funnel-like part resembles a throat that opens into a mouth, giving it a signature for communication and expression — the fifth-chakra center. The sweet nectar at the end of the funnel reminds us of our highest good; from that place we apply our own sweet nectar as we communicate and express ourselves.

Helpful suggestions

Find a cozy spot for doing the following exercise:

Get a large bowl of warm water, a bath towel, and a bottle of Crimson Monkeyflower essence. Put your bare feet into the warm water. Add several drops of Crimson Monkeyflower essence to the bowl and place several drops of the essence under your tongue. Get into a comfortable position and close your eyes. Allow yourself to relax and breathe all the way down to your feet. Feel the warmth of the water and begin to slightly wiggle your toes or move your feet gently in the water. Feel the gentle flow of movement in your body as you do this.

Get in touch with how you have been feeling over the past month or so. What deep emotions are you holding on to? Where did they come from? How did they begin? Let yourself experience them. Breathe into the experience. You may want to continue moving your feet or still them, whatever is most comfortable to you.

Take your experience into the mouth of the crimson-colored monkeyflower.

Taste the bitterness of its petals and the bitterness of your experience. Gradually find your way to the mouth of the flower and slide down the funnel to its sweet nectar. Take a sip of the nectar and notice how you feel. Take as much as you need, letting go of some part of your bitterness with every sip. Imagine the nectar at the core of your being and see yourself taking a sip of your own sweet nectar as you are embraced by the core of the flower. Hold on to the feeling that it gives you — or, rather, that you are giving yourself. Gather your courage and strength and claim your personal power as you slowly find your way out of the flower's mouth. Stay with your experience as you open your eyes and dry your feet.

Repeat this exercise visually or physically throughout the month as often as you can.

Affirmations

- "I express my anger from my place of highest good."
- "I let go of sticky relationships or friendships that I no longer want."
- "I swim in my sea of emotions, continuously moving and flowing."
- "I am the power that is within me."

Case History

Soma, age forty-eight, took the Crimson Monkeyflower essence for eight days with the intention of resolving old anger and the desire to respond more positively in his life. Each day, he engaged in a conscious meditation when he took the flower essence. He also had a photo of the Crimson Monkeyflower next to him that he could gaze into. He found the Crimson Monkeyflower essence to be calming, nurturing, softening, strengthening, and peaceful.

Soma felt that this essence strengthened his communication, writing, teaching, and speaking skills in an immensely powerful and creative way. He commented that this essence had an effect on his thought patterns, causing "a definite shift from personal worries to calmness, clearness, and creativity of thought." He also experienced "a release of encoded old anger from my body, which was replaced with creativity and elevation."

LFE's Research Provers' Project Findings

PHYSICAL SYMPTOMS

CRAVINGS: None

SENSATIONS: None

PAIN: None

MODALITIES: None

HEAD: None

EYES: None

FACE: None

EARS: None

STOMACH: None

ABDOMEN: None

BOWEL CONDITION: None

URINE: None

FEMALE: None

MALE: None

EXTREMITIES: None

BACK: None

SKIN: None

EMOTIONAL SYMPTOMS

PATTERNS OF BALANCE: "I felt more relaxed," "worked through the ending of a cycle of old anger and rage associated with the last essence I took," "feeling more balanced and at ease," "focused on my emotional well-being more," "felt more calm," "this essence brought my mental and emotional bodies back to a more normal state of being," "helped me be more patient," "offered a feeling of cleansing and healing," "I felt I experienced a breakthrough," "I felt more centered," "I felt more creative"

PATTERNS OF IMBALANCE: "experienced old anger and rage, especially related to the last essence I took"

MENTAL SYMPTOMS

PATTERNS OF BALANCE: "I thought about all the anger and rage I felt while taking the last essence and realized how powerful it was for me," "focused on thoughts more," "reflections of the past," "I took time to think about past behavior," "this essence allowed me to have some perspective on my life; it was gentle, not strong," "it gave clarity about my misunderstandings," "had more insight into things," "more receptive toward understanding"

PATTERNS OF IMBALANCE: "impatience," "misunderstanding," "thoughts of anger and rage," "tension"

SPIRITUAL REFLECTIONS

"I prayed for people I argued with while taking the last essence," "I asked for forgiveness and also gave it to others who had conflicts with me," "this essence helped me feel at peace and calm"

DREAMS/NIGHTMARES

No dreams reported.

DESERT LARKSPUR

(Delphinium scaposum)
PRIMARY QUALITY: GRACEFUL PASSAGE

FAMILY: Buttercup (Ranunculaceae)
OTHER NAMES: Wild Delphinium, Barestem Larkspur, Espuelita, and Naked Delphinium. There are numerous species of larkspur. "Delphinium" is derived from the Greek word *delphis,* which means "dolphin" and refers to the shape of the flower; Dioscorides called the flower "dolphin-head."
WHERE FOUND: open desert, hillsides, knolls, and mesas in Arizona, Utah, Nevada, New Mexico, Montana, Wyoming, and Colorado
ELEVATION: low deserts up to 7,000' in the pine zone
ENERGY IMPACT (CHAKRA CORRESPONDENCE): fifth and sixth chakras
KEY RUBRICS FOR POSITIVE HEALING PATTERNS: ease in communication, positive attitude toward life changes, imagination, clarity
KEY RUBRICS FOR SYMPTOMS AND PATTERNS OF IMBALANCE: difficulty expressing self, resistance to change, lack of awareness
OTHER RUBRICS: anger, anxiety, awareness, birds, breakthrough, brow chakra, calm, change, cheerfulness, children, confidence, creativity, death/dying, denial, discernment, dolphin dream imagery, ease, flexibility, flight, freedom, grace, guidance, harmony, healing, heart imagery, impatience, insight, inspiration, intuition, loneliness, love, motivation, mouth, nerves, patience, psychic, right-brained, security, self-empowerment, spiritual, throat chakra, transition, transmutation, understanding, visualization

Traditional use

Medicinally, various species of larkspur have been used to kill scabies, pubic crabs, and head lice by grinding the seeds and steeping them in either rubbing alcohol, vinegar, or tincture of green soap, depending on the ailment.

Blackfoot women used a species of larkspur (*Delphinium bicolor*) as a blue dye for quill work and to shine and straighten hair. Hopi Indians grind the flowers with corn to produce blue cornmeal; they use this sacred blend in religious ceremonies.

Because the larkspurs contain delphinine and other toxic alkaloids, they are known to be poisonous to livestock, especially sheep and cattle. Larkspur is most poisonous in its earliest stage, decreasing in potency with age.

Homeopathic use

Unknown to author.

positive Healing patterns

- Gives guidance toward higher spiritual truths and ways of living.
- Offers gracefulness in communication and ease in life transitions, such as rites of passage, spiritual initiations, and changing of life cycles.
- Ignites a spark of inspiration that stirs excitement within, tapping into our personal gifts and awakening our potential to embrace higher opportunities and to dance with life.
- Enhances the power to use imagination and clarity of thought to transmute that which serves our highest good. Crystallizes the present and captures the moment.

symptoms and patterns of imbalance

Desert Larkspur may be an appropriate flower essence for those who

- Lack spiritual direction
- Resist change and feel challenges and struggles while facing life transitions
- Lack inspiration, creativity, imagination, guidance, and grace
- Are unaware of their personal gifts and talents
- Lack grace and ease in communication.

features of the original flower-essence water

ODOR: full and sweet
TASTE: full and sweet

SENSATIONS: cooling and soothing in throat
WATER COLOR: clear

physical makeup

ROOT, STEM, LEAVES/LEAFLETS, HEIGHT: Desert larkspurs are showy, erect plants with long, thin stems whose blossoms emerge on a leafless stalk that rises from a cluster of fine or coarse, dark-green, angled leaf blades. They have a woody root stalk. The leaves are palmately divided into lobes and with rounded tips. The seed pods are oval and hollow. Other plants that resemble larkspur are monkshood (aconite), columbine, and shooting star. Larkspur grows in sizable colonies, intermingling with other spring flowers and contributing their bluish purple hues to the colorful bouquet of spring flowers. The average height is 1 to 2 feet, and 2 to 3 feet for the larkspur species in general.
FLOWER COLOR: Royal blue and violet-purple with whitish centers
FLOWERS: The five-petaled, royal blue blossoms are triangular with a pronounced violet-purple backward spur. Inside the spur is a hint of white with purple lines. Their prolonged upper seal also looks similar to the spur of a bird. There are five sepals, and the flower heads are approximately 1 inch in diameter, grouped on a spike-like raceme with yellow stamens and followed by a three-part seed capsule.
BLOOMING PERIOD: March to May

Doctrine of signatures

- The shape of the flower is very bird-like and gives a sense of freedom, grace, ease, and flight. The structure of the plant is very light and gives a definite feeling of being a highly evolved plant.

- The royal blue color is linked to the fifth or throat chakra (communication); that chakra and the Greek name "dolphin," for the shape of the spur, both refer to breath and the understanding that easy and intelligent communication is based on pattern, rhythm, and sound. The purple colors of the flower correspond to the sixth or brow chakra, relating to the process of imagination, inspiration, and creative visualization.

- When drinking the flower-essence water, a powerful cooling and soothing sensation is felt in the throat, which again highlights the throat chakra.

Helpful suggestions

If you like dolphins and can relate to what it would be like to be a dolphin, try this exercise: Take three to four flower-essence drops, then close your eyes and imagine yourself as a dolphin swimming freely in the ocean. You have the freedom to swim where you wish, and you can swim close to shore if you'd like people to swim and play in the water with you. Find your rhythm as you ride the waves of the sea.

Listen to your breath as you take a dive in the water and come up for a new breath. Listen to the tone of your voice as you play and communicate with your other dolphin friends. Listen to the sounds of the ocean within and without. Observe your patterns and stay with those patterns. Feel your freedom and be yourself.

Another exercise is similar to the above: Choose a favorite bird, such as an eagle, hawk, or raven, and imagine yourself to be that bird. Take flight as the bird and feel the grace and ease of swooping and flying. Spread your wings: Extend your arms and, with open hands, move your arms gently up and down as if in the wind. Imagine how it feels to be flying in the air, the personal freedom and empowerment, the insights, the messages, the lessons learned. Use your voice to make a sound like the bird. Receive the gifts of the bird and apply them to your life situation. Remain in the feeling of the true expression and freedom of flight, and embrace who you have become as you enter your new life situation. Look at the opportunity being given to you and welcome it.

Affirmations

- "I am open to the gracefulness of change as I ease into a new life passage."
- "Light shines all the way through me and all around me as I take flight on my journey."
- "I communicate with ease and grace, listening to my breath, rhythm, tone, pattern, and sound."

case History

This flower essence has been given to a variety of people experiencing life transitions. It has been used consistently with much success for young teenage girls entering the rite of passage into womanhood. It has also been used for boys entering manhood, although not as consistently. It has been used for those facing changes in lifestyle, partnership, death and births, initiations, and life cycles. The reports are very positive in helping people to accept and face their life challenges or transitions gracefully, and to feel more at ease with their personal freedom and in expressing and communicating that freedom with self and others.

LFE's Research provers' project findings

PHYSICAL SYMPTOMS

CRAVINGS: Fruit
SENSATIONS: Pulsing at back of throat; a feeling of "expansion" inside of mouth
PAIN: Piercing pain at base of neck on right side; felt that "something was changing"
MODALITIES:
  WORSE: Tired in early evening
  BETTER: None indicated
HEAD: None
EYES: None
FACE: None
EARS: None
STOMACH: Felt more relaxed
ABDOMEN: None
BOWEL CONDITION: None
URINE: None
FEMALE: None
MALE: None
EXTREMITIES: None
BACK: None
SKIN: None

EMOTIONAL SYMPTOMS

PATTERNS OF BALANCE: "calming," "patience with self and others," "felt happy and more relaxed," "eased emotional stresses," "positive feelings," "desire to comfort others," "felt more secure," "was feeling rejected until I communicated," "felt more trust"
PATTERNS OF IMBALANCE: "loneliness," "felt heavier emotionally," "annoyed with daily restrictions and routines," "longing for freedom," "desire to communicate," "was more restless"

MENTAL SYMPTOMS

PATTERNS OF BALANCE: "awareness of changes in the earth as well as in myself," "thinking of various symbols related to dream imagery," "positive attitude and thoughts," "relaxed my fleeting analytical way of thinking about situations which were personal for someone else," "mentally felt good with more clairvoyance; more intuitive, higher understanding or knowing," "increased memory," "more right-brained and less left-brained," "more creative," "letting go of thoughts of the past," "urge to communicate thoughts"

Spiritual Reflections

"I felt a huge trust in destiny, in purpose, in God," "realization and understanding of a Higher Power," "experienced an awareness and understanding of the larger plan for us in the universe and being guided by Divine directions," "we are being cared for and helped through the changes taking place," "it is a comfort to know that, in spite of massive shifts in consciousness and in the environment, we are just where we're meant to be in time and space and we will be cared for," "felt freedom of transformation and forming a new life," "I think this is a remedy to assist people in times of crisis or transition"

Dreams/Nightmares

Increased dream imagery and symbols. Dreams of butterflies and birds. One prover had agitated dreams, while other provers had more peaceful, vivid dream images.

DESERT MARIGOLD

(Baileya multiradiata)
Primary Quality: Flexibility

Family: Sunflower (Compositae)
Other Names: Woolly Marigold, Wild Marigold, Desert Baileya, *Baileya del Desierto,*
Hierba Amarilla, Mary's Gold (in honor of the Virgin Mary)
Where Found: desert areas, slopes, roadsides, and sandy, gravely areas of the South-
west, from Utah and Nevada to southeastern California and Sonora
Elevation: to 5,000'
Energy Impact (Chakra Correspondence): third chakra
Key Rubrics for Positive Healing Patterns: willingness to flow with life's cir-
cumstances, balance of wisdom and intellect
Key Rubrics for Symptoms and Patterns of Imbalance: controlling, overstructured, rigidity, overly intellectual, lack of intuition
Other Rubrics: acceptance, appreciation, attachment, awareness, calm, centeredness,
clarity, confidence, contentment, crown, dreams, emotions, empowerment, environment, flexibility, harmony, insight, nurturing, peace, perspective, purification, quietness,
receptivity, refreshed, relaxed, sleep, solar plexus chakra, taste, trust, uplifting, worry

traditional use

Unknown to author.

homeopathic use

Unknown to author.

positive healing patterns

- Heightens our emotional awareness;
  reminds us to ease the mind, relax
  the senses, and tap into our center
  in order to become empowered.
- Teaches us to be more accepting
  and flexible, less attached to outcomes, and willing to flow with
  life's journeys.

- Helps us to balance intellectualism
  and wisdom.
- Reminds us to take time to cuddle,
  to nurture ourselves, and to find
  softness in our own presence.

symptoms and patterns of imbalance

Desert Marigold may be an appropriate
flower essence for those who

- Are rigid, overstructured, needing
  to be in control
- Are unwilling to try new things, generally feel stiff, hold on too tightly,
  and are overly attached to outcomes

- Tend toward intellectualism rather than trusting intuition.

Features of the original flower-essence water

ODOR: subtle, sweet smell
TASTE: similar to the smell; very subtle
SENSATIONS: a feeling of gentleness, softness, and quietness throughout the body; a subtle tingling sensation in the throat to the solar plexus, then through the upper chakras and out the top of the head
WATER COLOR: clear

physical makeup

ROOT, STEM, LEAVES/LEAFLETS, HEIGHT: Blooming sporadically over a long period of time, the desert marigold is one of the showiest common bloomers of the sunflower family. Its presence graces the desert roadsides, and its long woolly stems and golden-yellow flowers brighten the dry, sandy washes. The velvety soft, well-divided lobed leaves are mostly clustered at the base of the fuzzy, pastel-greenish-grayish-hued stems. The long stems grow in a clump, and each stem bears a single flower.
FLOWER COLOR: Golden-yellow
FLOWERS: The flower heads are daisy-like and about 2 inches in diameter, with a golden-yellow center. The outer rays often bleach out in the sun and turn papery with age. To identify this flower, make sure the seeds have withered ray flowers attached to them. Paperdaisy, a similar member of the sunflower family, grows and blooms at the same time. It is difficult to tell the two apart, except that the paperdaisy has small leaves that grow along the entire length of the stem.
BLOOMING PERIOD: March to May, August to October

Doctrine of signatures

- The intensity of this plant's bright golden-yellow hue corresponds with the third chakra, the solar plexus, and brings a mental awareness that allows for one's rational mind to work more effectively. One's intellect, full of facts and knowledge, is a useful tool to have. Yet beyond the intellectualism lies the wisdom of knowing and intuiting the beauty of life and embracing that beauty in everyday living.
- The golden-yellow color heightens our emotional awareness, energizing and empowering us to break free of old patterns. The center is strong, the color is bright, the petals soft and delicate. Taking time to relax and fill ourselves with this golden-yellow radiance brings us to our center.
- The flow and flexibility of this long fuzzy spinal stem is yet another reflection of the wisdom of flowing with life.

Helpful suggestions

1. Take the time to find a quiet spot to be alone or do this exercise prior to bedtime. Take three to four drops of the Desert Marigold flower essence with the intention to connect with yourself and find your center. Ask

yourself if there is something you are overly attached to. Do you have a desire to understand how to deal with your attachment? Be honest with yourself. In what ways are you rigid? In what ways are you unwilling to negotiate? Is there something you are overly attached to but you don't know how to deal with that attachment?

Identify the attachment. Pick it up and look at it. Turn it around some more. What is your investment in this attachment? How do you know if this attachment serves you?

After you have taken the time to identify, talk to, and look at whatever you are attached to, tell the attachment you are going to put it on hold and ask for guidance in how you can change your relationship with the attachment. Sleep on this and take your time to watch how your relationship with your attachment unfolds while you continue to take the essence over a period of time. When you feel your rigidity, ask yourself if there is something you can learn to replace the rigidity with. Work with this and pray to understand and act upon the ebb and flow of life's graces.

2. Visualize yourself as the tall, flexible stem of the desert marigold plant. See yourself bend softly in the wind. Stand up and actually be the stem; bend back and forth as if the wind were gently blowing on you. Imagine how the breeze would feel. Will you freeze up and not bend, or will you move with the sensations of

the breeze? Allow the wind to carry you. Listen to its sounds and tones. Visualize the golden-yellow flower blossom opening from the top of the stem. Look at its color; notice the neat folds of the petals and bright golden-yellow center. Put yourself in the center. Feel its softness. Reach out and touch the soft, delicate petals. Imagine that softness within yourself. Feel the softness within yourself. Take a deep breath and blow it out as if you were the wind.

Affirmations

- "I honor my ability to be flexible and to flow with the challenges presented to me in my daily life."
- "I trust the wisdom that comes from deep within and I act according to the wisdom as I intuit and understand it."
- "I give thanks to Mother/Father God/ Spirit for all that is given me and for blessing the power of my wisdom."

case History

Mary, a woman in her fifties, came to me for flower essence therapy with several different symptoms. Some of her symptoms included a very busy internal dialogue regarding where to live. She had moved to the Verde Valley of Arizona several months before and had felt some stress in selling her former home. Now more changes were occurring, and she was confused about where to build a new home. Mary said that she was overly attached to what she thought she wanted and wasn't sure if her attachment was serving her best interests or the larger picture. She had been lying awake at night, worrying about what to do and trying to figure out ways to control her future.

I recommended the Desert Marigold to Mary to help her relax, find her center, and be at peace with herself so that she could bend more easily and become more flexible in response to the guidance that would be presented to her. I also suggested some helpful exercises and affirmations to do at bedtime and when she woke up at night. Within two weeks, Mary reported that not only was she sleeping better, but she found herself being more flexible in solving everyday problems and was more willing to go with the flow."

Life's Research Provers' Project Findings

Physical Symptoms

Cravings: None

Sensations: Mouth felt refreshed and improved in taste

Pain: None

Modalities:
  Worse: None
  Better: Daytime, mealtime, sleep

Head: None

Eyes: None

Face: None

Ears: None

Stomach: Calm and relaxed

Abdomen: None

Bowel condition: None

Urine: None

Female: None

Male: None

Extremities: None

Back: None

Skin: None

Other: Taste in mouth was refreshing; sense of smell was keener

Emotional Symptoms

Patterns of Balance: "calm," "content," "comfortable," "neutral," "relaxed," "sadness yet excitement for new beginnings," "quietness," "strength," "uplifting"

Patterns of Imbalance: No comments from provers

Mental Symptoms

Patterns of Balance: "a knowing that I'm responsible for repeating patterns," "viewed things and people around me with a more calm and relaxed attitude," "thoughts and emotions were slowed down so I was able to understand things better," "calm," "quiet mind," "comfortable," "thankfulness," "letting go and starting new," "helped put things into perspective," "helped to see clearly," "trust," "mentally stable"

Patterns of Imbalance: No comments from provers

Spiritual Reflections

"Overall sense of calm, trust, and knowingness"

Dreams/Nightmares

Dreams were very colorful, bright, and animated. Sleep improved. No specific dreams recorded.

DESERT WILLOW

(Chilopsis linearis)
PRIMARY QUALITY: THE EMPRESS

FAMILY: Bigonia (Bignoniaceae)
OTHER NAMES: *Mimbre, Flor de Mimbres, Catalpa linearis,* Desert Catalpa, Jana, Flowering Willow
WHERE FOUND: along desert waterways and washes, grasslands, foothills, and mesas from Redlands, California, east through the Mojave and Colorado deserts, in Arizona deserts, in New Mexico and western Texas along the Pecos and Rio Grande basins to southern Nevada, and in northern Mexico
ELEVATION: 1,500' to 5,500'
ENERGY IMPACT (CHAKRA CORRESPONDENCE): first, third, fourth, fifth, and seventh chakras
KEY RUBRICS FOR POSITIVE HEALING PATTERNS: abundance, appreciation, beauty, communication, feminine sexuality, nourishing, nurturing
KEY RUBRICS FOR SYMPTOMS AND PATTERNS OF IMBALANCE: closed down sensually or sexually with self or partner, lack of love and nurturing
OTHER RUBRICS: arms, breakthrough, breasts, brow, calm, change, cheerfulness, chest, cleansing, clarity, crown chakra, enthusiasm, eyes, faith, feet, femininity, freedom, genitals, gentleness, hands, healing, heart chakra, home, insight, inspiration, love, mind, mindfulness, nose, pelvis, positive imagination, positive thought, prosperity, opening, psychic, purification, receptivity, root chakra, self-empowerment, senses, sensitivity, sensuality, sexuality, simplicity, solar plexus chakra, spiritual, strength, thankfulness, thinking, throat chakra, tingling, transition, trust

traditional use

A tea or moist, hot poultice made with the flowers treats coughing with a flushed face; it also treats chest and lung fatigue with a thin, fast pulse. The leaves, bark, and flowers made into a tea or tincture can be used as an antifungal and anti-Candida agent to treat infections of the intestinal tract and such symptoms as foul burping, acid indigestion, abnormal stools, hemorrhoids, rectal itching, and varicose veins. The crushed leaves and bark can be sprinkled on scratches, scrapes, and minor sores. Native Americans used the wood to make bows. The beauty and grace of this flower catches the eye of those who cultivate it is as an ornamental.

homeopathic use

Unknown to author.

positive Healing patterns

- Nurtures, nourishes, restores, and empowers feminine energy and the power of positive thought and imagination, whether male or female.
- Offers appreciation of beauty, simplicity, and abundance.
- Teaches us to "go with the flow" in life, being receptive and intuitive while letting our hearts open and be touched by faith.
- Encourages the freedom of openly expressing love and sexuality within yourself and with your partner.
- Teaches manifestation from within to without, allowing us to tap into our innermost sensations, thoughts, words, and feelings.
- Opens us toward song and praise.

symptoms and patterns of imbalance

Desert Willow may be an appropriate flower essence for those who

- Are out of touch with their feminine side (male or female)
- Need help in discovering their inner beauty and in loving themselves
- Need nurturing and nourishment
- Feel closed down sexually or sensually within themselves or partners.

features of the original flower-essence water

ODOR: sweet, full, and sensual
TASTE: strong and earthy, somewhat bitter; doesn't taste like it smells

SENSATIONS: eyes opened wider, awareness highlighted, hearing more acute, energized
WATER COLOR: clear

physical makeup

ROOT, STEM, LEAVES/LEAFLETS, HEIGHT: Desert willow is an upright large shrub or a small tree that can reach up to 25 feet tall, with roots that reach 50 feet or more into the ground. The dark-brown trunk is scaly and ridged and can grow to 1 foot in diameter. The long, narrow (6 to 7 inches long, $3/_8$ inch wide) slightly green leaves alternate along the stems and are smooth, untoothed, and somewhat curved with a waxy coating that prevents loss of moisture through the leaf's outer layer. Desert willow is a deciduous tree, dropping its leaves and becoming dormant in hot weather and then forming new tree sprouts and leaves when the summer rains begin.

FLOWER COLOR: Pink to lavender, tinged with whitish yellow and magenta colors

FLOWERS: The pinkish violet, sweet, spicy, sensual fragrance of desert willow and the flower's artistic beauty are unique. The large, showy, sensual flowers are a soft deep pink or lavender, orchid-like and trumpet-shaped, and grow up to $1\,^1/_2$ inches long in 3-to-4-inch terminal clusters. The flower petal has three upper segments and two lower segments, with three pairs of magenta-colored streaks and two yellowish stripes between the magenta streaks. The flower is sprinkled with dots, streaks, and blotches of all the colors in the spectrum. Hiding deep inside the flower are five white stamens with soft yellow anthers. The flowers are followed by long, narrow, brown seed capsules that split lengthwise when mature and remain dangling from the tree long after the leaves and flowers have fallen. **BLOOMING PERIOD:** April through August

Doctrine of signatures

- The soft colors, elegance, and beauty of desert willow's flowers demonstrate a sensual, flowing, loving compassion that is very feminine and nurturing.

- The artistic beauty of the flower also represents an appreciation of beauty, simplicity, and abundance.

- The posture of desert willow's flowing branches, leaves, and flowers represents its ability to come forth in abundance and flow.

- The trumpet-like shape and deep throat of this flower indicates the fifth chakra and, along with all of the above signatures, represents an ability to go into our inner depths of hearing and listening and tune into our deepest energies and vibrations. It also gives an urge to sing out loud and to praise life and all its wonders.

- The deep magenta color of the desert willow flower corresponds with the root chakra and is indicative of our connection to the Earth Mother and our sensuality and power. The pinkish color of the flower also corresponds with the fourth or heart chakra; there is an intertwining of passionate, sensual energy of the root or kundalini currents with the creative, loving force that emanates from the heart chakra. The yellow and white colors relate to the third and seventh chakras, which tap into higher wisdom, intrinsic knowing, and conscious living.

- The taste of the flower essence is very earthy.

Helpful suggestions

When is the last time you took a candle-light bath by yourself or sat under a tree in complete silence or took time to clear your energy by smudging yourself with sage? Desert willow beckons you to love, nurture, and nourish yourself. Take time to be with yourself in a way that you know deep inside serves you best. Prepare a nutritious food or beverage that is relaxing and nourishing to you. Find a place to be alone, be it a candlelight bath, a nature setting, or your favorite couch or chair — whatever place you find to be relaxing and nurturing. Read a book, write a song or poem, listen to your favorite music, or close your eyes and just be with yourself. Enjoy what you give yourself and the way you nurture yourself. Then complete the activity with the food or beverage you prepared — or maybe you started out that way!

Here is a short journey to experience:

First look at the photo of the desert willow and capture her image. Imagine being in the center of her opening and taking in her full sweet fragrance. Feel the scent surround you and invite you to reach deeper inside. Look around you and see her deep magenta colors against the soft pink and lavender petals. Take in all that you can: the beauty of her simple elegance, the movement of her sensual flow, the strength of her abundance, and the wonder of her creative life-force energy. Let your heart and voice sing out to praise life and all its wonders.

Feel the passionate, sensual energy that emanates from your heart center. Give thanks for all that is good in your life!

Affirmations

- "I nurture, nourish, and love myself every moment of every day."
- "I honor my ancient sensual and sexual nature and allow myself to freely express it."
- "I fertilize my thoughts and feelings with an abundant flow of compassion and beauty."

Case History

Cheryl, a woman in her forties, wanted to heal and honor her "feminine side," work toward being a softer person, and tap into a deeper level of intuition, love, compassion, and inner strength with softness. She acknowledged the pain relating to her feminine issues and that for a long time she had been in denial about that pain. She wanted to bring her femininity into balance within herself and with her partner.

I asked Cheryl to do a simple exercise each time she put the essence drops in her mouth: See yourself wearing a sensually soft magenta gown, sitting inside the flower as an empress, leaning against the velvety softness of the flower petal. Breathe in the sweet, spicy fragrance, letting it fill your lungs and your entire being. As you feel the embrace of this sensual aroma, feel the gentle sweetness and strength inside the petal. Listen to your deepest sounds and words. Listen to your breath. In a soft, quiet voice, sing a gentle song that touches your heart. Then sing the song openly to your heart's content. Feel your energy level. Tune in to the power of your vibration. Be with it, stay with it, carry it with you wherever you go.

Cheryl, along with many other women and men, have enjoyed Desert Willow's flower essence and the powerful nurturing that it offers. It helped her become more in touch with her femininity, softer with her partner, and much more appreciative of her body. She discovered that she was able to honor her beauty, within and without, and to freely express herself.

Life's Research Provers' Project Findings

PHYSICAL SYMPTOMS

CRAVINGS: Hungry in general

SENSATIONS: "Felt a great amount of energy passing through my body, as if the channels inside had become widened," tingling in hands, feet, and spine

PAIN: None

MODALITIES:

  WORSE: None indicated

  BETTER: Improved sleep and felt better all day long

HEAD: None

EYES: Increased depth perception: "I see light with ever-so-soft hues," "I saw streaks of light at the horizon at moonrise, which no one else I was with saw."

FACE: None

EARS: Increased sound perception

STOMACH: None

ABDOMEN: None

BOWEL CONDITION: None

URINE: None

FEMALE: Consistently heightened sexual energy; hot energy all day long

MALE: No males in this survey

EXTREMITIES: Leg cramps, tingling, and energy flow in hands and feet

BACK: Tingling and energy through spine

SKIN: None

OTHER: "I felt that I got in touch with my energetic body more strongly than ever before. I felt it as electric currents and tingling sensations and that they were very present in my awareness." "Previously trapped energy is now moving."

EMOTIONAL SYMPTOMS

PATTERNS OF BALANCE: "calming," "balancing," "good feelings," "emotional breakthrough: 'out with the old, in with the new,'" "desiring to feel open and new," "letting go of an old sadness and accepting something new and exciting," "emotionally stable," "aware," "happy and sad," "I feel a sense of taking care of myself first (rare for me)," "I feel a calming balance of truth and serenity," "inner peace," "inner trust," "made me take a good look at myself," "this essence generally made me feel good; I became aware of any negative emotions and was able to reverse them," "felt more empathetic toward others," "able to tap into personal truth," "had the ability to transform sadness into a joyful flow," "crying had a satisfying/transforming feel to it — was cleansing," "I felt appreciative and thankful"

PATTERNS OF IMBALANCE: "irritable with myself when I became judgmental"

MENTAL SYMPTOMS

PATTERNS OF BALANCE: "open mentally," "alert," "patient," "mentally clear," "a judgmental part of me was analytical and critical — and then I become more aware of what I was doing and was boosted by my instincts," "gave me clearer thinking and control of my thoughts," "more aware," "I wanted to take time out to read more," "mental energy less controlling"

PATTERNS OF IMBALANCE: "a bit spacey"

SPIRITUAL REFLECTIONS

"Divineness is all around us," "feel connected to Spirit with this essence," "in times of trial, I feel a trusting that Spirit will watch over me," "am more thoughtful spiritually," "I really loved how this essence helped me spiritually; I was given a lot of information on spiritual development that I feel will always stay with me," "I established deeper contact with what felt like my spiritual body," "I felt new energy sensations like I'm lighter," "I felt that I made new connections with an essential part of myself that has been trying to emerge for some time," "I had a channel of spiritual vision and energy"

DREAMS/NIGHTMARES

"I was in a state between waking and dream. My partner had his hand on my chest. I felt a pulsing in my heart like an orgasm of the heart, and then a cord of light streamed out of my heart. This was a real, bodily felt experience — An incredible opening."

ECHINACEA

(Echinacea angustifolia)
PRIMARY QUALITY: REJUVENATION

FAMILY: Sunflower (Compositae)

OTHER NAMES: Kansas Snakeroot, Black Sampson, Purple Coneflower, Rudbeckia, Spider Flower, *Brauneria angustifolia;* derived from the Greek word *echinos,* which means "hedgehog," referring to the prickly receptacles and scales. Linnaeus named the plant "Rudbeckia" after Rudbeck, father and son, who were his predecessors at Upsala.

WHERE FOUND: Native to the United States, *E. angustifolia (augustifolia)* generally grows west of the Mississippi in dry, open areas, roadsides, fields, and prairies (this is the echinacea used in LFE's Echinacea flower essence). *E. purpurea* grows in areas east of the Mississippi.

ELEVATION: most U.S. climate zones as described above

ENERGY IMPACT (CHAKRA CORRESPONDENCE): first, second, and sixth chakras

KEY RUBRICS FOR POSITIVE HEALING PATTERNS: vitality, cleansing and elimination of old patterns, understanding

KEY RUBRICS FOR SYMPTOMS AND PATTERNS OF IMBALANCE: confusion, exhaustion, rejection, repression, blocked emotions, thoughts, and insights

OTHER RUBRICS: abdomen, aggressiveness, anger, anxiety, appreciation, awareness, binding, brain, brow chakra, calm, challenged, change, communication, consciousness, dreams, emotions, groundedness, head, healing, impatience, mind, nerves, perspective, purging, rejuvenation, relief, repression, revitalized, root chakra, solar plexus, spleen chakra, stomach, surrender, tension, transition

Traditional use

Echinacea was used medicinally by the Plains Indians more than any other plant. They used it to treat the bites of snakes and rabid dogs, fevers, stings, septic sores, and poisoning. They smoked echinacea to relieve headaches, and horses with distemper were treated by blowing smoke into their nostrils. The root was chewed or made into a powder for toothaches, mouth and gum sores, and swollen glands, such as in rheumatism, arthritis, mumps, and measles. Other Native Americans made a juice of echinacea to treat burns and added the juice to water that was sprinkled over coals in "sweats" for purification. Some Indians even used the juice to desensitize their hands, feet, and mouths to help them walk on hot coals during fire rituals.

The early settlers used echinacea as their choice home remedy to cure colds, indigestion, and influenza, and by 1920 it was among the most widely known pharmaceutical herbal drugs in the U.S. Echinacea is still considered one of the best blood cleansers, known today as the "king of the blood purifiers." Echinacea is a natural antibiotic that works like penicillin in the body and is used to build the immune system and to treat exhaustion, lymph glands (when sluggish), infections, fevers, congestion, colds (especially in children), viruses, syphilis, gangrene, gonorrhea, cancer, leukemia, AIDS, eczema, pimples and boils, dull, tired eyes, tonsillitis and mouth sores, prostate glands, peritonitis, poisonous bites and stings, and indigestion.

CAUTION: Overuse of echinacea can cause the very symptoms that it cures.

Homeopathic use

The homeopathic tincture is derived from the roots. It is recommended more in material (lower) doses, rather than in potencies, due to the pathogenic symptoms the higher potencies produce. Echinacea is used as an immune-booster and for blood poisoning, and used to treat conditions similar to those mentioned above in "Traditional Uses." Some symptoms that indicate treatment with an echinacea remedy are confusion, depression, postnasal catarrh, receding gums, mouth sores, ulcerated sore throat, purple tonsils, sour belching and heartburn, painful pectoral muscles, septic conditions from snake bite, gonorrhea, and foul ulcers; all discharges are foul smelling. It is also used to treat suppressed menstrual discharges, recurring

boils, chilliness, nausea, cold flashes, fevers, and the last stages of cancer to ease pain.

positive Healing patterns

- Helps us eliminate old patterns, old thoughts, and old actions, finding new ways to restore and revitalize the true inner nature of Self.
- Stimulates our emotional/mental/ spiritual energies toward purging.
- Helps us foster a new place of growth within ourselves, becoming and being that which is already inherent within.
- Opens us to spiritual insights, clearer understanding, and a deeper perspective on ourselves; helps us internally see our dreams, memories, thought-forms, and imaginings.

symptoms and patterns of imbalance

Echinacea may be an appropriate flower essence for those who

- Feel emotionally, mentally, or spiritually toxic
- Feel rejected and out of touch with themselves
- Need to eliminate unwanted built-up emotional/mental/spiritual patterns
- Feel confused, worried, or concerned about personal inadequacy — who are frustrated and want to understand and release dysfunctional personal patterns
- Lack the ability to access spiritual

vision, intuitive perception, and new ideas, and who lack cohesiveness of thought.

features of the original flower-essence water

ODOR: aromatic and pleasantly strong (not sweet)

TASTE: full and strong, mildly tart yet pleasant (not sweet)

SENSATIONS: feel refreshed, energized, more overall energy; cooling effect

WATER COLOR: clear

physical makeup

ROOT, STEM, LEAVES/LEAFLETS, HEIGHT: Resembling black-eyed Susan, echinacea has a strong erect stem that is coarse, hairy, and bristly and it grows up to 3 feet high. The pale- to dark-green leaves are thick, rough, hairy, and broadly lanceolate, pointed, and coarsely toothed. The leaves grow from 3 to 8 inches long and are mostly basal, with the upper leaves shorter and narrower. The long black taproots take several years to mature. The root and leaves taste sweet at first, with a slightly bitter aftertaste and a tingling sensation in the mouth.

FLOWER COLOR: Lavender/purple

FLOWERS: A solitary composite flowerhead emerges from the stem; it is about 3 to 4 inches across and has a faint musty fragrance. The flower has a cone-shaped center that is petaled with orange-reddish-purple tubular florets with a prickly sunflower-like center, encircled by twelve to twenty light lavender-purplish spreading ray flowers or petals. Each petal typically has four creases. The flowers have a faint aroma and a slightly sweet taste that leaves a tingling sensation in the mouth. In the late fall, when all the petals have fallen off, the stiff seed heads are still visible until they eventually drop off.

BLOOMING PERIOD: July to October

doctrine of signatures

- The coarse, rough, bristly stem and leaves and the stiff center of the flower symbolize our tendency to be coarse, stiff, and rough within ourselves and to externalize such behavior until we become more aware of who we are and work toward eliminating it.

- The deep taproot, taking several years to mature, represents our own growth patterns of developing learned behaviors, habits, emotions, and personality traits over time; as we become more conscious of who we are, it takes time to undo what we have learned and to let go of what we no longer want to be. By exploring and uncovering our own taproots, we are able to restore and revitalize our true essence.

- The orange-reddish center of the flower head also symbolizes the lower chakras (first and second), influencing our roots and where we came from, promoting life-energy, and detoxifying ourselves emotionally and mentally as well as physically. The core protrudes outward and its fiery colors are also symbolic of the sun.

- The lavender/purple ray flowers represent the sixth or brow chakra, which is linked to the immune system, sinuses, ears, eyes, and face. Spiritually, the brow chakra serves as an opening to spiritual insights and creative imagination. It gives us the ability to see our memories, dreams, thought-forms, and imagination. Emotionally and mentally, this center helps us deal with worries, rejection, lack of individuality, and inadequacies.

Helpful suggestions

Take three to four drops of Echinacea flower essence. Notice how it tastes and how it makes you feel. Take some time to sit quietly and check in with how you are feeling. Ask yourself if there is something that stands out — a thought, a feeling, a situation, or another person that holds you back or brings you down. Get in touch with what that is and how it affects your energy and wellness. Now close your eyes and place the issue in a circle filled and surrounded with the colors of orange and red. For example, if it is a feeling, imagine your feeling surrounded and filled with these colors. If it is a situation, visualize the situation filled and surrounded with reds and oranges.

When you have captured the visualization, hold onto it for several minutes. Take several deep breaths, breathing into the fiery circle and then breathing out of the circle. As you breathe in, imagine that you are filling the circle and the situation (feeling, thought, person) with good feelings and positive energy. As you breathe out, imagine that you are releasing any bad feelings or negativity. Continue to breathe with this concept in mind several more times, with each breath becoming deeper and deeper. See your image slowly fade away.

Now imagine purple ray flowers extending outward from the circle of reds and oranges. The purple rays form a crown around the inner circle of glowing fiery colors. Imagine the purple rays stretching from the circle where you have placed your issue to your head. Imagine the purple color all around you. Notice anything you see or feel. Breathe the purple color slowly into your throat, hold your breath, and then slowly let it go. Now let the purple rise to your brow chakra. Breathe in and through the brow chakra, hold your breath, and slowly let it go. Next take the purple all the way up to the top of your head. Breathe it in and let it dissolve out of your head. Again notice how you feel. Allow yourself some time to sit quietly and be with your experience before you reenter your world.

Affirmations

- "I am the power of rejuvenation, change, and new growth."
- "I am eliminating that which holds me back and I am moving forward."
- "I find deep satisfaction in letting go of the old and bringing in the new."

case History

Sheila, age twenty-one, was attracted to taking the Echinacea flower essence. Her work at a coffee shop was stressful for her, especially on busy days. While taking the essence, she felt that her "energy and spirits were lifted up," she slept more deeply at night, her breathing patterns improved, she had more clarity, and she generally felt less burdened emotionally. She also stated that she felt "more connected to a different plane of consciousness — still in the present one, but in a new and more elevated one at the same time." When Sheila wasn't taking the essence, she found that her energy level decreased, she was more emotional, and she experienced back pain.

LFE's Research provers' project Findings

Physical Symptoms

CRAVINGS: Drank more water, craved less sugar, more protein cravings, appetite increased

SENSATIONS: Tightening in throat, tingling and numbness under tongue

PAIN: None

MODALITIES: Inconsistent

HEAD: Headaches — "waves of pain in my brain"

EYES: None

FACE: None

EARS: None

STOMACH: Vomiting

ABDOMEN: None

BOWEL CONDITION: None

URINE: None

FEMALE: None

MALE: Relief of prostatic constriction

EXTREMITIES: None

BACK: None

SKIN: None

OTHER: "Lack of sleep at night, yet lots of energy throughout the day," "slight increase in physical exercise," "intense headache and vomiting the third day of taking the essence; the last day I had an unobstructed productive flow of energy," "experienced a deep gut cleansing," "tension in muscles and nervous system intensified, reaching a point of major stress, and then I began breathing more easily and becoming more calm," "decrease of energy when I stopped taking the essence," "major energy boost"

Emotional Symptoms

PATTERNS OF BALANCE: "felt a rapid clearing of feelings and an increase of 'emotional light,'" "release of emotional tension helped ease physical stress," "seemed to make tasks easier as emotions mellowed," "felt refreshed, released, and settled," "ease of stressors," "feel more organized and settled," "felt comfortable and released," "breakthrough of emotional energy leading to communication and creativity on a higher level," "emotions heightened," "felt a breakthrough allowing me to feel calm and flowing," "felt more grounded," "some old trapped energy/charge seemed to be making its way out of me; the vomiting wasn't related to the flu or a food problem, just a deep moving of energy at a gut level," "deeper calm," "helped me find a quiet place," "craved time to be alone," "more aware of my emotions," "more flexibility"

PATTERNS OF IMBALANCE: "felt more anger and frustration, which led to a breakthrough," "uncomfortable expression of anger," "emotionally and physically stressful," "intense," "unacceptance of life's circumstances," "difficulty making adjustments," "anxiety," "felt I was going to scream," "heightening of emotions from laughter to tears," "irritability"

MENTAL SYMPTOMS

PATTERNS OF BALANCE: "easier to concentrate," "calmer, more removed or observant of the situations at hand," "realized the force and intensity needed to move out old energy patterns," "active wondering and questioning," "quieting of mind," "more observing of self and seeking in a more intense way than usual," "brought issues to consciousness," "more clarity," "mind more active," "more clarity of thought," "more grounded," "intellectual clarity"

PATTERNS OF IMBALANCE: "thought about what to do or what needed to be done when I couldn't sleep at night, felt 'heady,'" "confusion and trying to figure things out," "more difficulty concentrating," "stress due to mental focus on normal life stuff," "spaciness"

SPIRITUAL REFLECTIONS

"Made general meditation easier," "I have great volumes of energy moving through me; it seems I was better able to track it and stay conscious of my inner workings," "felt more creative"

DREAMS/NIGHTMARES

"I am with a man who has been an important teacher for me in the past. We are facing each other, standing and looking into each other's eyes. He is telling me how to work with the new energy, rather than letting it scatter and disperse out of my head."

Most provers had an increase of dream awareness. Dreams helped them work out stress-related feelings.

EVENING PRIMROSE (WHITE)

(Oenothera caespitosa)

PRIMARY QUALITY: INNER STRENGTH

FAMILY: Evening Primrose (Onagraceae)

OTHER NAMES: Tufted Evening Primrose, White Stemless Evening Primrose, Rockrose, Sandlily

WHERE FOUND: native to North America; grows on dry, stony, and rocky slopes, roadsides, railway embankments, and ponderosa forest clearings throughout the West

ELEVATION: 3,000' to 7,500'

ENERGY IMPACT (CHAKRA CORRESPONDENCE): fourth and seventh chakras

KEY RUBRICS FOR POSITIVE HEALING PATTERNS: awakening, purity, self-identity, healing issues related to mother, nurturing, bonding

KEY RUBRICS FOR SYMPTOMS AND PATTERNS OF IMBALANCE: depression, rejection, unclear identity, unclear values, issues with mother

OTHER RUBRICS: aches, anxiety, ceremony, crown chakra, earth, emotional wounds, feet, feminine, gentleness, hands, heart chakra, hidden, link, meaning of life, moon, nervousness, powerful, prayer, reevaluate, root, self-identity, sensitivity, sexuality, strength, subtleness, suppression, tingling

Traditional use

There are many and varied evening primroses, and the entire family is known to be useful in many ways. The Blackfoot Indians boiled the leaves and stems and dried the roots as food during the winter. Crushed seeds and leaves were made into a poultice to treat wounds and bruises. Navajo Indians use the white-stemmed evening primrose in a lotion to treat boils, and they use the entire plant as a poultice to treat spider bites. The plant is also used as a medicine by the Navajo in the Bead Way, Big Star Way, Red Ant Way, and Blessing Way ceremonies.

The evening primrose family has also been known to treat spasmodic asthma, whooping cough, gastrointestinal disorders, irritated bladder, and chronic diarrhea. The seed oils contain fatty acids required for healthy skin and are very high in essential oils, especially gamma-linoleic acid, which eases PMS, lowers blood pressure, and rebuilds red-blood-cell mobility in people with multiple sclerosis. Other uses include the treatment of alcoholism, allergies, hyperactivity, dry and flaky skin, dandruff, schizophrenia, heart disease, cancer, psoriasis, anorexia nervosa, nervous sensitivity, and Parkinson's disease. Hildegard of Bingen recommends gathering a bouquet of primroses and bandaging the bouquet onto the heart like a compress during sleep to calm the nerves and to bring happiness.

homeopathic use

The mother tincture is prepared from the fresh plants and is used to treat *Cholera infantum,* diarrhea, and hydrocephalus.

positive healing patterns

- Encourages us to participate in ceremonies honoring the earth and the moon; by doing so we will find, gather, and nurture our inner strength.
- Helps us uncover hidden emotional wounds, especially related to our mothers, and to bond with our feminine nature including sexuality issues.
- Aids depression, rejection, sexual suppression, and nervous and anxiety disorders through prayer and meditation.
- Helps us to reevaluate and reconnect with the meaning and value of life.
- Brings a sense of purity and calm throughout our being.
- Helps us tap into the depths of our own sweet nectar or core essence, linking and awakening our physical, emotional, mental, and spiritual selves.

symptoms and patterns of imbalance

Evening Primrose may be an appropriate flower essence for those who

- Lack inner strength and are overly sensitive
- Are prone to depression, nervousness, anxiety, rejection, or sexual suppression
- Have unhealed childhood issues that relate especially to the mother, have not bonded with the mother, or feel rejected by the mother
- Are confused about their identity.

features of the original flower-essence water

Odor: subtle and sweet, yet potent

Taste: subtle, not very flavorful although it tastes like fresh spring water

Sensations: light-headed, refreshed, flutter in heart, feeling quiet, experienced a "clearing"

Water Color: clear; flower petals became translucent in the water

physical makeup

Root, Stem, Leaves/Leaflets, Height: The root is yellowish with a white inner flesh. The sturdy bluish green leaves grow in a basal rosette that comes directly from the root crown. The soft, hairy, velvety leaves are variously toothed and range from $1\frac{1}{4}$ to 4 inches long, emerging from a petiole almost equal in length.

Flower Color: White

Flowers: The pleasantly sweet-scented white flowers open in the evening and close soon after the sun shines on them the following day. The flower grows up to 3 inches across, with four large, showy, overlapping petals that appear very delicate. The petals emerge from a slender floral tube that rises from a tuft of narrow leaves and contains a sweet nectar. Only long-tongued hawkmoths can get to the nectar. The thin flower petals have slight veins, and the center of the flower is yellowish with eight long, delicate, whitish stamens and yellowish anthers. Each flower lives for only one night, and the following day it turns pink as it wilts.

Blooming Period: March to June, September to October

Doctrine of signatures

- The flower emerges from a tuft of leaves that grow directly from the root crown, and the significance of the white flower (seventh or crown chakra) demonstrates a magnetic healing flow of energy from the root crown to the crown at the top of the head, thus linking consciousness of the physical body, emotional body, and mental body with spiritual consciousness. The flower wilts to a gentle pink color, corresponding with the power, compassion, and love of the heart or fourth chakra.
- The soft yet strong velvety, hairy leaves symbolize gentle strength.
- The flower appears delicate, yet it's stronger than it seems; its nectar is deep and sweet, yet it can grow from dry, rocky ground. This is symbolic of having a strong foundation or connection to earth,

taking in earth's nectar and giving it back to Spirit. The physical vitality of the flower lasts only one night, giving the flower a full appreciation of valuing its short life.

- The flowers bloom toward evening, all evening long, and in the early morning before being hit by the sun. This is a significant signature of its relationship to the moon, the feminine, and the mother.

Helpful suggestions

Make a commitment to take at least a month to observe and experience how you value yourself and the way you live. Take Evening Primrose flower essence on a daily basis at least twice a day throughout your selected time period. Ask yourself how you are like your mother in ways that you do and don't like. Identify any old emotional wounds that have been hidden over the years, which pertain to your relationship with your mother or a mother figure. How has your relationship with your mother, and your relationship with yourself in response to your mother, affected who you are and how you live? What are you willing to accept in your relationship with your mother? What are you willing to change within yourself and your response/s to your mother? How has this relationship influenced who you are, your relationship to yourself, your relationship to others, and how you live? If there has been an absence of a mother in your life, how has this affected you? What have you accepted and not accepted? Evaluate and tap into the core of these questions through-out this cycle. Seek professional therapy, counseling, body work, or whatever is needed to help you uncover any emotional wounds that reach out for healing.

During the full moon(s) of this cycle, spend an hour or so outside under your favorite tree or spot, either by yourself or with a friend or a circle of friends. Thank Spirit for the earth and the moon, and for all that you have and are in this life.

Say a prayer of thanks and honor for your mother and for all the things she has shown you. Say a prayer of thanks for yourself and for the ways that you have listened and what you have learned. Ask for guidance to help you to further heal old wounds and issues related to your mother and to yourself in response to your mother. Keep your intention clear, and stay focused on your desire to heal.

affirmations

- "I am guided by the Light to the doorway of my soul."
- "I happily and freely celebrate my cleansing and renewal."
- "I honor and embrace my mother and myself unconditionally."

case History

Shana, age forty-two, took the White Evening Primrose flower essence as a med-itation to help her get in touch with her relationship to her mother. She felt that if she could understand that relationship more clearly, she would understand herself

and her own femininity better. Because Shana didn't live near her mother, she called her about every week to check in and see how she was doing.

While taking the essence, Shana found that she was better able to hear her mother speak, and she learned things about her that she hadn't known before. She became more sensitive and receptive, not only to her mother's needs, but about her mother's life experiences and the wisdom she has gained. Shana found herself softening toward her mother and felt her heart open. She had a greater realization of who her mother is, without judgment and criticism, and she accepted the part of her mother that is "human" and that appears "limiting." Not only did Shana nurture and change how she saw her mother, she also had greater insight in how she viewed herself. Shana comments that she made some "significant changes" within herself and is grateful for the Evening Primrose flower essence.

Lfe's Research provers' project findings

PHYSICAL SYMPTOMS

CRAVINGS: Spicy foods, water

SENSATIONS: Tingling sensations in hands and feet

PAIN: Neck and backaches

MODALITIES: None

HEAD: Holding stress in neck and head

EYES: None

FACE: None

EARS: None

STOMACH: None

ABDOMEN: None

BOWEL CONDITION: None
URINE: None
FEMALE: Increased sexual energy, more hot flashes in top half of body
MALE: None
EXTREMITIES: Tingling sensations in hands and feet
BACK: Backaches
SKIN: None

EMOTIONAL SYMPTOMS

PATTERNS OF BALANCE: "more relaxed and at peace with myself," "I feel nurtured"
PATTERNS OF IMBALANCE: "more irritated than normal by others who complain and are impatient"

MENTAL SYMPTOMS

PATTERNS OF BALANCE: "more calm," "peaceful," "relaxed"
PATTERNS OF IMBALANCE: "felt mentally blocked due to neck- and back-aches," "sensitive," "nervous," "anxious"

SPIRITUAL REFLECTIONS

"Felt stronger and closer spiritually, chanted more, increased meditation and yoga, felt a connection with sexuality and spirituality"

DREAMS/NIGHTMARES

None reported by provers.

HONEYSUCKLE

(Lonicera japonica 'Halliana')
PRIMARY QUALITY: HARMONY

FAMILY: Honeysuckle (Caprifoliaceae)

OTHER NAMES: Halliana, Hall's Honeysuckle, Japanese Honeysuckle, *jin yin hua*, Gold and Silver Flower

WHERE FOUND: A native of Japan, Korea, Manchuria, and China, this honeysuckle is cultivated in most areas of the United States with preference for full sun or part shade, growing along fences and hedgerows, tolerating poor drainage once started.

ELEVATION: all U.S. climates

ENERGY IMPACT (CHAKRA CORRESPONDENCE): third and seventh chakras

BACH FLOWER REMEDY: Honeysuckle (*L. caprifolium*) is used for those who tend toward nostalgia and homesickness, and who dwell on past events that were filled with happy memories. Honeysuckle resembles strength and wisdom, and the ability to let go of those attachments.

KEY RUBRICS FOR POSITIVE HEALING PATTERNS: balance, concentration, intimacy, integration, optimism

KEY RUBRICS FOR SYMPTOMS AND PATTERNS OF IMBALANCE: attachment, mental tension, nostalgia, lack of harmony with self and others

OTHER RUBRICS: ambition, anxiety, apathy, avoidance, balance, calm, charm, cleansing, communication, companionship, confidence, cooperation, creativity, crown chakra, emotional attachments, enthusiasm, focus, gentleness, grace, groundedness, healing, holding on, homesickness, imbalance, individuality, insight, letting go, light, loneliness, mental attachments, mental clarity, mutuality, opposites, partnership, purification, reconciliation, solar plexus chakra, spirituality, understanding, wisdom

Traditional use

Lonicera japonica was first recorded in the *Tang Ben Cao* in A.D. 659 and is still commonly used as an important Chinese cooling herb to clear heat, toxins or "fire energy," and poisons from the body. The flowers and stems make a cooling summer drink that can be used to treat diarrhea and to cool fevers. *L. japonica* has many properties in common with European species of honeysuckle, including such components as tannins, flavonoids, mucilage, sugars, and salicylic acid (from which aspirin was once made). Research has demonstrated the plant's ability to raise or lower blood pressure. Its antibacterial, anti-inflammatory, antispasmodic, and detoxifying properties are used to treat flu, coughs, catarrh, asthma, painful joints, laryngitis, boils, diarrhea and gastroenteritis (related to food poisoning), swollen lymph glands, the acute stages of rheumatoid arthritis, and the onset of a feverish cold characterized by sore throat, headaches, and thirst. The stems and branches are used to increase circulation of energy (or *qi*) by eliminating heat in the acupuncture meridians. The flowers can be used for perfumes and potpourri. *L. j. 'Hallianna'* is also grown as a ground cover and used for erosion control.

homeopathic use

The species *Lonicera pericylmenum* is used as a homeopathic remedy to treat marked irritability with violent outbursts.

positive healing patterns

- Brings together opposites (with self or others) in mutual balance, integration, and harmony.
- Highlights partnerships or companionship while maintaining individuality.
- Teaches charm and grace in expression of self.
- Helps us "purify" the past and stabilize the present by letting go of dreamy nostalgic and ungrounded memories that don't serve us.
- Helps us concentrate, focus, and increase keener mental activities, which in turn build confidence and optimism.
- Heightens hopes for new possibilities and the potential for happiness.

symptoms and patterns of imbalance

Honeysuckle may be an appropriate flower essence for those who

- Grieve the loss of a loved one, knowing that the happiness once experienced with that person cannot return in this lifetime
- Feel out of balance with themselves or with others, can't seem to be in "sync," and lack interest in present circumstances
- Have difficulty maintaining their individuality in partnerships and strive for balance, integration, and harmony in their partnership and within themselves
- Feel anxious, have too much mental tension, and are confused by and dwell on their past memories and experiences, which may or may not be reality-based, or on life goals that have not yet manifested
- Are out of touch with the "sweetness" of life and the "sweetness" within themselves due to old fears and the inability to let go in order to integrate the past with new memories and experiences of the present.

features of the original flower-essence water

Odor: powerfully sweet and aromatic
Taste: powerfully sweet and aromatic

SENSATIONS: Lightness in solar plexus, refreshing taste, uplifting; vital force feels stronger.

WATER COLOR: clear and slightly milky

physical makeup

ROOT, STEM, LEAVES/LEAFLETS, HEIGHT: Honeysuckle (*L. japonica*) is an evergreen vine or shrub and a vigorous twining climber. It can grow up to 15 feet high, covering 150 square feet. The stem is tough and slightly hairy. The slightly hairy, veiny, oblong leaves are shiny green on the top side with a duller green underside. They grow in opposites, and each leaf is connected to a small pair of leaves from which the flower emerges. The lower leaves are stalked, while the upper and smaller leaves underneath the flowers join across the stem, forming a disk. Following the flowers, poisonous black berries appear.

FLOWER COLOR: Opens white, then turns yellow

FLOWERS: The flowers carry a rich and powerful, sweet fragrance. The creamy white tubular flowers are borne in pairs and divided into five lobes that split into two diverging lips. The upper lip consists of four uniting lobes, and they look like little feet or hands with four toes or fingers. The lower, single lobe or lip arches backward. The corolla tube is from 1 to 2 inches long. Five long, white, spindly stamens with yellow anthers and one pale green pin-headed pistil emerge from the center.

BLOOMING PERIOD: June, July, August, September

doctrine of signatures

- The significance of the leaves growing in pairs (twice) and the flowers growing in pairs highlights the plant's signature of balance and partnership, bringing together opposites in harmony and cooperation. This signature also resembles the bringing together of one's own inner balance, peace, and joy.

- The sweet, powerful aroma, the taste of the flowers, and the flower's overall appearance bring an amazing feeling of grace and gentleness, highlighting imagination and perhaps longing for the sweetness in life once experienced. This signature treats that which it cures, offering sweetness and happiness in the present.

- The white color of the flower indicates the seventh chakra and a purification of past to present; it is cleansing and stabilizing to an individual's entire energy system. The yellow color of the flower represents mental activity, concentration, focus, intellectual abilities, and an awakening of greater confidence and optimism. It is also the color related to the third chakra, or solar plexus chakra, linking digestive, intestinal, and psychosomatic diseases that can be worked with through this center.

- The shiny upper side and the duller lower side of the leaves, as well as the joining of the leaves, also indicate the bringing together of opposites.

- The open hands and feet symbolize a balance of giving and receiving in harmony.

Helpful suggestions

What is it within yourself that feels "out of sync" and not quite in balance? In what way do you feel isolated within yourself? Are you aware of a part of yourself that you would like to integrate into your whole? What stands out in your relationship with your partner that doesn't feel balanced? In what ways are you and your partner opposite? How could you bring together your "opposite" with your partner's "opposite," toward integration and mutual harmony? Do you have a nostalgic memory in your past related to yourself, a previous partner, your present partner, or someone else that you are holding onto? How does this memory hold you back and interfere with your current direction in life or in your partnership? Are you ready and willing to integrate and reconcile your parts?

Take three to four drops of Honeysuckle flower essence and ask yourself the above questions. Tune in to your thoughts and feelings. Is there something in your mind or a previous experience that comes up? Do you have an "opposite" issue with your partner that you need to come to terms with? Close your eyes and imagine the sweet fragrance of honeysuckle embracing you. Take in the aroma at its fullest. Breathe into the aroma and stay with it for a while. Then imagine drinking honeysuckle's sweet nectar. Feel its refreshing taste at the back of your throat. Feel the liquid nectar reach down into your solar plexus. Take another few deep relaxing breaths. Tune into the effect this has in your solar plexus. How do you feel? Stay with your feeling and openly express to yourself how you feel. Release this feeling as much as possible in this moment, then ask yourself if you are ready to do something else.

When ready, tap into the sweetness of the nectar in your solar plexus and take that sweetness into your entire being. Smell the sweetness, taste the sweetness, feel the sweetness, have a dialogue with the sweetness. Ask for clarity in your situation. Find out how you can make use of the sweetness of this essence and integrate it into your present situation. What are you willing to let go of? What do you need to feel balanced and whole? In what way can you compromise? Again, take some deep breaths and just be with yourself in this exercise and see where it takes you.

Gather what you have learned, let go of what you have released, and open your eyes. The next step is up to you. Do this exercise or make up one of your own while you take the Honeysuckle essence as many times a day, or days in a row, as you can for a month or so.

Affirmations

- "I am the power to integrate all that I am and all that I am becoming."
- "I am willing to reconcile with my opposites and bring harmony and balance from within."

- "I honor fond memories for how they have helped me be who I am today."

case History

Suzy, age forty-three, took the Honeysuckle flower essence to help her release old nostalgic memories. She took this essence four different times. Each time that she tried it, she "started getting nostalgic feelings, not all bad, that brought up past feelings about love life and intimacy." Suzy felt that the essence helped her work through some of these memories in deep emotional ways.

However, in the evenings, she would get severe headaches, stuffed-up sinuses related to her asthma, extremely swollen lymph glands, and arthritis up and down her spine and from the bottom of her neck to the top of her buttocks. Upon discovering the traditional uses of Honeysuckle that included the treatment of asthma, arthritis, headaches, and lymph glands, Suzy realized that her symptoms fit the symptom picture of Honeysuckle and what homeopaths refer to as "like treats like" or "the cure is like the disease." Suzy's symptoms were an expression of her body's inherent defense mechanism being called into action. She understood that the Honeysuckle flower essence provided a means to stimulate her symptoms, rather than suppress them, in order to influence a cure. Although her symptoms were provoked, she also felt that a cleansing and healing of these symptoms took place.

I find the correlation between the flower essence and the actual physical uses and treatment of the plant fascinating.

LFE's Research provers' project findings

PHYSICAL SYMPTOMS

CRAVINGS: Ate more with no particular cravings; drank more water and less coffee
SENSATIONS: Felt shaky all over for one day; could feel energy/tingling move from spinal base to abdomen to solar plexus to heart and upward and outward
PAIN: Muscle soreness and tension
MODALITIES:
  WORSE: During sleep
  BETTER: Daytime
HEAD: None
EYES: None
FACE: None
EARS: None
STOMACH: None
ABDOMEN: None
BOWEL CONDITION: Slight constipation
URINE: Less frequent
FEMALE: None
MALE: None
EXTREMITIES: Muscle soreness and tension
BACK: Muscle soreness and tension
SKIN: None
OTHER: Physically invigorating and energetic — an energy boost. "Reminded me of more physical expression of energy, like when I was in my youth through twenties, that lasted for about an hour."

EMOTIONAL SYMPTOMS

PATTERNS OF BALANCE: "felt relaxed, calm, and invigorated," "increases positive emotional states and energizes them," "more enthusiastic," "very pleasant and comfortable," "felt better generally with more ambition," "increased emotional balance," "felt an opening of chakras"

PATTERNS OF IMBALANCE: "intensification of old fears of loss that have been present my whole life," "experienced crying and yelling that I didn't want to live in fear and hold onto things anymore — quite an emotional experience"

MENTAL SYMPTOMS

PATTERNS OF BALANCE: "more aware, my mind feels energized," "more active, relaxed, and able," "seemed to open cognitive paths some," "increased mental balance," "had more focus and concentration"

PATTERNS OF IMBALANCE: "when the emotion would strike, my mind would take off like a bullet creating scenarios that would support the fear," "my mind seemed out of control," "my mind was holding onto past stuff," "unable to redirect or focus my mind"

SPIRITUAL REFLECTIONS

"No major increase or change — helped me be 'reflective'"

DREAMS/NIGHTMARES

No significant dreams were remembered or recorded. Dream intensity or relationship to dreams wasn't indicated.

INDIAN PAINTBRUSH

(Castilleja chromosa)
PRIMARY QUALITY: CREATIVITY

FAMILY: Snapdragon or Figwort (Scrophulariaceae)
OTHER NAMES: Painted-Cup, Whole-Leaf Paintbrush, Desert Paintbrush
WHERE FOUND: dry, sunny places in woodlands and forests, roadsides, and clearings in ponderosa, pinyon, and juniper forests in Southwestern states
ELEVATION: 2,500' to 7,000'
ENERGY IMPACT (CHAKRA CORRESPONDENCE): first, second, fourth, and sixth chakras
KEY RUBRICS FOR POSITIVE HEALING PATTERNS: creative expression, family values, passion, resourcefulness
KEY RUBRICS FOR SYMPTOMS AND PATTERNS OF IMBALANCE: abandonment, anger, codependence, insufficient family system, lack of resourcefulness
OTHER RUBRICS: acceptance, artistic, beauty, breakthrough, brow chakra, calm, cheerfulness, clarity, connectiveness, dependence, depletion, dreamwork, emergence, energetic, exhaustion, family heritage, fiery, freedom, fullness, heart chakra, imagery, insight, inspiration, love, past life, receptivity, reflection, relaxation, revitalize, root chakra, self-expression, sensuality, sexuality, silence, spleen chakra, tiredness, warmth, vibrant, vision, vitality

Traditional use

There are two Native American legends about the origin of Indian paintbrush. The first legend[2] is about a Blackfoot maiden who fell in love with a wounded prisoner held captive in her camp. She discovered that the tribe was allowing her to care for him so that he would be well enough to torture later. The maiden helped the prisoner escape and they set up their own camp. Eventually, she became homesick for her old camp and returned to gaze upon it one last time. While hiding behind some bushes, she heard two braves discussing her betrayal and realized that she could never return again. She cut her leg with a stick, and with her blood she drew a picture of her old camp on a piece of bark and threw it away, returning to her lover's camp. As the legend goes, the first Indian paintbrush grew where the stick fell, dyed with the maiden's blood. Another legend is about a brave who was painting a prairie sunset; he became unsatisfied with his artwork and threw his paintbrushes down on the ground. Great Spirit grew the flowers where the paintbrush fell.

There are over 200 species of Indian paintbrush, making it difficult to identify. The flowers of Indian paintbrush can be eaten and taste pleasant. The long white corolla tube contains a sweet nectar at its base, and it can be pulled out and eaten. Hopi Indians traditionally ate the raw flowers and used the plant as a medicine and in ceremonies. The Tewa Indians also ate the raw blossoms and used the whole plant as a bathing solution for aches and pains, especially associated with long outdoor ceremonies. Navajo Indians make a tan dye from the blossoms and a greenish yellow dye from the stems and leaves. The plant is also known to have been mixed with minerals to make a black paint. At Jemez, New Mexico, the flower bracts were mixed with chile seeds to prevent spoiling of the chile seeds. The root is used to treat spider bites and horse ailments, and the leaves are used to treat stomach problems and burns.

Caution: A high selenium content is reported in Indian paintbrush, and only small doses should be eaten.

homeopathic use

Unknown to author.

positive healing patterns

- Encourages us to take time to be still and to relax in silence; through that silence we gain access to clarity.
- Through clarity we are guided toward higher vision and an awareness of our eternal nature; as we understand our eternal nature, we gain access to our past lives and who we really are as spiritual beings, resulting in an ability to creatively express who we really are

on the physical, emotional, mental, and spiritual planes.
- Stirs creative, inspirational, passionate, visionary, and artistic self-expression while feeling grounded and connected to our roots.
- Encourages us to find the needed resources to meet our survival needs so that we can live a fuller, more creative life.
- Promotes dreamwork and receptivity to visionary guidance.

symptoms and patterns of imbalance

Indian Paintbrush may be an appropriate flower essence for those who

- Are overstimulated, exhausted, low in vitality, and lacking in creativity
- Need help to stay grounded (meeting survival needs) while pursuing creative and artistic endeavors
- Lack vision and insight, especially related to their family roots and family systems
- Feel withdrawn sexually, especially related to emotional heart wounds and vulnerability, and who feel closed down in general.

features of the original flower-essence water

Odor: bitter
Taste: strong and bitter
Sensations: tingling sensation straight down to root chakra
Water Color: clear

physical makeup

Root, Stem, Leaves/Leaflets, Height:
Indian paintbrush is semiparasitic and lacks a well-developed root system. The underground root system of the plant has tubes called "haustoria" that burrow into the roots of a host plant, such as sagebrush, oak, or grasses; it depends on the host plant to supply water and nutrients by penetrating its tissues. Seedlings don't grow well or at all if a host is not found. The stem is purplish and slightly fuzzy, growing up to 16 inches tall. Often many flowering stems grow from the same plant. The lanceolate, somewhat narrow leaves alternate up the stem, and are more prolific toward the base of the stem. The reddish green, grayish-haired leaves are three-lobed; they look like a tiny hand, and they are fuzzy and soft growing up to 2 inches long. Fuzzy seed pods alternate along the stem all the way to the top. Inside, many seeds line each half of the pod.

Flower Color: Pale green flowers with fiery reddish orange bracts

Flowers: Pale-green flowers are borne in dense, leafy, bracted spikes. The flowers are hidden above brightly colored, reddish orange, leaflike, slightly hairy bracts that form a spike. It is the colorful bracts that highlight the inconspicuous flower blossoms. The flower-clustered spikes top the stems and are up to 3 inches long. Each individual bract has three fiery red petals that grow from a green base. Stamens appear to grow out of five to seven petals on the whole cluster, and they have reddish orange anthers.

Blooming Period: March through October

doctrine of signatures

- Indian paintbrush's dependency on other plants demonstrates its low vitality, physical weakness, and energy depletion. Even though the plant steals nutrients from host plants, it also has the ability to integrate with and give something to the plant that it has taken from. The host plants don't seem to suffer greatly by sharing their nutrients. Once Indian paintbrush's energy is "grounded" (by burrowing its own root system into the roots of the host plant), it has made a breakthrough to the "other side"; and no longer struggling for survival, it has the freedom to be creative and vibrant. As people, we often need compassion from others to assist us with survival needs (getting a job, locating resources, finding an affordable home, health and nutritional guidance, medical needs, etc.). Once those basic survival needs are dealt with, we can then feel the relief to live more freely and creatively. Also, the tendency to exhaust and deplete ourselves of energy without taking the time to ground ourselves takes away from our creative potential. This signature also shows our need to take time to relax, revitalize ourselves, and get help if we need it so that we can be creative and live life more fully.

- The significance of Indian paintbrush's roots burrowing into the roots of other plants and the reddish orange color of the bracts corresponds with the root chakra; this gives attention to understanding and identifying the roots that connect us to our spiritual heritage. From this vantage point, an awareness of dysfunctional patterns from this and past lives may surface for examination and dissolution. We are able to interpret life's challenges — past, present, and future — in a new light and act accordingly. The sharing of the host plant's vital nutrients, with seemingly no loss or harm to themselves, is an example of the law of supply: humble receiver and unconditional, compassionate giver.

- The hidden, pale-green flowers correspond to the fourth or heart chakra, and the brightly colored reddish orange bracts growing from a green base show a direct connection between the heart and the first or root and second chakras. It is a beautiful representation of exchanging and transmuting those chakras in their fullness of life, love, and beauty.

- The brightly colored reddish orange leaflike bracts growing upward on the spike are striking in desert and ponderosa landscapes. Their

appearance is highly artistic and the "paintbrush" style bracts give an incredible sense of emergence, creativity, inspiration, warmth, and vitality.

- The soft, fuzzy, delicate leaves (with their tiny hands) and flowers stretch outward as if to receive and give the life-force.

- The corolla tube inside the flower petal has a sweet nectar; when you eat a few flower petals and sit in silence, Indian paintbrush will provide visions, imagery, and spiritual insights if you are open to receive its gifts. This signature is indicative of the sixth chakra.

Helpful suggestions

Take Indian Paintbrush flower essence when you are prepared to be with yourself for at least thirty minutes and are willing to be silent from deep within. Your silence will guide you in this journey. Find a comfortable position and close your eyes. You may want to lie down to give yourself total relaxation and to eventually take a nap. If there is something in particular that you're seeking guidance with, give yourself a few moments to gain clarity and to set your intention.

Then take three to four drops of the flower essence and take several deep breaths. Relax. Shut out the world and any thoughts or duties that may enter your space. Ask any interference to leave, and let it be known that this is your time to enter the depths of your internal silence.

Slowly continue to breathe. Take a deep breath and hold it at the top of your head at the crown chakra (pineal), and eventually let it go. Repeat. Now take another deep breath and this time hold it in your brow chakra (center of your forehead), then gradually let it go. Repeat. Next take the breath to your throat chakra, hold it, and gradually let it go. Repeat. Keep taking breaths as deep and long as possible, and breathe and hold a breath in your heart chakra (upper thoracic: heart, lungs) and let it out. Repeat. Then take an even deeper breath and hold it in your solar plexus chakra (thoracic: stomach, liver, kidneys, adrenals, pancreas, gall bladder, small intestines, duodenum) and gradually let it out. Repeat. Take another deep breath and hold this breath in your spleen chakra area (lumbar: large intestine, sex organs, bladder, lower back) and gradually let it out. Repeat. Now breathe all the way down to your root chakra (sacral: coccyx, rectum, anus). Hold the breath at the base of your perineum and gradually let it out. Repeat. Finally, take another deep breath and let the silence take you on your journey. Notice any images, colors, words, or sensations that you experience. When you are finished or when you wake up, open your eyes and write your experience in a journal.

Affirmations

- "I breathe into the deep silence within, stirring my creative powers."
- "I honor all life before me, giving thanks to my mother and father, grandmother and grandfather, and all the great-grandmothers and great-grandfathers before them."
- "I love myself for who I am and, through love of myself, I creatively express compassion toward humanity and all of life on earth."

Case History

Curtis, age forty-three, says, "When I take Indian Paintbrush flower essence, I take a few drops several times daily until the bottle is empty. Somewhere between the first drop and the end of the bottle, I have an experience of the plant's gift. The first time I took the remedy, approximately two years ago, I was feeling inadequate and unempowered, stuffing my feelings especially in relationship to my spouse. I was experiencing doubts and concerns about expressing many of my true feelings for fear of upsetting her. I'm sure this related to my nonconfrontational approach to life that was a deep-rooted dysfunctional pattern related to fear of abandonment. This was a pattern of codependency that had a profound effect on my self-image, freedom of expression, and creative intimacy in my marriage. Within three days, I began feeling more assertive about my feelings, and within seven days I simply expressed and asserted myself from a place of personal power and the foundation of my own being. As a result, I have more intimacy with my spouse and I'm feeling more creative in my life.

"I also had a profound but different kind of experience after eating a raw

Indian paintbrush flower while on a quest in my favorite wilderness retreat. This experience provided me with insight through visual images while in a meditative state. Exhausted from a two-day hike, I sat on my perch overlooking Sycamore Pass. Nearby was a small Indian ruin that was special to me. I was having no success focusing my mind. This was unlike my usual meditation, in which I could silence my mind more easefully. I decided to eat a raw Indian paintbrush and lie down until the sun came close to the horizon. As I lay down and closed my eyes, I was able to completely let go. Within a few minutes I began to arrive at a state of inner silence. I was between a conscious and a sleep stage. A powerful image of a colorful Indian man wearing a red headband and dressed in ceremonial attire appeared in the ruin. One moment he was there, and then he disappeared. I sat up while maintaining my inner calm. A voice in my head that was not of my own but that of a Native American began giving me wisdom about the path I was about to take. The image of the Indian coming out of the ruin was powerful, colorful, magnetic, and peaceful. Certainly the Indian paintbrush had a role in facilitating this experience."

Lfe's Research provers' project findings

Physical Symptoms

Cravings: More fruits and fruit juices; drank more water
Sensations: Related to visual imagery
Pain: None

Modalities:
  Worse: Inconsistent reporting of sleep patterns
  Better: None
Head: None
Eyes: None
Face: None
Ears: None
Stomach: Stomach upsets, upset digestive system
Abdomen: None
Bowel condition: Constipation, then diarrhea
Urine: None
Female: None
Male: None
Extremities: None
Back: None
Skin: None
Other: Physically tired, insomnia; had a feeling of heaviness (weight or pressure) in the heart area that lifted after a short time

Emotional Symptoms

Patterns of Balance: "an emotional mood lift — made me feel lighter," felt emotionally uplifted, had feelings of peace and sunlight that seemed to relate to something 'cosmic,'" "had a peaceful feeling, more in moments of being still," "a sense of a deep need to celebrate"
Patterns of Imbalance: "felt sad and emotional about relationship problems," "mildly depressed," "fearful of future and of living arrangements," "emotionally unbalanced," "lack of confidence," "lack of calm," "a sense of not caring, indifference"

MENTAL SYMPTOMS

PATTERNS OF BALANCE: "more creative," "more understanding," "more right-brained," "kept getting sensations of seeing butterflies, and feelings of butterflies in my stomach," "more philosophical and reflective," "dream images," "mental clarity," "this remedy sparked images that made me curious," "had yin/yang imagery," "simple reflections in a quiet way on the meaning of all the earth changes and cosmic vibrations we are experiencing at this time," "heartfelt reflections," "conscious reflection of the meaning of symbols that appeared to me," "images of sunlight," "I seem to understand more of what is going on around me," "I am more excited about my kids and my job in my thoughts"

PATTERNS OF IMBALANCE: "worrying about survival issues: where will I live? can I take care of myself?" "fear of the dark, fear of being alone"

SPIRITUAL REFLECTIONS

"I prayed a lot to ask for support in getting through whatever changes will be coming for me. I also said a lot of protection prayers for myself and, especially at night, experienced imagery and a sense of growing into a more harmonious and cosmic life of peace and brotherhood; felt love of fellow men," "could be taken by a group to encourage creative reflection on earth changes or for experiencing mutual peace and sunlight"

DREAMS/NIGHTMARES

"Work was being done in dream state," "my dreams were very clear in their meaning to me," "I had more lucid dream images."

LUPINE (silverstem Lupine)

(*Lupinus argentus*)
PRIMARY QUALITY: PATHFINDER

FAMILY: Pea (Leguminosae)

OTHER NAMES: Silvery Lupine, *Azee' bi ni'i*, which means "wondering about medicine" (Navajo)

WHERE FOUND: coniferous forest meadows and clearings

ELEVATION: 7,000' to 10,000'

ENERGY IMPACT (CHAKRA CORRESPONDENCE): sixth and seventh chakras

KEY RUBRICS FOR POSITIVE HEALING PATTERNS: appreciation of the moment, uplift, spiritual guidance

KEY RUBRICS FOR SYMPTOMS AND PATTERNS OF IMBALANCE: struggle in the past or future, inability to access a higher purpose in life

OTHER RUBRICS: anxiety, avoidance, balance, blame, brokenheartedness, brow chakra, burden, calm, change, clarity, confused, consciousness, contentment, courage, crown chakra, death/dying, depression, dreams, evolutionary, faith, fear, freedom, giving, grief, grounding, healing, insight, intellect, intimacy, intuition, irritability, light, love, misunderstanding, openness, paranoia, pathfinder, patience, peaceful, positive, protection, quieting, receptivity, release, repression, sadness, sensitive, silence, spacey, stability, strength, surrender, tension, thought, transformation, transition, transmutation, understanding, vision, willingness

Traditional use

Lupine is a Latin word meaning "wolf." This name was given to the plant because it was believed that lupines robbed the soil of its nutrients. Like the wolf, however, the lupine has been misunderstood. With help from certain bacteria, the lupine's root nodules actually put nitrogen that they obtain from the air back into the soil. This common trait of the pea family improves the soil. Some lupines are known as "green manure crops" because they absorb excess pesticides and other soil poisons, although several other species have seeds that contain alkaloids that are dangerous to livestock, especially sheep.

The seeds of *Lupinus albus* and *Lupinus polyphyllus* are made into a powder that is used to treat skin problems such as scabby pores and blemishes, and it is added to facial steams and skin masks to revitalize dull skin and to diminish oiliness. The seeds of certain species are roasted to extract toxins and made into flour or used as coffee substitutes. The leaves are made into a lotion by the Navajo to treat poison ivy blisters. The Navajo also use lupine in the Male Shooting Way and Evil Way ceremonies.

Some species of lupine were planted near Chernobyl, Ukraine, to help absorb radiation following the nuclear disaster there.

Most lupines have showy flowers of white, pink, lavender, purple, or blue, causing some species to be made into ornaments.

Homeopathic use

Unknown to author.

positive Healing patterns

- Opens our ability to step beyond ourselves and be filled with Light energy.
- Shows us the silence or space of being, allowing us to acknowledge and be in that space without looking ahead or behind, and to be guided by intuition and a natural flow of energy. This is the experience of a pathfinder (lupine's primary quality).
- Prepares us for our next cycle of change or life passage, allowing it to take place between what was and what will become.
- Helps us attain our visions and aspirations and bring them into practical application, thus enriching ourselves and others and the way we live. It teaches us to balance our physical, emotional, and mental aspects to support our spiritual goals and to ground ourselves in the world.

- Offers spiritual inspiration, clarity, calmness, balance, openness, and positive direction.
- Helps us surrender to our highest good.

symptoms and patterns of imbalance

Lupine may be an appropriate flower essence for those who

- Lack physical/emotional/mental balance to support their spiritual goals and vision, and who need or desire encouragement to help relieve imbalances such as sadness, grief, anxiety, tension, guilt, or misunderstanding
- Are unable to access spiritual vision, intuitive perception, clairvoyance, or a higher wisdom
- Are unable to or struggle to internally see memories, dreams, ideas, or insights, or feel disturbed by old memories
- Lack a higher life-purpose, spiritual vision or guidance, cohesiveness of thought and planning, and inspiration
- Have abnormal sleep patterns, sensitivity to light, frontal sinus infections, or inability to maintain body temperature.

features of the original flower-essence water

Odor: sweet and subtle
Taste: mellow, smooth, and sweet

SENSATIONS: Gentle cool tingling and calming of energy went down to solar plexus then root chakra, and then spread up and out through the crown chakra. Gives a feeling of calmness, centeredness, peacefulness, and balance.

WATER COLOR: clear

physical makeup

ROOT, STEM, LEAVES/LEAFLETS, HEIGHT: The silverstem lupine has root nodules that put nitrogen obtained from the air back into the soil. This improves the soil and the land on which they grow. Silvery hairs grow along the stem, and the stem appears graceful and flexible. The slightly hairy leaves alternate along the stem. They are darker green above and lighter green below. They grow up to 3 inches long and 3 inches wide, with seven to nine divided, fingerlike leaflets that are palm-shaped. The center of the leaflets hold water after a rain. The palm-shaped leaves face the sun, following it throughout the day.

FLOWER COLOR: Lilac/lavender and white

FLOWERS: The colorful, showy flowers are pea-like in their appearance. The flowers grow in terminal clusters toward the top of the stem. The flower consists of two petals. The broader upper petal is slightly hairy on its back and seems to fold backward, and the smaller petal folds closed. If you open up the inside of the folds, you will see five or six tiny stamens with golden-orange anthers. The flower grows about $^1/_2$ inch long and is followed by a 1-inch green, fuzzy pod. You can see the impression of little peas or beans inside the pod. One white spot appears on each fold of the upper petal. The lower petal is solid lavender in color. The flowers carry a sweet, pleasant fragrance.

BLOOMING PERIOD: June to October

doctrine of signatures

- A distinct signature of the lupine is the open-palm-shaped leaflets that face the sun throughout the day. When our hands are open and not clenched, we are able to feel the power of Light enter and energize our bodies. Open hands also depict giving as well as receiving, balance, openness, and willingness to surrender. The leaflets' trough-like center holds water and nurtures the plant.

- The lupine's broad, folded flower petals offer an impression of openness with protection. The lavender color of the lupine represents the sixth chakra and, along with the plant journey and plant experience, the flower carries a deep sense of inner vision and of following one's path to higher evolvement. Sitting in a field surrounded by lupines, my friends and I all felt an incredible opening in our sixth and seventh chakras. We were filled with visionary aspirations. This plant opened our ability to step beyond ourselves and to be completely filled with Light energy. It awakened our intuition and insights at a deep level. Through the relaxation of our sixth or third-eye chakra, each of us (there were four of us in one setting, and two in another) consistently experienced an incredible silence. This flower was showing us the silence or space of just being — looking neither ahead nor behind. It's about being in that silent place, acknowledging the place, and allowing yourself to be guided by your own energy flow.

- The misunderstanding that lupines rob the soil of nutrients rather than give nutrients back to the soil is a fascinating signature. The nodules of the roots actually obtain nitrogen from the air, which enables them to enrich the soil. I believe this signature symbolizes our ability to attain our visions and aspirations and bring those visions into practical application, thus enriching ourselves, others, and the way we live. It is about bringing a physical/emotional/mental balance to support our spiritual goals, and grounding ourselves in the world.
- The fragrance and taste of the flowers — both naturally and in the flower-essence water — is sweet, pleasant, and calming.

Helpful suggestions

Find a quiet, meditative spot. Take several drops of the Lupine flower essence and close your eyes. Imagine yourself as a Native American, walking on an old road in a ponderosa forest. Suddenly you hear a deep-bellied bugle-like call that sends a tingling rush of excitement through your body. You turn to the noise and see two large male elk (elk resemble the moose and are smaller) standing about thirty yards from you. You notice how big and long their anthers are. Only somewhat startled, they begin to move in another direction. Astounded by their magical presence, you watch as their powerful bodies fade off into the distance. You have a short conversation with yourself about what it meant to you to come into the elk's path, and you realize that the elk represent strength, power, stamina, and the ability to pace themselves. You marvel at what this may mean in your own life as you continue to walk down the road, in search of a new adventure.

You see a clearing ahead in the forest, and you notice that the sun is glistening above the clearing. So you head toward the clearing and, as you approach it, you see acres and acres of purple lupine and other wildflowers. You are delighted to see such an elegant bouquet in this field of wildflowers. The sweet fragrance of the lupines fills you with a gentle sweetness, and you find yourself calm and peaceful. You seek a spot in which to sit with these beautiful flowers.

You find a grassy area under a small pine tree toward the edge of the clearing. Sitting in your spot, you sit in wonderment with open hands, thanking Spirit for having led you to such an enriching, beautiful place. You thank the lupines for being there for you as you continue to marvel at their presence. You close your eyes as you feel the spiritual abundance that the lupines are giving you. With your eyes closed, you realize that you are without thoughts, that you are simply in the moment, feeling the moment. An incredible silence is felt throughout your body, mind, and soul. It is a silence that you find nurturing and peaceful. Tears gently stream from your eyes and down your face. The stillness is so precious and endearing to you, and you realize how much you need this in your life.

You continue to sit for a long time, unaware of time and space, past and future, within and without. Your entire being is filled with the sweet fragrance and presence of the lupines. You feel an opening within yourself and a lifting of your energy from the crown of your head. You also feel an incredible Light and warmth come through your body from the crown of your head and your brow chakra, encircling your face, then moving downward all the way to your toes. You slowly open your eyes, and once again you give thanks. Filled with the presence of the silence and the Light, you get up and start on your journey home, feeling thankful that the Pathfinder is now within you and always available to you.

Affirmations

- "I open my hands to receive the power of Light."
- "My pathway is illuminated by my intuition and inner silence."
- "I honor my personal growth and surrender to my highest good."

Case History

Bruce, age thirty-nine, was in a confused emotional state and not feeling connected to himself. He had a general feeling of dissatisfaction and imbalance in his life, and he was experiencing anxiety that he couldn't relate to a cause. He felt that he might have an unresolved issue, yet he couldn't identify it. He asked for God's help in seeking higher guidance while taking the Lupine flower essence. At the end of two weeks, Bruce felt a lifting of his mood and a general well-being. He felt that he had found a silence from deep within that helped him feel at peace with himself. He also found that his anxiety was gone. Bruce's comments about taking Lupine were: "I felt a general lifting of mood out of a negative space, which helped me feel more balanced and quieted my internal dialogue. The quieting of my mind was positive, grounded, and balanced, and I had more clarity of thought in my ability to carry out tasks. I also realized that I was more organized at work than I thought I was, and that felt good."

LFE's Research Provers' Project Findings

PHYSICAL SYMPTOMS

CRAVINGS: Water, tomatoes, juice
SENSATIONS: Calming, relaxing effect
PAIN: None
MODALITIES: Provers were inconsistent in sleep and wake patterns.
HEAD: Headaches
EYES: Heightened vision and depth perception

FACE: None

EARS: Senses are more acute.

STOMACH: Stomachaches

ABDOMEN: None

BOWEL CONDITION: None

URINE: None

FEMALE: Hot flashes (unusual)

MALE: None

EXTREMITIES: None

BACK: None

SKIN: None

OTHER: Some provers felt more tired, while others experienced an energy boost.

EMOTIONAL SYMPTOMS

PATTERNS OF BALANCE: "became more aware of the irritability of others and wasn't comfortable being around it, both from an emotional and a spiritual point of view," "felt more emotionally sensitive," "helped me to remain calm during a crisis with my girlfriend; she was in shock and I didn't panic, which I thought I normally would have done," "helped me feel grounded," "I felt this was a good essence to use to have more control of emotions during a stressful period or situation," "the stronger intuition and emotional control was healing to me," "I felt closer to nature," "I get things done that need to get done," "I experienced a curious mixture of anxiety about old issues and also a sense of contentment and freedom from those issues — a paradox," "felt nourished, grateful, and emotionally consoled," "felt peaceful and fulfilled," "I experienced a release of sadness in relation

to the past on the fourth day of taking this essence," "I felt a stableness to get through feelings of grief and sadness related to a reflection of some memory," "felt strong," "got in touch with old feelings and was able to move through them with resolution," "felt strongly sensitive," "more patient"

PATTERNS OF IMBALANCE: "wanted to run away from irritability caused by others," "felt guilt," "I felt sad even though I kept getting a sense of new beginnings; my feeling was in relation to completing the old," "sadness," "grief," "avoidance," "anxiety," "broken-heartedness," "repression," "tension"

MENTAL SYMPTOMS

PATTERNS OF BALANCE: "more aware of wanting to stay in balance," "I wrote a lot of notes while taking this essence about how it affected me and what was happening in my life," "was more clairvoyant and intuitive," "more understanding," "I feel this could make someone's reaction to an undesirable situation better and easier to get through," "I seem to remember more things, especially at work," "enjoyed a wise-woman sense," "reflected on how fortunate I really am," "'new beginnings' was the message that I kept drawing in when I took this essence," "sharp, sensitive, and strong," "experienced a thoughtful, gentle awareness," "I decided to make a choice to get in touch with my needs and to let the past go"

PATTERNS OF IMBALANCE: "old memories were disturbing," "misunderstanding," "paranoia," "guilt"

Spiritual Reflections

"I said a lot of protection and healing prayers for my friend and for myself," "when I looked at the sky and the sun was coming down between the clouds, I could see sunny rays hit the ground and I found this peaceful and relaxing," "felt a connection between spiritual expression vs. spiritual regression which questioned my spirituality and helped me to accept it in new ways"

Dreams/Nightmares

"I had a dream in which I was explaining to someone that if you take a class the changes won't happen unless you practice. I realize that was a message for me, as I just finished a class and wasn't doing the exercise. I needed a new beginning."

Provers in general had more dream imagery and dreams, although not always remembered.

MEXICAN HAT

(Ratibida columnaris)
PRIMARY QUALITY: RELEASE

FAMILY: Sunflower (Compositae)
OTHER NAMES: Yellow Coneflower, Prairie Coneflower
WHERE FOUND: roadsides, fields, dry sandy grassy areas, open meadows, and clearings in pine forests throughout the West
ELEVATION: 5,000' to 8,500'
ENERGY IMPACT (CHAKRA CORRESPONDENCE): first, second, and third chakras
KEY RUBRICS FOR POSITIVE HEALING PATTERNS: self-empowerment, letting go of undesirable situations and people
KEY RUBRICS FOR SYMPTOMS AND PATTERNS OF IMBALANCE: abandonment, abuse, anger, addiction, fear, grief, hopelessness, suppressed emotions, holding on to the above
OTHER RUBRICS: achiness, anxiety, apathy, avoidance, blame, bowel, breakthrough, burden, clarity, calm, cleanse, confusion, control, denial, depression, doubt, earth, emotions, feelings, groundedness, guidance, guilt, healing, heart, mindfulness, mother, mystery, nerves, nourishment, nurture, protection, rage, release, resentment, root chakra, solar plexus chakra, sorrow, spleen chakra, stomach, support, surrender, tears, tension, unknown

traditional use

Native Americans made a pleasant-tasting tea by brewing the leaves and flower heads. No other uses found.

homeopathic use

Unknown to author.

positive healing patterns

- Teaches us to let go of or surrender that which we have no control over.
- Helps us release certain feelings and emotions that we have held onto for a long time.

- Helps us release emotional situations that cannot be worked out with those involved due to their lack of availability, physically, emotionally, mentally, and/or spiritually.
- Reminds us to nourish our earth mother as we nourish ourselves, and to ask her for guidance and support in ways in which we need nurturing and nourishment.

symptoms and patterns of imbalance

Mexican Hat may be an appropriate flower essence for those who

- Hold onto situations/events/people they have no control over
- Hold onto emotions and feelings that aren't understood and can't seem to be identified
- Hold tension and anxieties related to fear, anger, grief, and sorrow that is preventing them from healing
- Need to get outdoors, connect with our earth mother, and find ways to nourish themselves.

features of the original flower-essence water

Odor: slightly fruity
Taste: bitter, strong, pungent "green"
Sensations: Feels like belly may explode; upset stomach
Water Color: slightly yellow

physical makeup

Root, Stem, Leaves/Leaflets, Height: The roots pull out easily, even in dry soil. The strong, fibrous stem is very slender, slightly rough, and small. It grows from 1 to 4 feet in height. The small, green, hairy, narrow leaves alternate and open pinnately into odd-numbered (five, seven, or nine) narrow segments that are about 4 to 6 inches long. The plants usually grow in groups.
Flower Color: Yellow and reddish orange-brown
Flowers: The terminal flower head is about 3 inches wide, with yellow and reddish to purplish brown ray petals that droop to the ground like a badminton shuttlecock. The petals are about $1\frac{1}{2}$ inches long, and each petal is slightly divided at the edge. At their center is a purplish-reddish-brown tubular disk that covers a cone-shaped or thimble-shaped column up to $1\frac{1}{2}$ inches long.
Blooming Period: June to October

doctrine of signatures

- The drooping petals reach down toward the earth, signifying the plant's ability to surrender and its need to be connected to the earth. This signature relates to our own need to let go, to surrender ourselves, and to let our highest good take over. The plant's droopiness also demonstrates a mystery that requires only surrender, since there is nothing we can really control but we have everything to let go of. It also reminds us to listen to Mother Earth's messages and to reach toward or connect with the earth to help us in our healing process.
- The yellow and reddish orange-brown colors represent the third or solar plexus chakra, second or spleen chakra, and first or root chakra, related to deep-seated emotions, feelings, and fears that, as already indicated, are unknown or not yet identified.
- The simplicity of Mexican hat's individualism shows that each flower is a separate unit yet connected to the whole and, with the above signatures, represents the fact that each of us has certain emotions that cannot always be shared with the people these emotions

relate to. The group consciousness of this plant demonstrates a unity between its members, yet acknowledges that each individual plant has its own healing process to work with and to eventually surrender.

Helpful suggestions

Take some time to be in nature and to be with our earth mother. Find a spot that you are drawn to and that helps you feel safe and secure. Sit on the ground and take three to four drops of Mexican Hat flower essence. Close your eyes and place your hands on the earth and feel the earth holding you as you are touching her. Ask her to help you surrender any emotions, situations, or people that you are holding on to and that no longer serve you. Keeping your eyes closed and your hands on the earth, allow the earth to take you on a journey and give you the nourishment you need. When you finish your journey, thank Mother Earth for providing for you and embrace the gifts she gives you in your daily life.

Affirmations

- "I surrender [my grief] and turn it over to God."
- "I let go of [situation or person] and pray for my/our highest good."
- "May the burdens I carry be released."

Case History

Eight years ago, a fifty-four-year-old woman came to me for flower essence consultations. She had a traumatic history of childhood sexual abuse, and at age four she had witnessed a murder. She also had some medical problems, including past breast cancer and multiple chemical sensitivity. She had been in counseling with a psychiatrist for several years to help her deal with her anger, fears, and grief. She wanted help in bringing up memories and feelings that she had suppressed over the years because she felt it would help her release things she had been afraid to let go of, including unidentified fears.

I gave her several remedies besides Mexican Hat, and each were taken individually in their own period of time. Her response to Mexican Hat was: "I feel that Mexican Hat helped me to get in touch with myself. No other essence yet has affected me so profoundly. It allowed me to get past a level of fear that's been holding me back, and it helped me to release some grief that I've been holding on to for a long time."

LFE's Research Provers' Project Findings

PHYSICAL SYMPTOMS

CRAVINGS: Chocolate, water, protein

SENSATIONS: Felt shaky, achy, and tired after tearful episodes; experienced involuntary "energetic/electrical impulses," especially in big toe

PAIN: None

MODALITIES: No consistent indications

HEAD: None

EYES: None

FACE: None

Ears: None
Stomach: Upset stomach after emotional release
Abdomen: None
Bowel condition: Better bowel movements (two or three a day instead of one), but more gas
Urine: Urinated more frequently
Female: None
Male: None
Extremities: None
Back: None
Skin: None

Emotional Symptoms

Patterns of Balance: "I felt that the out-of-control experience served to bring me ultimately to a much more clear and peaceful space by letting go of the clutter of dammed-up emotions inside," "realized how much emotional tension I was holding on to and felt all these emotions surfacing," "helped me to release these emotions," "had calming effects on my nerves and stomach," "felt relaxed," "helped me to feel healed emotionally," "felt emotionally uplifted"
Patterns of Imbalance: "felt isolated, lonely, separate, and found myself in uncontrolled tears and emotion; I felt as if I was in menopause all in one day; after dumping it all out, the feelings began to ease and then I could think and feel more balanced," "I experienced an intense magnification of all the things I have struggled with in my life," "emotions were all internal, not triggered outwardly; experienced intensifications of sadness, hopelessness, and isolation that couldn't be controlled or stopped; my emotions wouldn't begin to fade away until after they crashed on the South Pacific shore," "I got angry with my Mom when she tried to point out that the things I was feeling weren't true," "felt out of control emotionally," "fear of letting stuff be released," "deeply hidden anger, rage, and resentments"

Mental Symptoms

Patterns of Balance: "more clarity and realization of the need to change old habits and thought patterns," "brings issues to the surface and understanding to release them," "allows mental state to be in a controlled, protective state of being without being confrontational or argumentative in situations that wouldn't serve," "cleansing of old thoughts and concerns, especially related to family," "helped me to be a good listener," "felt mentally uplifted"
Patterns of Imbalance: "mental confusion, wondering why all these emotions had such a grip on me," "mental dialogue is negative and fearful; afraid to let go"

Spiritual Reflections

"Showed me how deeply I can be gripped by the drama of life's emotions," "I felt the energy of something protecting me and realized my higher self or Spirit was there for me"

Dreams/Nightmares

"I'd taken a job as a waitress in an exclusive restaurant just opening up. My first day, I figured I'd be feeling well. I've done it so much I thought it would be easy. It was a day from hell! I kept mixing things up, forgetting things such as which people to take the orders to. The manager, who had a very disappointed look on his face, came up to me and said I could pick up my things and go. I went home, and my son and boyfriend (played by Sean Connery) were there. They were sympathetic and soothed my bruised ego. As I was walking down the hall in the house, I said to "Sean" in his Scottish accent, 'It furthers one to have somewhere to go.' I woke up with that phrase in my ears and thoughts and lay there thinking about it. I think I was done with the old way of living and I need to live differently."

OTHER COMMENTS

"This essence brought up some deep family issues for me. My oldest sister and I haven't been on speaking terms for four years. We got together on the second day of taking this essence and spent two hours talking. I realized a lot of things about myself, her, and our family. The essence helped me relax my nerves or anxieties I had before, during, and after my meeting with my sister."

MORNING GLORY

(Ipomoea purpurea)

PRIMARY QUALITY: LIBERATOR

FAMILY: Morning Glory (Convolvulaceae)
OTHER NAMES: Common Morning Glory, Blue Stars, Pearly Gates, Flying Saucers, Heavenly Blue, *Tlitliltzin, Badoh Negro*
WHERE FOUND: fields, thickets, and yards throughout the U.S.
ELEVATION: most U.S. climates
ENERGY IMPACT (CHAKRA CORRESPONDENCE): fourth, sixth, and seventh chakras
KEY RUBRICS FOR POSITIVE HEALING PATTERNS: clarity, freedom, inspiration, love, new beginnings, vitality
KEY RUBRICS FOR SYMPTOMS AND PATTERNS OF IMBALANCE: closed down, not in touch with natural body rhythms, resistance to waking up
OTHER RUBRICS: breakthrough, brow chakra, calm, centered, cleansing, compassion, crown chakra, dreams, early, expression, fresh, guidance, heart chakra, higher presence, illumination, imagination, insight, liberation, light, morning, purification, rejuvenation, release, spiritual abundance, spiritual direction, surrender, unmotivated, vision, visualization

Traditional use

There are over 600 species of morning glory. Because of the wide variety of species and the different effects produced by the use of seeds as opposed to roots, it is difficult to document the plant's use as an herbal remedy. Some morning glory species, such as *Ipomoea violacea,* contain chemical substances closely related to lysergic acid diethylamide (LSD); the highest concentration is found in the seeds, which were used as a hallucinogen in sacred Aztec rituals. The seeds were mixed with ashes of poisonous insects, tobacco, and select live insects to rub on the body to give Aztec priests courage before sacrifices.

The whole plant, and in particular the roots of *Ipomoea hederaea,* is used as a purgative, and the dried seeds are also hallucinogenic and toxic; they are used in Asia to treat constipation, expel worms, promote menses, and as a diuretic. *Ipomoea mauritiana* is an woody vine that grows tonic tubers used in Ayurvedic medicine to treat nerves, spinal paralysis, rheumatism, liver, and urinary disease, and to tone circulation.

Ipomoea purpurea is a common cultivated garden plant that doesn't produce hallucinogenic effects. The roots have a purgative effect due to fatty-acid substances they contain.

Homeopathic use

The species *Ipomea convolvulus Duartinus* is a homeopathic remedy used to treat pain in the lower left side of the back when stooping, kidney disorders, and right-shoulder pain due to renal colic.

positive Healing patterns

- Offers a freeing or liberation of self that is guided by a Higher Power.
- Promotes spiritual vision, guidance, inspiration, imagination, purification, clarity, and abundance.
- Opens the heart toward an expression of love and compassion.
- Stimulates vitality and the feeling of rejuvenation. Helps us make a fresh start.
- Helps us break free of old habits and patterns through spiritual awakenings and liberation of self.

symptoms and patterns of imbalance

Morning Glory may be an appropriate flower essence for those who

- Are spiritually "lost" and seek spiritual guidance
- Aren't in touch with their natural bodily rhythms, tend to be sluggish, and have difficulty sleeping at night or getting up in the morning
- Can't seem to break through old patterns or habits, and need help making a fresh start
- Have hearts that are closed down, causing them to lose touch with themselves and with higher guidance.

Features of the original flower-essence water

Odor: subtle
Taste: stronger than smells; slightly sweet
Sensations: intensification of visually seeing brightness and colors of light; gives a feeling of depth and insight
Water Color: clear

physical makeup

Root, Stem, Leaves/Leaflets, Height: *Ipomoea purpurea* is a creeping or twining, high-climbing vine up to 10 feet long with slightly hairy stems and entire, broad, heart-shaped leaves. The leaves are prominently veined and feel very soft.
Flower Color: Violet-purple
Flowers: The trumpet-shaped flowers have five violet-purple rounded petals that create a soft, glowing, whitish pink star emerging from the funnel-like center and stretching into a deep magenta color toward the flower's edges. The underside color of the flower is a soft pink with a striking deep magenta-colored star. There are five whitish stamens with soft pink anthers at the center, and five small green sepals at the base of the funnel. The flowers average 3 inches wide; they bloom at their peak in the early morning and are usually open less than twenty-four hours. They have a subtle smell that is difficult to

detect, and they prefer early morning and cooler air.

BLOOMING PERIOD: July through October

Doctrine of signatures

- The main signature of this plant is in its name — "glory" — and the glorious whitish and pink-colored light emerging from the center of the flower. This impressive feature gives an illuminating spiritual signature of light and vision and an all-encompassing presence of Spirit. This presence gives off an incredible sense of liberation, spiritual abundance, and inspiration. The white light also relates to the seventh or crown chakra, representing surrender to our Higher Power and release.

- The star in the center of the flower also is a signature of the heavens, and with its upwardly climbing vine, both signatures give a feeling of liberation as they reach for the heavens. The star represents spiritual direction and guidance.

- The violet-purple and magenta color of the flower corresponds to the brow or sixth chakra, which is an opening of spiritual vision, imagination, clarity, visualization, and purification. This color is highly magnetic and very purifying in how we relate to our body-minds.

- Its name "morning" and the fact that the plant opens early in the morning is a signature of the plant's preference to open and make a fresh start every morning of its life. It also corresponds to an ability to learn how to live and function naturally in the body by rising with the sun.

- The heart-shaped leaves are a signature of the heart, and the pinkish color in the center of the flower also refers to the heart or fourth chakra, awakening a higher love, compassion, and expression in our lives.

Helpful suggestions

Take a good look at the colored photo of morning glory and notice the glowing shades of white and pink in the center of the flower, the deep magenta star that reaches toward the edge of the flower, and the violet-purple color of the petals. How do you feel when you look at morning glory? What do you see?

Take several drops of Morning Glory flower essence and close your eyes. You may want to do this exercise at bedtime for guidance in your dreams, or you may choose to take this essence upon waking as a way to begin your day. Imagine yourself inside the glowing center of morning glory and embrace the whitish pink light inside and all around you. See yourself glowing in this light. Feel the warmth of your glow. Notice any visions or images that you have. Take a moment to ask Spirit for any personal guidance that you are seeking while you are in your "glow state." Breathe and relax into your glow. Feel the safety and security that your glow provides you. Feel the peace and softness it gives you. Allow your heart to open. Stretch your arms and hands above you, and your legs and feet below you. Imagine your hands and feet touching God's glow or Spirit's glow. Let your own soothing glow be touched by God's glow and feel your connection. Visualize the colors: white, pinks, violets, purple, magenta. Let yourself journey with the glowing colors and whatever visualizations, feelings, and insights are given to you. When you are ready, open your eyes and maintain your glow as long as you can. Write down your experience in a journal. Remember your experience throughout the day, and try to stay connected with your glow.

affirmations

- "May the love in my heart flow within me and outside of me to every living thing."
- "May the Light within me shine forth and illuminate my path, and may my mind be clear and aware in this moment now."
- "I celebrate this day with a new thought, a new feeling, and a new activity."

case history

Melinda, in her mid-thirties, had flower-essence therapy to help her continue to break free of old patterns. She had a history of abusing alcohol, pharmaceutical drugs, and cigarettes, all of which were in her past. Melinda was given spiritual guidance to use flower essences as another

form of treatment and was drawn to making a fresh start.

She had difficulty getting up in the mornings and felt that she needed to be "revitalized." After taking the Morning Glory flower essence, she began to feel like a "new person." She began getting up earlier, and she was more enthusiastic about approaching her boss with some work issues; she came to the conclusion that she needed to speak from her heart and let herself be inspired and guided by Spirit.

LFE's Research provers' project findings

PHYSICAL SYMPTOMS

CRAVINGS: More water, started eating cheese, more spicy herbs

SENSATIONS: None

PAIN: Two provers had a sore jaw during one day of taking this essence

MODALITIES:

  WORSE: No indications

  BETTER: During sleep

HEAD: Headaches

EYES: None

FACE: None

EARS: None

STOMACH: None

ABDOMEN: None

BOWEL CONDITION: None

URINE: None

FEMALE: None

MALE: None

EXTREMITIES: None

BACK: None

SKIN: None

OTHER: Muscle aches

EMOTIONAL SYMPTOMS

PATTERNS OF BALANCE: "emotional releases; I liked the feeling this essence
gave," "relaxed and at peace," "had understanding in my heart about experiences
that I wanted to intellectually deny"

PATTERNS OF IMBALANCE: "affected my
feelings of physical security: somewhat
scared, being hard on myself and not
understanding why," "irritable"

MENTAL SYMPTOMS

PATTERNS OF BALANCE: "mental clarity,"
"created a lot of deep thinking," "more
compelled to keep a journal and especially
to write down dreams," "revealed an overall picture or description of my life,"
"increased awareness," "had insight into
my dreams," "more inspired"

PATTERNS OF IMBALANCE: "mind wan-
dered from issue to issue, person to person," "more mental dialogue"

SPIRITUAL REFLECTIONS

"Helped me look inside myself for
answers," "have focused on denial of inspiration," "suppression of joy or anything
that flows from my true self and is
oppressed by the dark clouds of self-
doubt," "increased meditation"

DREAMS/NIGHTMARES

"My dreams of a possible animal guide
were strong, and I had been having them
before taking this essence. The essence
brought more clarity to my dreaming.
One of the animals is winged and one is
four-legged. The winged one makes me
think of the "gypsy" side of how I've been
living, as if I'm flying around in my life
and from place to place. The four-legged
one tells me I need to ground myself. They
are both significant in my life right now,
and I like them a lot."

In general, provers were more aware of
their dreams and some kept a dream journal while taking this essence. Dreams
seemed to be more spiritually related.

MULLEIN

(Verbascum thapsus)
PRIMARY QUALITY: SECURITY

FAMILY: Snapdragon or Figwort (Scrophulariaceae)
OTHER NAMES: Velvet Dock, Velvet Plant, Flannel Leaf, Flannel Mullein, Blanketweed, Woolly Mullein, Candlewick, Candelaria, Torchweed, Torches, Donkey's Ears, Hag's Taper, Common Mullein, Our Lady's Candle, Gordolobo, Candle Flower. *Verbascum* is a Latin word, used in Pliny's writing, which comes from the word *barb ātus* and means "bearded." *Thapsus* was a town in Sicily, or the word may come from the isle of Thapsos, which is now Magnise. The Latin word *mollis* means "soft," and refers to its velvety leaves, on which the English name is based.
WHERE FOUND: Waste areas, river bottoms, along roadsides, railroad tracks, hedgerows, dry meadows and open grassy places, pastures, gravelly and chalky banks around settlements, and disturbed earth throughout North America. Can be found between juniper-pinyon and ponderosa belts in the West. Native to Europe and naturalized in the U.S.
ELEVATION: averages 4,500' to 7,000'
ENERGY IMPACT (CHAKRA CORRESPONDENCE): second and third chakras
KEY RUBRICS FOR POSITIVE HEALING PATTERNS: intimacy, listening, purpose, positive masculine energy, protection, security, sensitivity
KEY RUBRICS FOR SYMPTOMS AND PATTERNS OF IMBALANCE: lack of intimacy, lack of direction and purpose in life, insensitivity
OTHER RUBRICS: acceptance, abandonment, aggressive, anger, anxiety, appreciation, assimilation, awareness, calm, centered, change, clarity, cleansing, communication, confidence, conscience, courage, creativity, depression, discernment, fear, focus, gentleness, goals, groundedness, guidance, highest good, impatience, indecisive, inner self, inner truths, joy, light, nonacceptance, nurturing, optimism, overbearing, patience, personal space, phallic, quieting, sadness, self-acceptance, sexual expression, softness, solar plexus chakra, soothing, spleen chakra, strength, truth, unconscious, values

traditional use

Mullein is a powerful, multifacetated plant that goes back into ancient history. In Homer's *Odyssey*, Ulysses used mullein as a protection against the enchantress Circe. In Europe and India, mullein was used to get rid of evil spirits.

In medieval Europe, the tall dried stems were dipped in tallow to make tapers or torches and were used in funeral and religious processions. The Spaniards called it "candelaria," and the English named it "torchweed." The dried down on mullein's leaves and stem was used to make wicks for candles, hence the name "candlewick." "Hag's taper" is a country name referring to "hag" as witch and "taper" as hedge taper (candle); witches were said to have used hedges (where mullein plants grew) as their shelter and they, too, made use of the light provided by the mullein candlestick.

Pliny and Dioscorides suggested preserving food by wrapping it in mullein's leaves. Dioscorides used mullein to treat scorpion stings, eye complaints, toothaches, tonsillitis, and coughs. Galen wrote about mullein's use to aid digestion and cleansing, and Culpeper recommended it as a treatment for gout, obstructions of the bladder and veins, and inflammations of the throat. The Appalachian Indians made an infusion of the leaves to treat dysentery, and the early settlers tied mullein leaves to their feet and arms to cure malaria. The Hopi Indians dried the leaves and used them as a smoking tobacco and as a cure for people who were mentally unbalanced or "to revive the unconscious."

Mullein has also been recommended as a remedy for edema, based on its properties as an absorbent. Mullein flower oil has long been known as a German folk remedy to treat earache and to remove warts, and the use of oil prepared from mullein flowers dates back to the Renaissance. Dr. Constantine Hering, the "Father of American Homeopathy," took it with him to America as one of his few herbal remedies. According to Moore, the roots can be used as a diuretic, to treat inconti-

nence, and to tone the bladder following childbirth. The use of mullein leaves was included in the National Formulary in 1916–36. Rich in mucilage, mullein leaves were traditionally smoked to relieve chest complaints, lung congestion, and asthma.

Leaves and flowers are used as an antispasmodic, astringent, mild diuretic, mild sedative, demulcent, emmollient, expectorant, and tonic, as teas, extracts, tinctures, infusions, gargles, or as a syrup. Mullein is known as the "natural wonder herb"; it has narcotic properties that aren't habit-forming or poisonous. Herbalists use mullein to treat a wide variety of ailments, including coughs, colds and pectoral complaints, bronchitis, asthma and catarrh, coughing or bronchial spasms, nervous disorders, hemorrhages from the lungs, shortness of breath, diaper rashes, tonsillitis, migraines, earaches, colic, emphysema, glandular swelling, swollen joints, problems of the mucous membranes, pulmonary diseases, venereal disease, and whooping cough. Mullein is also a painkiller and can be used as a sedative to induce sleep.

The leaves, as an external woundwort, can be placed on burns, injuries, sprains, and broken bones to encourage healing and to relieve nerve pain. The leaves can also be placed in shoes when the soles are thin, or around a blister to prevent rubbing while walking, or as an emergency Band-Aid™. They are also a handy replacement for toilet paper when out in nature. The flowers can also be used in a facial cream to soothe the skin or as an infusion to brighten hair. Seed oil soothes chilblains and chapped skin, and the plant is also used as a dye.

homeopathic use

Tincture of the fresh plant is made from its leaves when it begins to flower. Dr. Samuel Hahnemann proved Verbascum as a "cough remedy" and generated a broad list of symptoms. Verbascum is primarily used to treat facial pains on the left side and trigeminal neuralgia (nerve pain in the face). It is also used to treat itching of the anus, incontinence, colic, earache, respiratory tract and bladder problems, catarrhs and colds, hoarseness, bronchitis, constipation, cough, deafness, hemorrhoids, and nerve pains.

positive healing patterns

- Promotes strength with softness, enhancing intimacy, humbleness, and gentleness.
- Is especially helpful to men who are seeking true intimacy and security in their relationships, or for women who want to strengthen yet soften their masculine nature.
- Guides us toward our inner light, encouraging focus and sense of purpose.
- Reminds us to listen to our inner selves and to others as they communicate their inner depths and feelings with us.
- Awakens our unconscious mind and heightens our conscience. Teaches us to live and act according to our inner truths and values.
- Activates creativity, sexual expression, joy, and optimism.

- Assists us in assimilating emotional and mental states that no longer serve us. Through the process of assimilation, we are able to incorporate our highest good and absorb it at the highest level possible.
- Soothes, calms, and nurtures our emotional and mental states.

symptoms and patterns of imbalance

Mullein may be an appropriate flower essence for those who

- Lack acceptance and awareness of their own inner worth and values
- Have feelings and thoughts of depression, fear, abandonment, sadness, irritability, anxiety, and/or impatience and who are unwilling or tired of listening to other people's problems, so they deal with others in a grumpy and impatient way
- Are overbearing and aggressive and who force issues with others
- Lack intimacy in relationships and want to soften their masculine nature yet stay strong in their positive masculine traits
- Lack incentive, focus, purpose, and direction and have lost touch with their own inner light and truths.

features of the original flower-essence water

Odor: slight honey-scented aroma is more profound in the water
Taste: slightly sweet

SENSATIONS: Soothing, cool, and gentle in the throat and in swallowing. Gives a relaxing, soothing feeling in the abdomen and solar plexus.

WATER COLOR: clear

physical makeup

ROOT, STEM, LEAVES/LEAFLETS, HEIGHT: Mullein forms a light-colored taproot and a basal rosette of large, soft, downy, woolly leaves that grow near the ground the first year of the plant's life. The second year, a tall, stout, thick, staff-like fibrous stalk emerges from the center of the basal rosette and can grow from 2 to 6 feet tall. The unbranched, woolly, phallus-shaped stalk produces large, thick, foxglove-like leaves that are soft and densely hairy, covering both sides with a flannel-like gray coat. The lower leaves are large and oval/lanceolate and have leafstalks. The upper leaves are stalkless and gradually become smaller and more ovate. The leaves alternate and have noticeable indented wavy veins. A unique feature of this medicinal mullein plant, compared to other mullein species, is that the leaves narrow at the base into two wings that pass down the stem. The leaves are highly absorbent and they pass rainwater down the stem and into the roots, allowing the plant to grow in dry places. The woolly down on the leaves also prevents the leaves from drying out. By placing the fresh leaves in your mouth and breathing in, a cool, moist, soothing sensation is felt. The fresh leaves have a slightly bitter taste. The soft fine hairs on the leaves and stalk also protect the plant from insects and grazing animals due to the irritation caused to the mucous membranes from the down. Mullein's average lifespan is two years, although some plants can survive up to three or four years. Propagation is by seed and the plant self-sows abundantly. New plants can usually be found near the old ones.

FLOWER COLOR: Lemon-yellow

FLOWERS: The slightly honey-scented, bright lemon-yellow flowers open randomly and are densely packed around the woolly cylindrical terminal spike for a foot or more. The tight flower buds, small lemon-yellow flowers, and round tiny-seeded pods all intermingle toward the top of the dense spike. The cup-shaped lemon-yellow flowers are stalkless, have five rounded slightly uneven petals, and are about 1 inch wide. They have five slightly orange stamens with deeper orange anthers.

BLOOMING PERIOD: July and August

doctrine of signatures

- Mullein's stalk is stout, thick, and tall, and its base is especially strong. The entire plant is soft, fuzzy, hairy, and velvety. The plant's character of strength along with its softness represents its ability to cut through coughing and bronchial spasms that damage the soft hairs lining the mucous membranes. The velvety soft, hairy, downy leaves resemble the soft hairs of the mucous membranes. The mullein's phallus-shaped terminal spike filled with flowers also represents strength with softness, promoting intimacy and gentleness.

- The densely packed lemon-yellow cuplike flowers, flower buds, and seeds are securely protected in the soft, woolly, phallic spike, demonstrating emotional openness yet a tightness offering security, protection, and personal space. This signature relates especially to men who are seeking true intimacy and security in expressing a soft, gentle, humble nature, or for women who want to strengthen yet soften their masculine nature. This signature also may refer to males with both strength with softness, or to helping males relate with others in strength and softness, learning to give lots of "warm fuzzies."

- Mullein's use as a torch or candlestick — in addition to the way the densely packed lemon-yellow flowers and buds circle around and upward toward the top of the spike giving off a yellowish light — is a signature of its ability to promote focus, purpose, and Light, thus guiding us toward our own inner selves and light and encouraging us to share our light with others in an effortless and steadfast way.

- The softly colored lemon-yellow flowers correspond with our third chakra and our emotional relationship with ourselves and others. These emotions may include depression, fear, abandonment, irritation, and sadness, yet with the ability to relax and let go. They also help us awaken and stir our unconscious minds which, in turn, heightens our consciousness and teaches us to live and act according to our inner truths and values. The orange stamens and anthers refer to our second chakra, or creative and sexual selves, activating feelings of optimism and joy.

- The woolly, earlike signature reminds us to listen to our inner selves and to others as they communicate with us.

- The incredible absorbency of mullein leaves is a powerful signature of the plant. They act as a relaxant, and they promote absorption in cases of cellular dropsy, chronic disease, pleuritic effusions, and similar accumulations of fluid. Perhaps, on another level, this signature can be related to a person's process of assimilating emotional and mental states that no longer serve the individual. Through the process of assimilation, the individual is able to take in and incorporate what he or she is able to absorb at the highest level possible.

- The taste of the leaves is slightly bitter and their temperature is slightly cool. The leaves have a mucilaginous quality, and the roots and flowers give off a soothing, aromatic scent. These qualities give a signature of the plant's physical ability to soothe irritated membranes, reduce fever, increase secretion, and clear the lungs. The flower-essence water is more aromatic than the flower itself, and the taste of the water is gentle, quieting, soft, and somewhat sweet. The sensation of drinking the water is soothing on the throat, and its gentleness and smoothness is felt all the way down to the abdomen and solar plexus.

Helpful Suggestions

Take several drops of Mullein flower essence and find a cozy spot where you can relax and "tune in." Imagine a soft, velvety blanket of leaves that form a rosette growing close to the ground. Take yourself into the center of the soft, thick leaves, lie against them, and feel the soft, woolly leaves touch your body. Gently take an edge of a leaf and place it between your lips. Breathe the fresh coolness and moistness into your mouth and throat, and take that sensation with you as you swallow. Breathe it in again and then breathe out slowly. See yourself emerge from the soft center, growing taller and stronger and with gentle determination. Breathe in the fresh leaves as often as you want and allow them to nurture and feed you.

Toward the top of your shoulders and around your neck and head, see and feel densely packed, five-petaled, lemon-yellow flowers with tiny orange anthers and buds all around you forming a spike at the top of your head. The flowers also are soft and fuzzy as they lie against your shoulders, neck, face, and head. They give off a soft brightness that allows your entire upper body to glow with Light. Inside, you feel your own inner light guiding you to listen to your inner voice.

Stay with your feelings, your thoughts, your images, your truths, and your light. See where they take you, how you feel, and what you experience. Embrace this entire experience and hold it with you as you step back into your ordinary world.

Affirmations

- "I allow myself to take time each day to know and understand myself and to appreciate my self-worth."
- "I am guided by my inner light and am focused toward a positive direction in my life."
- "I seek intimacy, security, and gentleness in my relationships."

Case History

Kristopher, age eighteen, was experiencing a major life change and crisis when he came to me for a flower-essence consultation. He had recently been involved in a robbery, had been temporarily put in jail, and was now given probation and allowed to live at home under the guidance of his parents. Kristopher lost his high school scholarship to a private school, and he lost his girlfriend. He was depressed, anxious, frightened, irritable, impatient, and angry at himself, and he felt abandoned and lonely.

Kristopher felt an effect of the Mullein flower essence within a few days after he began taking it. "I had a psychological effect from the essence. It helped me to feel more centered and calm. It also helped me to look deeper inside of myself and to be more introspective about myself and my values. It made me look closely at myself and the events which led up to the robbery. I've slowed down and take more time to look at things. I also began praying a lot."

Kristopher's mother made the following comments: "His personality is becoming softer. He's more open and intimate with family members, and he has a greater ability to focus."

Kristopher took Mullein flower essence for several weeks and came back for a refill because he liked taking it so well and it helped give him a new sense of purpose in life.

LFE's Research provers' project findings

PHYSICAL SYMPTOMS

CRAVINGS: Fruit, water, coffee (unusual for the prover who reported it), smoothies
SENSATIONS: None
PAIN: Soreness in left shoulder and neck
MODALITIES:
    WORSE: night with difficulty sleeping
    BETTER: daytime
HEAD: None
EYES: None
FACE: None
EARS: None
STOMACH: None
ABDOMEN: None

BOWEL CONDITION: None
URINE: None
FEMALE: Fewer hot flashes
MALE: None
EXTREMITIES: None
BACK: None
SKIN: None
OTHER: Waves of calm and clearing of lungs

EMOTIONAL SYMPTOMS

PATTERNS OF BALANCE: "the need to be alone," "quiet," "more intuitive," "feeling grateful for love and nurturing in my life," "felt more self-confident and with personal power," "felt in control of my life and experienced a positive field around me," "I feel like something was protecting me," "I cleaned out some closets — literally — and I felt more patience," "I feel like getting rid of the grime," "I felt caring yet unattached," "felt stronger," "I felt an emotional ease and lightness, an opening," "I felt a calming effect followed by extreme sedateness," "I felt lots of warm fuzzies"
PATTERNS OF IMBALANCE: "annoyed by others," "irritable," "impatient," "tired of listening to others' problems," "feeling out of sorts with the things I do every day and with people around me," "unable to relate to others as usual or to be as forgiving as usual," "felt sorrow in my heart," "low self-esteem," "felt grumpy and irritated," "feeling stuck"

MENTAL SYMPTOMS

PATTERNS OF BALANCE: "the need for personal space and time to reflect," "images that came to me were very bright so that I could see more clearly," "more clairvoyant and right-brained," "questioned myself in why I do what I do, asking myself how I can eliminate some of my responsibilities to find time for me," "I had a focus on work, security issues, money issues, and new business ventures," "was especially focused during this essence," "I saw some truths about myself and about other people," "was more clear," "had a greater understanding," "visualization of releasing blockage"

PATTERNS OF IMBALANCE: "longing to escape," "lack of creativity," "irritable," "annoyed," "impatient"

SPIRITUAL REFLECTIONS

"Awareness of a circle of light and wholeness, the self, mandala, and protection from evil," "I felt a gift to my inner self and the acceptance of my self-worth and acknowledgment of my own inner value," "I wanted more time to reflect and pray."

DREAMS/NIGHTMARES

"I had a dream that gave me a positive resolution of a problem with my stepson."

"I had dream images that included lovers, a star, family, nurturing, a circle of light, and children watching out the window of a red room."

Dreams were enhanced with most provers.

ONION

(Allium cepa)

PRIMARY QUALITY: MEMBERSHIP

FAMILY: Lily (Liliaceae)

OTHER NAMES: The Latin word *unio* means "one large pearl," and the Chinese name for onion is "jewel among vegetables."

WHERE FOUND: Native to Asia, onion bulbs grow throughout the world.

ELEVATION: many climates throughout the continent

ENERGY IMPACT (CHAKRA CORRESPONDENCE): fourth and seventh chakras

KEY RUBRICS FOR POSITIVE HEALING PATTERNS: belonging to a group, bonding, releasing grief and suppressed emotions

KEY RUBRICS FOR SYMPTOMS AND PATTERNS OF IMBALANCE: confusion, disinterest, grief, lack of belonging, sadness, withdrawal, difficulty crying

OTHER RUBRICS: abdomen, anger, anxiety, awareness, bowels, breakthrough, calm, challenge, change, clarity, cleansing, clear, confidence, courage, criticism, crown chakra, doubt, dreams, empathy, feminine, gas, group consciousness, guilt, harmony, heart chakra, home, idealism, impatience, irritability, leadership, masculine, membership, mindfulness, misunderstanding, nervousness, peace, planetary consciousness, positive, present, relaxed, restless, self-awareness, self-empowerment, self-esteem, spiritual, strength, tears, understanding, wisdom

traditional use

The onion is one of the world's oldest cultivated plants, honored in India, China, and the Middle East for its powerful healing properties. It appears in old Egyptian writings and tomb paintings. The concentric layers of the bulb were thought to represent the universe. Onion is also known as the remedy that Alexander the Great fed to his troops in battle to give them strength. In folk medicine, it was a custom to wear a piece of onion or garlic on a string around the neck to ward off colds and infections.

Medicinally, the onion contains antibacterial and antifungal components that, in a paste or juice form, can be used to prevent infection in wounds and burns. The bulb of the onion is also used as a stimulant, carminative, condiment, culinary seasoning, diuretic, and expectorant, and is used as a remedy in cases of cold or croup. A volatile oil in the onion stimulates the tear glands and mucous membranes of the upper respiratory tract, which causes the eyes and nose to water. The onion also contains sulfur, which causes the eyes to burn as well. Alliums are also used in ornaments, crafts, and dyes. The dyes are made from onion skins and produce yellows, oranges, and browns.

Homeopathic use

Mother tincture is prepared from the red onion. *Allium cepa* is a remedy used to treat illness in which the primary symptoms include streaming eyes, sneezing, and burning nasal discharge, such as in hay fever and colds. Early stages of laryngitis with hoarseness, and coughs triggered by cold air with a splitting sensation in the throat, are other indications of *Allium cepa*. The remedy is also used for either burning or neuralgic pain that shifts from side to side. It is effective in treating shooting neuralgic pain associated with earache in children, headaches behind the forehead that get worse upon closing the eyes, tearing pain in the larynx during coughing, and toothaches in molars. There are many other homeopathic uses for the remedy, but these are the main ones. One dose is recommended, rather than repetitive use.

positive Healing patterns

- For those who need to find supportive belonging and to love and feel loved within a group. Shows us that within ourselves we are an integrative system of energy and how each individual's energy system contributes to the larger system of energy — world membership.
- Teaches us the effectiveness of the power in bonding and how bonding brings out an individual's strengths, creating a desire for strengthening community support in relation to actions, thoughts, spirituality, and understanding of oneself.
- Helps release suppressed emotions, especially related to sadness or grief, by peeling off old layers and getting to the "heart" of matters. As the layers are peeled off, the heart has the capacity to expand and to radiate its creative force of energy and power.
- Creates peace within oneself and peace toward others.
- Helps us balance physical power with spiritual insight and wisdom. This essence represents expanded consciousness and oneness with the Infinite.

symptoms and patterns of imbalance

Onion may be an appropriate flower essence for those who

- Feel rejected, not very social, withdrawn, confused, and disinterested in life or in themselves
- Are needy, mistrusting, and lacking in a sense of belonging
- Have emotional entanglement and low productivity associated with the sadness felt in not understanding the self; this lack of self-understanding creates a loss of a sense of belonging with others
- Need or desire to peel off another dysfunctional layer of the ego in

order to gain a higher awareness and spiritual understanding of the self

- Have physical symptoms that include head congestion or headaches, heartaches, confusion, restlessness, anxiety, nervousness, or tension
- Find themselves suddenly crying, feeling sadness from deep within.

features of the original flower-essence water

ODOR: sweet onion smell
TASTE: sweet onion taste
SENSATIONS: Soothing and cool in the throat. Mind cleared. Feel relaxed in belly and mind and throughout the body.
WATER COLOR: clear

physical makeup

ROOT, STEM, LEAVES/LEAFLETS, HEIGHT: The onion grows from seeds or from a small bulb that is narrow-rooted. It shoots out an erect stem that carries an umbel of flowers. The larger and stronger the plants grow, the larger the bulbs become. There are four to six leaves at the base of the plant. The leaves are narrow, cylindrical, smooth, hollow, and blue-green. The plant can grow up to 4 feet in height. When the tops yellow and begin to fall over, the bulbs can be dug up. The bulb is made of many layers that can be peeled off one at a time. The outer few layers are made of a dry, thin, waxy skin. Onion contains sulfur and has a sulfur-like smell.
FLOWER COLOR: Whitish pink with green-striped center

FLOWERS: There are six petals or segments in each globe-shaped umbel, giving a star effect. Each petal has a green stripe in the center and there are six stamens with tiny yellow anthers. The umbels smell and taste sweet, like an onion.
BLOOMING PERIOD: June through August

doctrine of signatures

- The main signature is the odor and vapor that causes the eyes and nose to water and helps release sadness and open the heart, strengthening love and spirituality.
- The layers of the onion can be peeled away to reveal another layer of depth and self-realization. Each layer brings another level of clarity and understanding of oneself, which opens the heart, creating a better understanding and clarity of one's role in the community, with one's circle of friends, and as a planetary citizen.
- The bulb and its growth are symbolic of the Light already within that spreads to all the outer layers as it grows in the earth's darkness. The flower head represents the Light needed to shine forth on the outside as well as the inside.
- The color of the flowers — whitish pink with green stripe — corresponds to the seventh and the fourth or heart chakra. The heart is the center where the union of what is above (spirit, vision, light, wisdom, and communication) meets

with what is below (matter, survival, procreation, knowledge, and personality). When the upper and lower chakras are in harmony, their energy currents flow freely and without obstructions. As the layers of the ego or the layers of sadness and grief are peeled off, the heart has the capacity to expand and to radiate its creative force of energy and power. The onion is a universal symbol; its primarily white flower head corresponds with the seventh chakra, demonstrating the balance of its physical power (unique and strong odor) with spiritual guidance and wisdom. With its many layers, the onion demonstrates a thousandfold (many-layered) effect, symbolic of expanded consciousness and oneness with the Infinite.

• The umbel represents group membership with its segments of six, needing each individual segment in order to form a group. Each member or segment plays an integral role in the group as a whole. In relation to the seventh chakra, we learn how we are an integrative system of energy within ourselves, and how each individual's energy system contributes to the larger system of energy.

Helpful suggestions

Onion is a teacher of self-understanding and self-awareness that helps us come to peace with ourselves and understand how we fit into the whole. By experiencing a bonding with self and letting go of that which is suppressed, our hearts and minds are open to receive a higher awareness of spiritual truths. These truths will, in turn, help us understand our relationship to the whole, giving us what we need to find where we belong and how to become a member of that community.

Are you willing to peel off yet another layer without resistance and to discover a new depth of understanding about yourself? Are you confused or distracted about who you are and where you fit with others? Does your heart hurt, and are you holding onto old sadness or suppressed emotions?

Take three to four drops of the Onion flower essence and close your eyes. Imagine yourself sitting cross-legged, bent at the waist with your head and face to the ground. Imagine your arms stretched out over your head so that the palms of your hands touch the earth. Below, you feel the darkness and coolness of the earth. Above, you feel the light and warmth of the sun. Take a deep breath from the earth into your mouth and through your throat. Hold the breath and then gradually let your breath move down through your heart, stomach, pelvis, and genitals, releasing the breath back to the earth. As you release your breath, imagine that you are letting go of part of yourself that you no longer wish to have (an old unresolved emotion, an old sadness, an old dysfunctional ego trait). Send the part that you are releasing to the Light above you, feeling your body becoming lighter.

Take another deep breath from the

earth into your hands and up into your arms. Hold the breath and then gradually let your breath move from your arms to your shoulders, throat, brow, and the top of your head. Then release your breath to the Light above, while imagining that you are letting go of an unwanted part of yourself. As you breathe out, feel your body becoming even lighter and slowly stretch your arms above your head as you move your torso into a sitting position. Your hands are now open above you with your palms facing the Light.

Now take another deep breath and allow the Light to enter your hands and flow up through your arms. Imagine that the Light energy is simultaneously moving downward from your throat chakra at the same time that it is moving up toward the top of your head. See the Light release from the top of your head and back to the Light, while at the same time it releases from the base of your spine and down to the earth. Imagine, and feel if you can, the energy currents in your entire body flowing freely through you. Sit quietly in that feeling and visualization. You may continue this exercise for as long as you like, enjoying your journey.

This is a good remedy to consider taking with the Sweet Pea flower essence; Sweet Pea's compassionate, gentle nature teaches us to love ourselves unconditionally and gives us a sense of belonging.

Affirmations

- "May the Light within me fill my heart with peace."

- "As I peel off my inner layers, I am discovering a newfound freedom of giving energy to others."
- "I am embodied by the One who lives and breathes through me and I see all of the universe as an embodiment of our Creator."

Case History

Shandor, age three, was suffering as a result of his parents' separation (his father had moved out of the home). He felt very confused about who he was and where he belonged. He was very sad and withdrawn, and he had emotional outbursts (crying, anger, agitation, hurtful behavior toward others). His sadness and emotional wounds prevented him from engaging in healthy social play with other children, and he felt isolated, not knowing how to fit in with others. His mother was concerned about Shandor's lack of ability to "belong" and fit in with other children his age.

I gave Shandor the Onion flower essence to help him release his sadness, uncover his heart wounds, and establish a sense of membership within his family. Shandor responded positively to the Onion essence. His anger and agitation noticeably lessened, and he seemed to feel less alienated emotionally from family members. About a month later, I followed up with the Sweet Pea flower essence to help him further feel a sense of belonging outside his family and with his peers. His mother observed that Shandor had a "shift of energy," and he especially was less hurtful to others — a reflection of feeling less hurt inside himself (refer to the Case History for Sweet Pea for the rest of Shandor's experience).

LfE's Research provers' project findings

PHYSICAL SYMPTOMS

CRAVINGS: junk food, bagels

SENSATIONS: Warmth in throat and in swallowing

PAIN: None

MODALITIES:

WORSE: evenings

BETTER: more energy in the mornings, improved sleep

HEAD: Pressure and slight pain at side of head and side of forehead, headaches

EYES: Pressure behind eye

FACE: None

EARS: None

STOMACH: None

ABDOMEN: Warm sensations

BOWEL CONDITION: Laxative, looser stools, "explosive," " bad gas with foul odor"

URINE: More frequent

FEMALE: More sexually aroused

MALE: None

EXTREMITIES: None

BACK: None

SKIN: None

OTHER: Physical vitality

EMOTIONAL SYMPTOMS

PATTERNS OF BALANCE: "feelings of peace," "relaxed," "calm," "positive," "optimistic," "creative," "elevated energy," "more assertive, positive, and confident," "happy and rested" "more patient and relaxed with children"

PATTERNS OF IMBALANCE: "irritable," "critical," "agitated," "crabby," "annoyed," "angered with self and others," "very emotional with self with outbursts of tears for no reason," "frequent outbursts of crying," "emotionally inconsistent"

MENTAL SYMPTOMS

PATTERNS OF BALANCE: "increased mental alertness," "mental clarity," "self-image enhanced," "aware of thinking about what was changing and feeling different," "more relaxed mentally," "more at peace with myself"

PATTERNS OF IMBALANCE: "inconsistency with critical thoughts and pickiness," "this essence caused me to think about people around me and to let them aggravate me when they normally would not do so"

SPIRITUAL REFLECTIONS

"Temporary loss of intuition inconsistent with experiencing increased spiritual influence and intuition," "experienced more peacefulness," "the song 'Peace I Ask Of Thee, Oh River' came to me:

"Peace I ask of thee, oh river, peace, peace, peace.
When I learn to live serenely, cares will cease.
From the hills I gather courage, vision of the day to be,
Strength to lead and faith to follow, all are given unto me
Peace I ask of thee, oh river, peace, peace, peace."

Dreams/Nightmares

"I'm in England (in real life I've been there six times) walking over a bridge. I meet a guy I used to go out with and he's pushing a baby in a carriage. I get to the other side of the bridge, which seems to be a sleazy part of town — erotic movies, body builders in skimpy outfits. I'm very curious, but I keep a safe distance and choose not to be a participant." The prover felt that this dream was about being exposed to "disturbances" that she chose not to participate in, and that she needs to "keep her place," know herself, and understand who or what would serve her to participate with.

Some provers had more lucid dreams than other provers.

OX-EYE DAISY

(Chrysanthemum leucanthemum)
PRIMARY QUALITY: INNER KNOWING

FAMILY: Sunflower (Compositae)

OTHER NAMES: Field Daisy, Common Daisy, White Daisy, Moon Daisy, Horse Gowan, Maudlin Daisy, Dun Daisy, Butter Daisy, Horse Daisy, Goldens, Great Ox-Eye, Mauldlinwort, Mauldelyn, White Weed. Derived from the Greek words *chrisos* (golden) and *anthos* (flower); strictly speaking, this refers only to two indigenous species, Ox-Eye Daisy and Corn Marigold, in which the entire flower is yellow. The name "ox-eye" refers to "white flower" and is Greek in origin.

WHERE FOUND: Patches in meadows or fields, along roadsides, and in waste lands throughout the continent. Native of Europe, naturalized in the U.S.

ELEVATION: all climates throughout the continent

ENERGY IMPACT (CHAKRA CORRESPONDENCE): third and seventh chakras

KEY RUBRICS FOR POSITIVE HEALING PATTERNS: aloneness without feeling lonely, intuition, insight, optimism, understanding, wisdom

KEY RUBRICS FOR SYMPTOMS AND PATTERNS OF IMBALANCE: lack of trust in intuitive guidance, loneliness, misunderstanding, being overanalytical, worry

OTHER RUBRICS: abandonment, abuse, anxiety, balance, calm, children, clarity, complexity, confused, creativity, crown chakra, energetic, enthusiasm, fun-loving, harmony, inner child, inner knowing, intellect, light, nurturing, parenting, patience, peacefulness, playfulness, positive, purification, relaxation, release, simplicity, solar plexus chakra, spiritual, vision

traditional use

An old tradition in Somersetshire, England, relates the ox-eye daisy with the Thunder God, and it has been referred to as the "dun daisy." In early Christianity, the flower was named "maudelyn" or "maudlin" after St. Mary Magdalen. Gerard referred to this plant as "maudlinwort." The older northern name for the daisy was "Baldur's brow," and this species, along with others of the chrysanthemum family, was dedicated to St. John.

Tender offshoots of the plant are quite tasty and can be eaten in salads. The roots and young leaves can be eaten steamed or cooked. Linnaeus Carolus states that horses, sheep, and goats will eat the plant, but cows and pigs refuse it due to its acrid properties. The balsamic flowers and green parts of the plant are known as a tonic and antispasmodic in the treatment of chest problems, bronchial catarrhs, chronic coughs, whooping cough, asthma, and nervous excitability. The leaves, flowers, and stalks can be boiled and sweetened with honey to drink for these purposes, or an infusion can be made. The entire plant can be put in distilled water and filtered to soothe conjuctivitis, and the leaf and flowers can be used externally for wounds, bruises, ulcers, and some skin diseases.

Gerard documented that Dioscorides used as an infusion of the flowers to wash away cold hard swellings, and it is reported that the infusion can be drunk to cure jaundice. Culpeper referred to ox-eye daisy as "a sound herb of good respect, often used in those drinks and salves that are for wounds, either inward or outward," adding that it is "very fitting to be kept in oils, ointments, plasters and syrups."[3] The root of the ox-eye daisy has been used to treat those with tuberculosis in cases of sweating. According to Moore, a tea made of the plant is diuretic, astringent, and mildly hemostatic. It can be used to stop irregular blood in the urine, piles, and stomach ulcers. It also can be used to treat bleeding of the sigmoid flexure (the S-curve of the large intestine between the descending colon and the rectum). A douche can be made from ox-eye daisy to treat cervical ulcers, and it is cooling to the urinary tract. In fact, ox-eye daisy is considered to be a woman's herb and has been dedicated to the goddess Artemis since ancient times.

homeopathic use

The homeopathic remedy is used to calm the nervous system and treats right-sided temple and jaw pain, pain in the teeth and gums (better with warmth, worse with touch), insomnia, and night sweats.

positive healing patterns

- Offers a safe, comfortable feeling and a desire for aloneness, simplicity, and protection without being lonely.
- Provides deep relaxation, peacefulness, inner knowing, and deeper spiritual wisdom, offering inner joy and happiness.
- Teaches balance between intellect and intuition, providing greater wisdom in understanding, vision, and clarity about the whole picture.
- Helps us develop our creative intellectual skills and trust our creative intuition and inner knowing.
- Highlights a playful, optimistic, positive, fun-loving, nurturing nature that is especially supportive of our inner child or children in our lives. Helps one gain wisdom about how to be a positive parent and how to relate to children in creative ways, building harmony and trust. Also helps a parent see a child's world by releasing their own personal blocks.

symptoms and patterns of imbalance

Ox-Eye Daisy may be an appropriate flower essence for those who

- Feel lonely and unprotected, but need to experience the purity and simplicity of being alone and protected without being lonely
- Are confused, anxious, nervous,

and worried, and have difficulty relaxing and may lead emotionally bitter and mentally chaotic lives

- Try too hard to figure things out and aren't connecting with their intuition — who take life too seriously
- Are striving toward a deeper spiritual awareness, understanding, and wisdom
- Have difficulty connecting with their children due to their own wounded inner child.

features of the original flower-essence water

ODOR: strong and sweet
TASTE: full, pleasant, and strong
SENSATIONS: Tingling sensations downward to the belly, then to the root chakra and all the way back up through the chakras and out the top of the head. Gives a feeling of energy, vibrancy, and youthfulness as well as clearer insights and a deeper wisdom.
WATER COLOR: clear

physical makeup

ROOT, STEM, LEAVES/LEAFLETS, HEIGHT: Ox-eye daisy has a shallow root system that is somewhat creeping. The dark green stem is erect, round, smooth, bendable yet sturdy, and slightly branched. It grows from 1 to 2 feet high. The leaves are dark green, small, somewhat hairy, and coarsely toothed or pinnately lobed. The basal and lower stem leaves are spoon-shaped, some-what oblanceolate to spatula-shaped, and between 2 and 6 inches long, including the petiole with a scalloped margin that forms rounded teeth. The narrow upper leaves become smaller and sessile, oblanceolate to linear, merely toothed to incised.

FLOWER COLOR: White with yellow center
FLOWERS: Each stem has only one large, daisy-like flower head, known as a solitary flower, at the end of each branch. The ray flowers are white with a yellow disk that is depressed in the center. The flower head is about 2 inches wide. Underneath the flower head is a ring of green sheathing bracts, the involucre. The sheath of bracts protects and supports the bloom and prevents insects from biting their way to the honey below; the bracts contain an acrid juice that insects don't like. Stamens are short and light green, with yellow anthers. Fruits have about ten ribs.

BLOOMING PERIOD: May through October

doctrine of signatures

- Ox-eye daisy's solitary nature is a signature of the plant's simplicity and individualism. It represents a safe, comfortable feeling of being alone without feeling lonely.
- In spite of its simplicity, ox-eye daisy has characteristic mandala patterns that magnetically attract us to its yellow center, the color of which relates to the third and seventh chakras. The center is like a golden-yellow head with a white halo, giving a feeling of deep relaxation, peace, inner knowing, and a

deeper spiritual understanding or wisdom. It is somewhat trancelike to experience this flower, especially at its fullest; it gives a sense of deep inner joy.

- The white ray-flowers represent the purification and cleansing of the entire energy system, in particular the seventh or crown chakra. With the yellow disk depressed in the center like an image of an eye, the flower offers a balance and understanding between intuition and intellectualism, providing a greater understanding, vision, insight, and clarity about the whole picture. It helps us develop our creative intellectual skills along the way, while also trusting and stirring our creative intuition and inner knowing. This opens us to greater wisdom and understanding that is felt from our root chakra all the way to our crown chakra and out the top of our head.

- The pronounced sawtooth leaves are like a sharp knife; they are used externally to treat wounds and bruises. The leaves and stems are very acrid. On an emotional/mental/spiritual level, the flower essence is also used to purify and cleanse wounds on all these levels, such as mental confusion, worry, emotional bitterness, mental and emotional chaos, trying too hard to figure things out, or childhood or inner-child wounds.

- The ox-eye daisy plant has a childlike joyous, playful nature. The position of the flower is optimistic and its color, although white, is very bright and stands out in a field of wildflowers. The flower-essence water gives a feeling of energetic youthfulness, optimism, and insight.

Helpful suggestions

Choose at least an hour or longer to be alone. Get in touch with and reflect upon the present moment and the past few weeks or month. If you feel like it, write in a journal for the following exercise.

Have you felt in balance or in sync with what you know logically to be true and how that relates to your intuitive self? If you have been feeling out of sorts in any way, try to get in touch with the core issue and where the feeling comes from. Do you have a specific issue in your life with which you seek greater wisdom and understanding from a Higher Power?

Study the ox-eye daisy photo. Look intently in the yellow disk at the center of the flower. Then look at the whole flower. Just gaze for awhile and allow yourself to experience it. Now relax and take several drops of Ox-Eye Daisy flower essence and close your eyes.

Imagine yourself in the golden-yellow center of the ox-eye daisy. Feel the warmth of a golden-yellow halo of light all around you. Feel the light enter your being, awakening your senses and stretching your solar plexus. Feel your solar plexus area relax. Let go of any emotional or mental tension.

Breathe the golden-yellow light and its warmth into your belly. Breathe out any old emotions or thoughts that you would like to release. Again, breathe in the golden-yellow light and warmth, and breathe out the old emotion or thought. Let your body and mind be filled with the golden-yellow light.

Slowly extend your hands and arms, feet and legs outward into the white petals of the ox-eye daisy. Allow your hands and arms to merge with the petals. Allow your feet and legs to merge with the petals. The golden-yellow glow has become a soft white glow that has circled all around you. Allow yourself to bask in this white-light energy field, and feel the strength and cleansing of its healing qualities. Now take the white light with you as you go back to the golden-yellow center. You will see that the two lights emerge into a softer, glowing golden-yellow. Check to see if you have left anything unresolved and if you would like to repeat the exercise again. If so, repeat the exercise with the unresolved feeling or thought. If not, take several long, deep breaths and open your eyes. Notice how you feel.

Write your experience, images, feelings, and thoughts in your journal and begin to find ways to be more creative, positive, understanding, and insightful about who you are and who you are becoming.

Affirmations

- "My thoughts are a reflection of who I am. The higher my thoughts, the freer I feel."
- "May I walk in harmony with the natural rhythm I feel from within."
- "I honor and trust what I feel in my heart when I make decisions and life choices."

Case History

Yolanda, age forty-three, took the Ox-Eye Daisy flower essence. This is what she had to say about her experience:

"The flower essence Ox-Eye Daisy came into my hands at the time when I was having a creative block with performing on my piano. I felt that the energy just wasn't flowing out of my hands and my heart felt blocked. As I took the remedy, I began to feel a flow from my power center and a lightness. A realization came to me after having a healing session with some friends. I was planning to organize and play for a fund-raiser that I really wasn't ready for. I felt a nervousness and anxiety and my creativity was blocked. I feel the remedy helped to move the energy. My music provides deep relaxation, spiritual wisdom, and inner joy for myself and others.

"Also, in my healing work of cranial therapy, the child in me was transferred to my client who hadn't played like a child in a long time. We continued the session playing like five-year-olds and having fun.

"I discontinued taking the remedy for a few weeks, then picked it up again and definitely noticed an inspiration to want to play the piano. I do feel that the Ox-Eye Daisy flower essence assisted my emotional and psychological bodies so that I can be more in the now of things."

LFE's Research provers' project findings

PHYSICAL SYMPTOMS

CRAVINGS: None

SENSATIONS: Light sensations in entire body, warm sensation in heart

PAIN: None

MODALITIES: None

HEAD: Slight throbbing at top of head

EYES: Increased vision, seemed to see more clearly

FACE: None

EARS: More aware of sounds and voices

STOMACH: Pressure in solar plexus

ABDOMEN: None

BOWEL CONDITION: None

URINE: None

FEMALE: None

MALE: None

EXTREMITIES: None

BACK: None

SKIN: None

EMOTIONAL SYMPTOMS

PATTERNS OF BALANCE: "felt more peaceful," "experienced emotional release; made me want to dance," "felt playful and childlike," "sparkles the imagination to love, which frees up the individual inside of you," "felt a natural high," "made me giggle," "felt goofy and mischievous," "drawn to feeling and being more creative," "playful and optimistic," "felt joyful and in harmony," "felt nurtured," "released some past stuff," "worked toward staying grounded"

PATTERNS OF IMBALANCE: "abandonment issues related to inner child came up," "impatient," "uncomfortable in solar plexus," "pressure building up in solar plexus"

MENTAL SYMPTOMS

PATTERNS OF BALANCE: "mental clearing and mental activity more simplified," "experienced a silence of mind," "experienced creative imagery," "felt calm and quiet, at peace with myself," "had more visions and experiences of imagery," "stimulates the imagination," "saw light swirling energy," "gives direction to sense of self," "desire to be more creative," "positive mothering images," "gives more creativity and understanding in dealing with children and finding ways to connect with them," "felt I had a larger perspective of things going on in my life," "this essence helped me analyze and focus with a clearer frame of mind"

PATTERNS OF IMBALANCE: "disoriented," "confused," "anxious," "tired," "worry"

SPIRITUAL REFLECTIONS

"Helped me have the wisdom and to see ways to heal my wounded inner child in order to help my own children heal themselves," "helped me become more aware of a feeling I wasn't aware that I was holding," "helped me tap into my own inner happiness and be more optimistic about life," "enhanced my imagination and trust in a higher power"

DREAMS/NIGHTMARES

Some provers had dreams, while others didn't. No significant dreams documented.

PALMER'S PENSTEMON

(Penstemon palmeri)

PRIMARY QUALITY: SELF-EXPRESSION

FAMILY: Snapdragon or Figwort (Scrophulariaceae)

OTHER NAMES: Pink Wild Snapdragon, Balloon Flower, Scented Penstemon

WHERE FOUND: roadsides, washes, and shaded mountain slopes in Utah, Arizona, and California

ELEVATION: 3,500' to 6,500'

ENERGY IMPACT (CHAKRA CORRESPONDENCE): third, fourth, fifth, and sixth chakras

KEY RUBRICS FOR POSITIVE HEALING PATTERNS: speaking one's truth from a higher perspective, sensitivity, clairvoyance

KEY RUBRICS FOR SYMPTOMS AND PATTERNS OF IMBALANCE: anger, misuse of communication, verbally abusive, lack of confidence in speaking

OTHER RUBRICS: assertive, bitter, brow chakra, clarity, compassion, creativity, expression, heart chakra, imagination, intuition, jaw, lungs, mouth, passiveness, perspective, resentment, self-expression, solar plexus chakra, spiritual guidance, suppression, throat chakra, vision, withdrawal, worry

Traditional Use

There are over 250 species of penstemon native to North America in a variety of colors. Native Americans used the leaves to make a poultice for the skin, and as a wash to treat eye problems. A tea was made and drunk to treat constipation, bronchitis, kidney problems, and whooping cough. The fresh leaves, mixed with sweet almond, apricot kernel, or olive oil can be made into a salve as a skin dressing to treat irritations of the outer skin, anus, and lips.

Homeopathic Use

Unknown to author.

Positive Healing Patterns

- Helps us express ourselves from a place of compassion within our hearts.
- Inspires us to work on a new pattern of speech from a higher and more creative perspective when communicating or expressing ourselves.
- Helps us speak creatively and with sensitivity toward others.

- Transforms the expression of bitter feelings and thoughts into a higher way of communication and self-expression.

symptoms and patterns of imbalance

Palmer's Penstemon may be an appropriate flower essence for those who

- Are angry or verbally abusive, with tendency to hold this anger in the jaw
- Are suppressed in the way they communicate
- Tend to speak more from reactions of the mind or emotions
- Lack clarity in their speech or their communication patterns
- Misuse communication and lack compassion and understanding in expressing themselves
- Lack the confidence to speak up and express themselves, and who are learning to speak their truths.

features of the original flower-essence water

ODOR: sweet, full fragrance, even more so than the flower

TASTE: strong and bitter

SENSATIONS: There is a deep sensation in the back of the throat. At first it's hard to swallow due to the strong, bitter taste, then it gets easier to swallow. My husband, Curt, felt a "subtle tingling sensation and a presence" in the back of his throat and a slight penetration to his third eye.

WATER COLOR: clear

physical makeup

ROOT, STEM, LEAVES/LEAFLETS, HEIGHT: Palmer's penstemon's tall, slender stem grows up to 5 feet high. The stem is pastel green and fibrous on the inside. The grayish green, rubbery leaves are shiny and waxy with a blue coating. The toothed leaves grow in opposites, are larger at the base, and grow up to 5 inches long. The upper leaves are smaller at the top and pair around the stem.

FLOWER COLOR: Pinkish lavender

FLOWERS: The bright pink flower carries a full, sweet fragrance. It has a tubular shape with two upper petals flared backward and three lower petals flared downward. The open flower resembles a large mouth. The enlarged flower tube is somewhat short and grows up to $1\,^1/_8$ inch wide. There are lavender variegated lines on the lower petals that guide bees to nectar inside the short tube. Four stamens emerge from the roof of the "mouth" or from the center of the enlarged tube with large pink anthers. A fifth stamen, called a "staminode," has replaced its anther with a dense cluster of yellow fuzzy hairs; it zooms out from the center of the "mouth" or tube and looks like the flower's tongue. Young buds have a line through their middle that separates the upper and lower petals and resemble a tight jaw line. If you look at the photo closely, you will see this feature.

BLOOMING PERIOD: March to September

doctrine of signatures

- The blue coating on the leaves corresponds to the fifth or throat chakra, which is linked to the mouth, teeth, esophagus, and thyroid. The throat area relates to creativity, associated with the right hemisphere of the brain. The pink color of the flower relates to the fourth chakra or heart center, which stimulates compassion and positive self-expression. These chakras together are a signature of speaking or expressing ourselves from the depth of our hearts rather than through our heads and emotions.

- The bud of the flower has a line through its center that separates the upper and lower petals, resembling a tight jaw line. I have used this essence for myself and others in treating temporomandibular joint dysfunction (TMJ) due to this apparent signature. The flower itself, in full bloom, resembles an open mouth. The fuzzy yellow head looks like a soft tongue. Again this points to a signature of the mouth and throat.

- The hint of lavender brings a softness and clairvoyance to the plant's personality amidst the yellow solarplexus (third-chakra) emotional and mental energy. The lavender highlights the brow or sixth chakra, guiding us toward creative imagination and spiritual vision. Again, this speaks to communication more from the heart and the higher perspective, rather than through the mind or emotions.

- The flower-essence water smells sweet yet tastes strong and bitter. It reminds us to communicate our "bitter truths" from the depths of our hearts as a way of healing the bitterness, rather than communicating from emotional reactions out of blame, anger, or resentment.

Helpful suggestions

Get into a comfortable position, take several drops of the Palmer's Penstemon flower essence, and close your eyes. Rub your hands together and warm them up well, then place the palms of both hands on each side of your face over the jaw area. Hold your hands still and allow the heat to radiate into your face. Feel the energy there and hold it. Try to tune in to how your jaw feels and where it wants to be touched. Now open your mouth slightly and place your fingers on the outside of your face to explore your jaw lines. Beginning at the top of the jaw and using your fingers on both hands, begin to massage the jaw line. When you feel pain or discomfort, gently but firmly press your middle finger into the pain and hold it there until you feel a release. Then slowly open your mouth wide and close it. Repeat this at least two more times. Follow the jaw line with your fingers and continue to massage or press all the way down to the center area where the fingers meet below your lower lip. Press your fingers into that area and then release them.

Now, starting at the top of the jaw line again, move your fingers on both sides of your face, pressing in a downward-sweeping motion. Repeat this several times.

Now rub your hands briskly again and

warm them up. This time, cup the palms of your hands, bringing your wrists together, and place your hands around your throat with your palms in the front of your throat and fingers around the back of your neck. Hold the energy there. Feel the warmth from your hands softly warm your throat area. Repeat this exercise several times so that your throat can feel the warmth.

Now open your mouth and take a deep breath, hold the breath and chant an "ahhhhh." Then let release the breath. Take a long deep breath and again chant an "ahhhhhhhh," but this time increase your volume. Find silence within as you release the breath. Repeat again and chant an "ohmmmm." Repeat as often as you like, using any chant you want. As you're chanting, breathe into your heart and then into your solar plexus. Then breathe back into your heart, then your throat, and then your third eye. Continue to chant as you consciously breathe into these areas. When you breathe out, remember to take a moment to rest in silence and then take in a long breath, hold the breath and chant while the breath is holding, and then release the breath. Do this as long as you want.

When you finish the exercise, notice how you feel and what you observe about yourself. Slowly open your eyes.

Affirmations

- "I embrace the highest good of all when I speak my truths."
- "I am mindful of my bitterness and I create a new and positive pattern of self-expression."

- "I allow the air of my body to communicate from deep within my heart."

case History

Charlene, age fifty-one, was a soft-spoken, compassionate person who lacked freedom of self-expression and tended to hold back in her speech and overall communication. Charlene also had a fear of speaking in groups, especially in public. Charlene felt that her stifled communication style didn't fully represent who she truly was, and she wanted to build her confidence to help her speak her truths. She also had TMJ and wore a mouth appliance at night.

Charlene took the Palmer's Penstemon flower essence to help with all these symptoms. She found that the flower essence inspired her to establish more creativity and confidence in her ability to express herself more freely. She also gained a deeper understanding of herself, particularly as related to her communication abilities. Charlene feels that the Palmer's Penstemon flower essence planted new seeds in her communication awareness and opened a new doorway for continued exploration of herself. She feels grateful for the assistance of Palmer's Penstemon in directing her on her journey of self-expression.

LFe's Research provers' project findings

PHYSICAL SYMPTOMS

CRAVINGS: Chocolate

SENSATIONS: Clearing of lungs

PAIN: None

MODALITIES: None indicated

HEAD: Relieved head congestion

EYES: Relieved watery eyes

FACE: None

EARS: None

STOMACH: None

ABDOMEN: None

BOWEL CONDITION: None

URINE: None

FEMALE: Stirred passion and sexuality

MALE: No male provers

EXTREMITIES: None

BACK: Tingling of the medial side of both my scapula bones (wing bones on back)

SKIN: None

OTHER: "My family was sick with the cold/flu while I was taking this essence, and I became ill also. The significant thing for me was after two days of having a cold, I was completely well. This is a first for me. Usually it lasts for two weeks for me. I was amazed!" "My lungs were clearer."

EMOTIONAL SYMPTOMS

PATTERNS OF BALANCE: "joy, love, and playfulness," "surrender," "felt appreciation," "more creative," "loving," "passionate," "sensed more of a purpose," "receptive," "felt feminine energy," "more sexual," "heart energy," "childlike," "able to surrender my emotions and let go to have more fun," "emotional breakthrough"

PATTERNS OF IMBALANCE: None indicated

MENTAL SYMPTOMS

PATTERNS OF BALANCE: "felt more lightness and play," "I have been painting — expressing my creativity — and I don't normally do this," "stronger purpose," "able to surrender thought dialogue," "more clarity"

PATTERNS OF IMBALANCE: None indicated

SPIRITUAL REFLECTIONS

"I realize my path in this life; the Sacred feminine fills me with passion and I express this by creating beauty; this is how She touches others through me," "I experienced more connection with the Source, more prayer, and more joy"

DREAMS/NIGHTMARES

Dreams were more powerful. One prover dreamed more about her mother than usual.

PALOVERDE

(Cercidium floridum)
PRIMARY QUALITY: EARTH WISDOM

FAMILY: Pea (Leguminosae)
OTHER NAMES: Blue Paloverde. The word *paloverde* means "green stick" in Spanish.
WHERE FOUND: washes, valleys, desert slopes, desert plains and grasslands, and depressions with underground water in southeastern California, Arizona, and Sonora
ELEVATION: 500' to 4,000'
ENERGY IMPACT (CHAKRA CORRESPONDENCE): first, second, and third chakras
KEY RUBRICS FOR POSITIVE HEALING PATTERNS: amend-making, groundedness, self-awareness, strength, survival
KEY RUBRICS FOR SYMPTOMS AND PATTERNS OF IMBALANCE: avoidance, blame, emotional miseries, being judgmental, lack of inner strength
OTHER RUBRICS: anger, anxiousness, appreciation, challenge, change, cleansing, compassion, confusion, consciousness, doubt, earth, emotions, fear, greed, healing, heart, insight, jealousy, love, protection, purification, release, rigidity, root chakra, sensitivity, solar plexus chakra, sorrow, spleen chakra, stomach, understanding, vision, wisdom

Traditional Use

Native Americans ground the seeds to make into a meal; birds and other wildlife also eat the seeds. Some animals eat the branches and pods.

Homeopathic Use

Unknown to author.

Positive Healing Patterns

- Helps us to be grounded and connected with the wisdom and gifts that the earth provides and that which is already inherent within ourselves.
- Teaches us the ease of survival and protection within a harsh environment.
- Helps us build emotional bridges within ourselves and close the gaps of unhealed emotional wounds.
- Offers gifts of unity and the healing of unhealed wounds within ourselves and with others. Gives us the insight and strength to make amends with others when possible and to make amends within ourselves.
- Opens our hearts to love, compassion, and awareness that help us be more sensitive toward ourselves and one another.
- Opens us toward a higher consciousness, inner silence, and ways of living based on wisdom and love.

symptoms and patterns of imbalance

Paloverde may be an appropriate flower essence for those who

- Lack a connection and relationship with the earth as a provider and resource, not only in physical form but in all forms
- Dwell on jealousy, greed, self-doubt, blame, possession, fears, and negative emotional miseries and insecurities
- Are rigid, clingy, anxious, analytical, judgmental, and tend to avoid their true feelings and thoughts
- Have closed-down hearts
- Lack the wisdom, insight, and inner strength to heal emotional wounds within themselves and with others.

features of the original flower-essence water

ODOR: very full, sweet fragrance
TASTE: sweet and tangy, vegetable-like flavor
SENSATIONS: Gives a very full feeling of being grounded; tingling sensation goes all the way down to the root chakra and then moves upward through the chakras and leaves out the third-eye chakra.
WATER COLOR: light yellow; flowers wide open in the water

physical makeup

ROOT, STEM, LEAVES/LEAFLETS, HEIGHT: The greenish blue color of the branches and trunk is a distinguishing attraction of this desert tree, which can grow up to 30 feet tall. The trunk grows up to $1\frac{1}{2}$ inches in diameter. The bark is smooth and thin, and becomes brown and scaly with age. The bark provides the sugar-making functions for the tree and does not depend on its leaves, as most trees do. Twigs produce a $\frac{1}{4}$-inch spine or thorn at each node at regular intervals. The leaves are rather small and inconspicuous; they appear after the winter rains and fall off when the soil has dried out late in the spring, then may reappear during a rainy season in July or August. The leaves are a dull green-blue and grow up to $1\frac{1}{2}$ inch long. They are compound and made up of small oblong leaflets divided on each side of a common leafstalk, resembling a feather. The leaflets are about $\frac{3}{16}$ inch long.
FLOWER COLOR: Bright yellow
FLOWERS: The flowers are made up of five bright yellow petals with a reddish orange spot at the base of the upper petal. They are about 1 inch wide, and four or five flowers grow in a 2-inch-long cluster. In full bloom, the flower petals spread open. Once the petals are formed, seeds develop in flattened seedlike pods that grow up to 3 inches long. The pods are yellowish brown with short-pointed ends. The seed pod and a cluster of about ten erect green stamens with brownish orange anthers emerge from its center.
BLOOMING PERIOD: Late March to May

doctrine of signatures

- It's a glorious sight to see the paloverde in full bloom! Their bright yellow flowers and attractive bluish green bark offer a gift of beauty and inspiration in the desert landscape. The tree's ability to survive in the desert, especially during seasons of little rain, is phenomenal. The tree's bark is able to produce food by taking over the sugar-making functions usually performed by leaves. These signatures demonstrate the paloverde's ease of survival and protection in a harsh, dry desert landscape. They also show the tree's groundedness and connection with the earth.

- Paloverde's smooth bark with spiny thorns at regular intervals is also a fascinating signature. It reminds us that even when our lives are going smoothly, we need to keep in mind that there will be times when thorns or challenges will be presented to us. By connecting with the earth and grounding within ourselves, we will be better able to meet our thorns and challenges.

- The yellow flower corresponds to the third or solar plexus chakra, which is associated with the digestive system, the adrenals, stomach, liver, gall bladder, and the left hemisphere of the brain. Many emotional and mental illnesses can be relieved by working with this center. The orangish red spots on the upper yellow petal correspond to the first or root and second or spleen chakras, which are associated

with our life-force, conscious creativity, sensations, and emotions. Paloverde gives us a message: "Reach out toward healing. Make amends with whomever you can, and make amends within yourself. Work toward healing any wounds that you know deep inside of you are unresolved. By building emotional bridges within yourself, you close the gaps of emotional wounds. Take responsibility for your personal choices. Share and embrace a higher vision within yourself. As you do, you will build a lightness of character that doesn't take life so seriously. This will help you tap into higher energies and rid yourself of the old negative patterns that hold you back. Accept and embrace the wisdom and gifts that the earth provides. Go sit on her lap and lean against a tree. Allow yourself to just be and you will see that she will take you beyond any judgments, and beyond your personality self. The gift that I bring to you is to remind you to ground yourself, explore your inner depths, and embrace your higher wisdom that is already inherent within yourself."

Helpful suggestions

Find a quiet spot and give yourself some quality time to do this exercise. Take several drops of Paloverde flower essence and close your eyes. Visualize yourself squatting. You are face-to-face with the smooth bluish green trunk of a paloverde tree. Look into the bark and examine it closely with your eyes and then with your hands. Take your hands and follow the smooth lines on the tree and feel its bark. Then look up and notice that above you are many bright-yellow (with hints of reddish orange) flower blossoms hanging on the ends of blue-green branches. Take in the bright yellow color as it swarms above your head.

Find a cluster of flowers near you and study an open flower. Notice that there's a reddish orange spot at the base of the flower's upper petal, and that the five almost-equal petals spread wide open. You can see a tiny flattened seed pod emerge from the center of the flower along with the cluster of short, erect, green stamens. Looking the flower over carefully, breathe its presence into the top of your head and take a long, deep breath all the way down to your root chakra. Repeat this several times, allowing the breaths to become longer and deeper.

Then shift to a sitting position and wrap your legs and arms around the tree while you lean against it with your chest and embrace the tree with a hug. Now breathe "into and out of" the paloverde's trunk. Imagine the breath and presence of the tree as one with your breath. Place your forehead against the trunk as you continue to hug the tree, and simply breathe and hold the tree or let the tree hold you.

Now breathe into the tree's roots and imagine its roots extending below you and building a bridge that connects to the base of your spine. Feel what it feels like to be connected and bridged with the earth and with paloverde's roots. Follow the roots deep into the ground and find the roots of other paloverdes in the area. Notice that the roots of the paloverde trees are connected. Notice the larger and more scaly roots that are older, and the tender and younger shoots that are beginning to grow new trees.

Again, build a bridge between those roots and your own. Feel into the powerful connection that the paloverde's roots and the earth give to you. Now notice your forehead and how it feels against the tree. Notice your neck/throat and chest/heart area and how it feels to be hugging the tree. Notice how your belly feels up against the tree. Breathe it all in and breathe out.

Now slowly release yourself from the paloverde's roots, let go of the tree, and sit. When you feel ready, open your eyes and hold the energy you just received for as long as possible.

Affirmations

- "Mother carry me in the wisdom of your deep blue sea,
  Mother hold me in the wisdom of humility,
  Mother carry me in the wisdom of your deep rich earth,
  Mother hold me in the wisdom of my new birth."

- "I see the higher truth in all things and I exist as an equal to all of life."

- "I allow the earth of my body to nurture me."

case history

Kumari, a woman in her late thirties, expressed the following intention regarding her need for a flower essence: "I am in the process of enduring the impact of an auto accident that happened with my nineteen-year-old daughter. I have experienced extreme emotions, emotional drain, sharpness, awareness, love, strength, and family. I wish for clear, strong, healthy, and positive growing learning wisdom!"

I gave Kumari Paloverde flower essence to help her during this challenging time in her life. Her comments about taking this essence are as follows: "In taking Earth Wisdom, at first I felt two things very clearly: cruel/loving. Now I've moved to more of a deep sense of strength, groundedness, firmness, and balance. I looked forward to the drops under my tongue because I love the ritual of stopping to listen and to acknowledge Mother Earth and then feel the thankfulness in my heart. Then discernment hit like it was very much in my face. What is this situation? What do I feel in my gut? I found myself being mad. Even if I had a good cause, it motivates me to go inside and look more closely. I felt an incredible sense of anger, confusion, and anxiousness, but then an eager anticipation to gain access with my higher inner wisdom to work it out."

life's research provers' project findings

PHYSICAL SYMPTOMS

CRAVINGS: Water, oatmeal and more easily digested foods, beer

SENSATIONS: Lightheadedness

PAIN: Stiffness and tension in jaw

MODALITIES:

    WORSE: None

    BETTER: Very deep sleep

HEAD: Lightheadedness and disorientation at times

EYES: Lost sight in left eye; was temporarily blurry and light around the edges, which was moving in a circular pattern

Face: None

EARS: None

STOMACH: Discomfort

ABDOMEN: Discomfort

BOWEL CONDITION: Irregular bowel movements

URINE: None

FEMALE: Increased sexual energy

MALE: None

EXTREMITIES: None

BACK: None

SKIN: None

OTHER: "I had more physical strength to do things. For example, I was able to move sandstone blocks without much trouble." "I felt I needed more physical activity," "I felt in touch with my body."

EMOTIONAL SYMPTOMS

PATTERNS OF BALANCE: "I experienced powerful releases," "I had an energy boost," "my sexual energy was increased and my heart center was able to let in higher doses of love," "a few times I felt my heart opening; trust played a role in this, and so did love," "I felt an opening of my heart that guided me toward loving myself," "I trusted my intuition more," "I experienced cleansing," "I felt more sensitive and aware of others' needs," "I felt an intensity in my solar plexus," "intense emotional feelings more than usual; more feeling on the verge of tears and more sensitive to other people, too," "helped bring up old emotional patterns that were self-destructive that needed release and healing and caused a great deal of self-examination," "I felt grounded and balanced and was able to observe myself through the currents of emotions," "I felt a lot of sadness, like a current or tide coming in and out; I felt it but didn't really go into it"

PATTERNS OF IMBALANCE: "more intense emotions; pain in my solar plexus all day long," "felt alienated from others," "brought up and intensified emotional hurts and old stuff from when I was younger that I haven't experienced in years," "I experienced intense negativity toward myself that really upset me, and I had fear of telling other people my true thoughts and feelings," "I felt some pretty wide emotional imbalances," "brought up fears"

MENTAL SYMPTOMS
PATTERNS OF BALANCE: "I saw visions through my third eye," "I had visions and past-life memories," "felt stimulated to write music," "I am becoming more aware of negative patterns and determined to notice and change them," "gained more insight and awareness of self," "was able to observe myself more clearly," "helped me be aware of basic fundamental patterns such as my roots and physicality, connections with parents and teachers in my past," "more sexual feeling," "my mind was clear, grounded, and focused," "increased concentration and follow-through"

PATTERNS OF IMBALANCE: "lack of clarity," "disturbed memory," "too much stuff in my head; need to get rid of it," "thoughts went round and round in circles trying to figure things out," "anxiety," "avoidance"

SPIRITUAL REFLECTIONS
"I realized all the love that is being given to me through so many different sources," "helped to remember the free will of choice and to ask for what I want," "my sensitivity and awareness is heightened," "I'm noticing more those things that I need to clear from my consciousness in order to be more my true self," "my spirituality begins in my body"

DREAMS/NIGHTMARES
Most provers reported that dreams were clear and vivid. However, no significant dreams were documented.

PEACE ROSE

(Rosa peace)
PRIMARY QUALITY: GIFT OF THE ANGELS

FAMILY: Rose (Rosaceae)

OTHER NAMES: The name "rose" comes from an ancient root *wrod*, the modern translation of which is *vard*, an Old English word meaning "thornbush."

WHERE FOUND: The rose is cultivated as an ornamental throughout the United States.

ELEVATION: most U.S. climates

ENERGY IMPACT (CHAKRA CORRESPONDENCE): first, fourth, and seventh chakras

KEY RUBRICS FOR POSITIVE HEALING PATTERNS: compassion, forgiveness, inspiration, joy, love, uplifting

KEY RUBRICS FOR SYMPTOMS AND PATTERNS OF IMBALANCE: burdens, depression, despair, facing death, grief, loss of a loved one

OTHER RUBRICS: anxiety, beauty, courage, crown chakra, diseases, faith, freedom, healing, heart chakra, illness, judgment, light, pain, protection, release, root chakra, self-pity, sorrow, suffering, surrender, trust, unforgiveness, worry

traditional use

The rose began its long European history in Greece, where its legend goes back to the Greek historian Herodotus. Its cultivation then spread to southern Italy, and from there to Persia and China. For over 3,000 years the rose has been the "queen of flowers." People of all lands have honored and cherished the rose. Cleopatra enticed Mark Anthony knee-deep in rose petals on her palace floor to gain his affections. The Romans crowned bridal couples with roses, and Roman banquets were decorated with rose centerpieces. Roses were a sacred flower to Aphrodite, the Greek goddess of love and beauty. Even as early as the tenth century, rose water (made by

simply placing rose petals in water) was prepared as a purification.

The Muslim conqueror Saladin had the Omar mosque purified in rose water upon entering Jerusalem in 1187. In the sixteenth century, an essential oil called an "attar" or "otto" was prepared from rose petals; its production has been a prominent industry in France ever since. The rose became known as the "gift of the angels" due to its safe, soothing healing qualities. Rose water became popular for cooking, and is an ingredient in a candy called "Turkish delight." Wine prepared from rose petals was made in ancient Persia, and rose petals have historically been used in jams, vinegar, and pies, and as a garnish.

American Indians gathered the wild

rose for ornaments and for medicinal uses. They used rose petals with bear grease to treat mouth sores, and they made a rose powder to treat fever sores and blisters. Sore eyes were treated with rose water, made with rain, and the inner bark of the rose root was used to treat boils. In 1699, William Penn brought eighteen cultivated rose bushes with him when he returned to the colonies from England. Both George Washington and Thomas Jefferson had affection for the rose, but John Adams was the first president of the U.S. to plant rose bushes near the White House.

Medicinally, rosehips are recommended in a tea as a source of vitamin C and as a mild laxative and diuretic. The petals offer a flavor to medicines in the form of a syrup and have been used in tonics and gargles to treat catarrhs, sore throats, mouth sores, and stomach problems. Roses are considered cooling and are used for soothing the mind in Ayurvedic medicine.

The petals are also common in potpourris. One of the most popular, best-loved fragrances is that of the rose. Its soothing aroma is associated with love and femininity and is found in perfumes, bath oils, soaps, hair tonics, skin lotions, ointments, creams, and air fresheners. One of the most costly oils is made from damask roses, which are cultivated in Bulgaria.

The peace rose is a hybrid tea rose that was introduced to the U.S. in 1945. It's the world's most common rose and is a parent of many other known roses. The peace rose is an exhibition winner of most of the world's top rose awards, including the National Gold Medal Certificate; it's one of ten roses with an almost perfect American Rose Society rating of 9.0.

Homeopathic Use

Rosa damascena is used as a homeopathic remedy at the onset of hay fever. It is also used to treat tinnitus, hardness of hearing, and eustachian catarrh; a patient may have symptoms of watery eyes, itching nose and eyes, and frequent sneezing.

Positive Healing Patterns

- Helps us come to terms with what is of value within ourselves.
- Inspires us to open our hearts to receive love, peace, joy, and beauty.
- Gives us the courage and faith to face our pains and suffering.
- Helps us release sadness and grief, allowing ourselves to emerge into fullness.
- Helps us release judgment and unforgiveness.

Symptoms and Patterns of Imbalance

Peace Rose may be an appropriate flower essence for those who

- Are suffering depression, especially in grieving or in the loss of a loved one; also for depression related to illnesses or diseases of self or others
- May be faced with their own death or a part of themselves that is no longer present

- Feel shut down in their heart
- Lack courage and faith, and who tend to reside in their pains and sufferings.

features of the original flower-essence water

ODOR: more aromatic in the water; very pleasant smell

TASTE: pleasant; tastes like a rose smells

SENSATIONS: soothing in mouth and down throat; heartwarming energy throughout the body

WATER COLOR: clear

physical makeup

ROOT, STEM, LEAVES/LEAFLETS, HEIGHT: The peace rose is a strong, spreading bush of medium height, growing up to 6 feet tall. It is a deciduous bush with long, prickly, reddish green, sturdy stems. The leaflets grow in opposites along smaller prickly stems and form a compound or cluster of three leaflets toward the end of the stems. Up to nine leaflets may appear on a single stem. The glossy, deep-green leaves are slightly toothed and oval.

FLOWER COLOR: Whitish yellow (soft creamy yellow) with pink to reddish rimmed tips

FLOWERS: The peace rose has an ovoid, or egg-shaped, bud that is full at the base and narrows to a rounded end. The bud unfolds into splendid extra-large whitish yellow blossoms with subtle translucent pink-rimmed tips. The layered effect of the blossoms includes about forty to forty-five petals, and the flower head can grow up to 6 inches wide. The layers appear tighter in the center and looser around the edge of the flower. The flowers are long-lasting, although the bush itself doesn't usually produce an abundance of blooms. However, the blooms it does produce are nearly perfect. The blossoms of peace rose carry a subtle rose scent.

BLOOMING PERIOD: Spring through fall

doctrine of signatures

- The peace rose bush has numerous branching stems covered with prickly thorns. It's easy to get caught off guard and prick your finger on the thorns when you least expect it — just like life itself. But that doesn't prevent us from picking or smelling the beautiful flower that emerges from within all those prickles. Isn't it amazing that within all the thorns — all the blows in life, our pains, sufferings, challenges, and hard work — that a beautiful, endearing, gentle flower can appear from nowhere? The flower certainly is a "gift of the angels." Just as in life, when we least expect it — we've lost all hope, feel out of touch with love, and feel pricked to death by our pains and challenges — somehow we're able to gather our courage, find our faith to go deeper inside our pain, and discover that even within the deepest pain, there is love. There is the flower, the angel, giving us the gifts of beauty, love, courage, and peace that we can produce within ourselves. And then we begin to unfold and to emerge into the flower, committed to becoming that which we have decided is of value, inspired by the opening we feel in our heart, inspired by the love we feel for ourselves, inspired by love itself, inspired by the love we feel toward others. We have set our hearts free. We have become the rose. We are able to love, to find our beauty, to live in courage and faith, and to find peace within ourselves amidst all the thorns, amidst all the setbacks, amidst all the grief, the pain, the suffering. We are love.

- The many layers and folds within the flower blossom are similar to the layers we experience in ourselves. The outer layers are looser, bigger, and easier to see, and the inner layers are tighter, smaller, and harder to see inside. In fact you have to tenderly push the inner layers back in order to find the center of the flower. The center is soft and vulnerable, yet its core essence — which is the essence of the flower's soothing aroma — is gentle but strong.
- The soft yellowish-whitish color of the flower relates to the seventh or crown chakra, offering purification and awakening to the entire energy system. Its color contains all the other colors of the spectrum, offering intensified and deep healing. The pink-rimmed tips of the peace rose correspond with the fourth or heart chakra, and relate to positive feelings of love, as well as emotions such as grieving the loss of a loved one, feeling a lack of love for life and self, and perhaps feeling self-pity and self-despair. The darker red-colored tips relate to the first or root chakra, which gives us the courage and strength to allow ourselves to unfold and emerge as the flower.

Helpful suggestions

This is a special time for you to make a commitment to yourself to find what is of value inside you that will allow you to become the flower. It is time to no longer be held back by life's thorns. How many more times do you need to prick your finger — to see, feel, and experience the blood dripping on your hand — in order to realize that it is no longer what you want? Nothing remains the same. Sad to say, in this great mysterious cycle of living and dying, that we can't hold onto the way we once loved people. Nor can we hold onto parts of our lives that we loved but are no longer here. Nor can we hold onto parts of ourselves that lead us to misery if we choose to change. Not all things in life are fair or easy to accept. There is always a bigger picture that God has planned to help us grow, love, let go, grieve in our sorrow, and feel the pain, so that we can again become the flower. Just like the rosebush, the flowers bloom according to the season. We too, bloom in relation to our life cycles. Sometimes there are fewer blooms on one rosebush; at other times there are many more. So it is up to you to make your choice to emerge and be the flower. If you're ready, let's go.

Take several drops of the Peace Rose flower essence into your mouth. Hold them there, move the liquid to the back of your tongue, and swallow. If you have a specific intention in relation to a feeling, another person, or within yourself, take a few moments to sit in silence to gather that intention. For example, if you have been ill or if you have had to face death within yourself or with a loved one, get clear on what you need to heal within yourself in relation to your experience. Be as clear as you can. If you aren't able to identify anything in particular, and you have an overall feeling of depression or sorrow, just feel into what you are feeling.

Imagine yourself as the rosebush. Visualize the prickly thorns on the long stems. Go to one thorn and identify that thorn in your life now. How does that thorn prevent you from being the flower? Look that thorn over carefully. How does it make you feel? Are you tempted to be pricked by it? Are you ready to let it go? If so, tell the thorn that you no longer need it in your life. Thank it for how it has helped you and how you have grown from it. Then say good-bye to it. You probably don't have to go very far to come upon another thorn. Look at this thorn closely. How has this thorn affected your life? How

has it helped you grow? What can you tell this thorn about the gift it has given you? How can you change your response to this thorn's gift? Can you let this thorn go? If so, thank it for how it has helped you, then tell it that you don't need it anymore. Say good-bye and bless it on its path. Repeat this exercise with as many thorns as you need until you reach the end of the stem and find yourself at the bottom of the bud.

The bud has a gentle, pleasant fragrance. It beckons you to come. Are you ready? If so, enter the bottom of the bud and feel around inside. Feel the soft, tightly closed petals preparing for their opening. Now take the bud and place it in your heart. Breathe into the bud as deeply as you can. Take long, slow breaths. Breathe the rose scent into your heart as well. Watch as the bud slowly begins to unfold its petals. Feel your heart opening and warming with the sun as the rose petals slowly emerge. Allow the petals to take their time. Let your heart open as one with the flower. Visualize a soft, glowing pink light around your heart flower. Let it open wider, and wider, and wider. See the petals unfold. Feel the warmth in your heart. Stay with the pink glow and let the glow circle all around you. Rest in this heart space and remember how it makes you feel. You have given yourself a beautiful gift. You are the flower and you can become the flower whenever you wish.

Affirmations

- "May I honor the beauty of all of life and all of life's passings."

- "May my pains and sufferings be inspired by hope and love."
- "My heart is a vessel of love, my mind is a vessel of truth, my body is a vessel of healing."

case History

This is a letter I received from Phil, a man in his forties:

Dear Rhonda,

I had been dealing with malignant lymphoma for three-and-one-half years prior to receiving the flower essence entitled 'Peace Rose.' I had recently been hospitalized for nearly three months, and had low energy and was very foggy in the head from all the drugs administered while hospitalized and after. I believe that I was depressed when I received the essence. My body and soul had been traumatized by my circumstances.

The essence was thankfully received and taken daily. I feel that the essence helped me lighten up and begin to focus on life and living again. I felt my heart open more and I was able to express more feelings, love, and joy. I was able to stop focusing on death and start expressing living and loving feelings and thoughts.

Initially, when taking the essence, I felt more energy. As time went on, I no longer felt increased energy, although my stamina has increased overall. I feel that the essence has helped me recover from the hospital trauma and increased my liveliness and courage to go on with life. I am now in the process of moving to Tucson without having a source of income. This thought had been scary to me in the past, yet now feels okay to go and be in Tucson with a lot of unknowingness. I do not feel as scared or judgmental as in the past. I am a lot more trusting that opportunities will present themselves more easily than in the past. I open to possibilities and have more faith and loving feelings in all that I do.

Thank you so much for assisting me in my healing process. This experience has been invaluable.

With much love,
Phil

Lfe's Research provers' project findings

Physical Symptoms

CRAVINGS: None

SENSATIONS: None

PAIN: Mouth sores

MODALITIES: None

HEAD: None

EYES: None

FACE: None

EARS: None

STOMACH: None

ABDOMEN: None

BOWEL CONDITION: None

URINE: None

FEMALE: None

MALE: None

EXTREMITIES: None

BACK: None

SKIN: None

EMOTIONAL SYMPTOMS

PATTERNS OF BALANCE: "this essence gave me the courage to change my mind," "I felt protected in a circle of light when taking this essence," "I am more allowing for changes to happen," "I felt peace and relief with this essence," "felt a sense of freedom and protection," "experienced healing," "felt my feminine inner beauty"

PATTERNS OF IMBALANCE: "lots of sadness," "depression," "burden"

MENTAL SYMPTOMS

PATTERNS OF BALANCE: "warm reflections on the newly found power of the feminine," "I feel more aware of watching for an effect of this remedy," "I made an important decision during this time that changes my path a little — finally realizing what my own needs are," "I feel this remedy helps in making powerful decisions"

PATTERNS OF IMBALANCE: "worrying," "anxiety"

SPIRITUAL REFLECTIONS

"By reflecting on the meaning of dream symbols, it seemed to bring the quality of the essence into the light," "I felt a newly found power from within"

DREAMS/NIGHTMARES

"I had dream images that produced a circle of light. I saw a beautiful woman inside of the circle (representing my power of feminine healing), hands holding a letter (which felt like I was receive a healing message), a snake (representing temptations and spiritual power), and a frog (representing personal transformation and healing). I felt that the circle of light implied protection from evil."

PINYON

(Pinus edulis)
PRIMARY QUALITY: PATIENCE

FAMILY: Pine (Pinaceae)

OTHER NAMES: Pinyon Pine, Rocky Mountain Nut Pine, Nut Pine, Colorado Pinyon Pine, Two-Leaf Pinyon, Mexican Pinyon Pine, Pino Pinonero

WHERE FOUND: Mesas, plateaus, and foothills, among juniper trees or ponderosa pines, and in dry mountainous regions and lower mountain slopes of New Mexico, Colorado, and Arizona. Native to the U.S.

ELEVATION: 4,000' to 9,000'

ENERGY IMPACT (CHAKRA CORRESPONDENCE): first, fourth, and sixth chakras

BACH FLOWER REMEDY: *Pinus sylvestris* is used for those who suffer from guilt and self-reproach, and who tend to take the blame for others' mistakes. These people tend to feel unworthy, inferior, and undeserving. They set unrealistic expectations for themselves and are usually introverted. Pine essence is taken to balance self-responsibility and to live more in the moment without dwelling on the past.

KEY RUBRICS FOR POSITIVE HEALING PATTERNS: appreciation, gentleness, introspection, purification, honoring death and dying

KEY RUBRICS FOR SYMPTOMS AND PATTERNS OF IMBALANCE: burdens, guilt, impatience, lack of perseverance, regrets, restlessness, shame, struggles with death and dying

OTHER RUBRICS: anxiety, approval, balance, blame, brow chakra, calm, clarity, cleansing, compassion, depression, dreams, emotions, female, femininity, fertility, fortitude, freedom, groundedness, harmony, heart chakra, insight, inspiration, introspection, love, mother, nurturing, oversensitivity, patience, peace, psychic, purpose, rejuvenation, release, root chakra, self-appreciation, self-responsibility, shortcomings, simplicity, sleep, solar plexus chakra, understanding, vision, vitality

Traditional Use

In prehistoric times, pinyon provided various Indian tribes with food, fuel, building materials, tools, and medicine. Pinyon nuts contain over 3,000 calories per pound and were a valuable source of winter plant food for the prehistoric people living in the pinyon-juniper habitats. The pinyon nut contains the twenty amino acids that make up a complete protein. Pinyon nuts were eaten raw, roasted, boiled, or ground into a flour. The Navajo made a tasty butter (*'athlic*) from pinyon similar to peanut butter to spread on corn cakes. To this day, pinyon nuts are still gathered to eat and to sell. Pinyon nuts can be used in a variety of foods, including cookies, candies, turkey stuffing, and pancakes. Also, the seeds are important wildlife food for songbirds, quail, squirrels, chipmunks, black bears, mule deer, and goats.

Navajo, Pueblo, and Hopi Indians boiled the pitch of the pinyon tree with sheep and goat hooves to make a glue. They then used the glue in their jewelry work, cementing turquoise into silver settings and sinew to the back of bows. Pueblo Indians also made a red pottery paint by mixing resin of old and new trees. Pitch was also mixed with sumac leaves and yellow earth to make a black inklike dye for coloring wool and blankets. One of the most important uses of the pitch was making it into a melting gum to waterproof basketry water jugs.

Medicinally, pitch was used as a dressing to treat open wounds by both Native Americans and white settlers; it is still used this way today in rural areas of the Southwest. The smoke from burning gum was also inhaled to treat head colds and earaches. The buds were chewed and then spit onto burns. The inner bark of the pinyon can be boiled slowly to make a tea, and then sweetened with honey to drink as an expectorant after the passing of a feverish chest cold. A small piece of the pitch can be chewed and eaten to soften the bronchial mucus; this is especially helpful for children. Pitch can also be melted and applied to splinters, glass, and other skin invaders. A Hopi grandmother told a friend of mine that the Hopi ate the sap of the pinyon to break up gallstones.

Fresh pinyon needles make a refreshing tea, which can be used as an astringent, stimulant, diuretic, or aromatic. The tea is used to treat rheumatism, fever, coughs, and delayed menses. It also stimulates the heart and respiration. Pinyon was also used in ritual practices and in many Native American ceremonies, and the pitch was used as a form of cleansing and purification for the deceased and the survivors.

Today, incense is made from the resin of pine and pinyons to clear negative energy from a place. Members of the Sword Swallowers order of the Great Fire Fraternity within the Zuni Indian tribe had yet another powerful use of pinyon medicine: following a ceremony, the young men would eat the young shoots of ponderosa pine if they wanted their wives to bear a son; they would eat the young shoots of the pinyon if they wanted their wives to bear a daughter. Interestingly, the pine was sacred to the Druids, who carried pinecones to represent fertility.

homeopathic use

A fresh tincture of *Pinus sylvestris* is made of leaves and young twigs. Symptoms include chilliness alternating with flushing, chilliness and sensitivity to touch, face alternating between red and pale, and general itching. It is also used to treat conditions such as bronchitis, constipation, diarrhea, weakness of the lower limbs, swollen glands, gout, heart palpitation, stiff joints, pains in kidneys, enlargement of the liver, rheumatism, and tinnitus.

The homeopathic remedy *Pix Liquida* (pine tar) acts on the mucous membranes and is used to treat itchy skin so persistent that one must scratch until it bleeds, cracked skin, bronchial irritation after the flu, hair loss, and constant vomiting of blackish fluid with stomach pains.

positive Healing patterns

- Provides an appreciation for peace, simplicity, introspection, gentle strength, and fortitude.
- Helps us feel freedom in who we are without shame, guilt, past burdens, or regrets, or needing approval by others. Helps us overcome oversensitivity in how we are affected by others and to focus on living in the present.
- Helps us take on a new responsibility for ourselves, to discover our essence, and to free ourselves and others of shortcomings.
- Offers gentle nurturing, endurance, perseverance, patience, and strength, highlighting the softer features of feminine qualities.
- Provides cleansing, purification, and rejuvenation. Is helpful in prayers or ceremony in dealing with the death of another, the death of a friendship, or releasing an old part of the self that no longer serves.
- Inspires us toward a higher spiritual vision and understanding.

symptoms and patterns of imbalance

Pinyon may be an appropriate flower essence for those who

- Need to take time to be with themselves and gather strength, introspection, and appreciation of self
- Hold onto past burdens or regrets, need approval from others, and are oversensitive about how they are affected by others
- Tend to be impatient and restless, and have difficulty living in the moment
- Have poor social skills and lack the ability to hold their own in the company of others
- Need cleansing and purification, and who may be struggling with the death of another or a death inside themselves
- Have lost their spiritual inspiration and whose heart is closed down
- Lack fortitude and perseverance, and who feel stuck in ways that no longer serve.

features of the original flower-essence water

ODOR: refreshing pine scent
TASTE: even more refreshing, smooth, and soothing
SENSATIONS: A tingling from the head to the root chakra, with heaviness in the solar plexus that seemed to churn. Then the tingling sensation goes back up through the heart and third eye. There is a light tingling energy that loops from the third chakra to the other higher chakras. Temples relax and feel more expansive, and an overall calmness is experienced. The lungs also experience an opening and a soothing in

the throat. This essence is highly energizing and rejuvenating.

My stepdaughter Jenny, age twelve, says the flower-essence water made her feel refreshed and awakened, and she felt a tingling in her lungs. Our friend Lauren, age thirteen, also said it was refreshing and reminded her of the woods and being in nature. She felt movement in the esophagus. She said, "My senses are awakened yet I feel peaceful, calm, and alert." Sarah, my then three-year-old daughter, said, "I feel something here (pointing to her heart), and it makes me feel good. I like it, Mom."

Water Color: clear

physical makeup

Root, Stem, Leaves/Leaflets, Height: Pinyon is a small and somewhat irregular-shaped tree that grows up to 40 feet high, but is commonly shorter. The short trunk grows up to 30 inches in diameter, and the dark, thin, rough bark is gray to reddish brown and furrowed into scaly ridges. Pinyon is many-branched. The lower branches tend to hang low and sweep the ground. The middle and upper branches spread out and are full. The short bluish green needles are slightly curved and stiff with sharp points, and are only about 1 to 2 inches long, clustered in twos. The needles are very fragrant.

Flower Color: Conelets are from dark red to pinkish purple

Flowers: Pinyons develop new branches by stretching out their buds in the summer. The buds are dormant throughout the winter and are protected by a cover of scales until the next spring. The buds emerge into tender conelets that look like spiny little pincushions. The male conelets are dark red, and the female conelets are pinkish purple. Both grow at the ends of branches in clusters, and they are about $^1/_2$ inch in diameter and about $^1/_4$ inch long (it is at this stage when the flower or conelet essence is made). The conelets then bear two tiny ovules on the upper surface of each scale that may be potential seeds. Soon after the conelet emerges, its scales are spread to capture windborne grains of pollen from its own tree or nearby pinyon trees. Once the pollen has been captured in the ovules, the pollinated conelet's scales close and the pollen grains are protected within. It takes nearly twenty-six months and three growing seasons for mature pine nuts to grow in stages as part of their developmental process.

Blooming Period: April to July

doctrine of signatures

- The tree stands firm, in strength and fortitude, graceful yet persistent and enduring. It gives a sense of being rooted and a sense of self in relation to the whole. The leaves are light and delicate, yet spiny and strong, giving an impression of firmness and persistence in a non-burdened way. Sitting under the pinyon tree and listening to the wind blow through the leaves and branches is a cleansing, restful, freeing, uplifting experience. The pinyon provides an appreciation for simplicity, peace, introspection, endurance, and gentle strength. A sense of self is restored and the heartstrings are opened.

- The pinyon has a mother-earthy feminine appearance as her full branches flow and dance with the wind. Although the young buds or conelets appear phallic, they are also soft and tender; this gives a nice balance between the male and female qualities, which highlights gentle strength, nurturing, and fertility. The way the needles are clustered in pairs is also a signature of the tree's balance. Interestingly, the Apache Indian woman would place her daughter's outgrown cradleboard in the crown of a young pinyon tree on the east side and say, "Here is the baby-carrier. I put this on you, young and still growing. I want my child to grow up as you do."[4] The Zuni Indian men would eat a young bud of the pinyon tree so their wives would bear a daughter. Both of these stories are examples of the pinyon's symbol of fertility and strength.

- The scent of the pinyon's pine needles and resin is fresh, cleansing, and rejuvenating. The taste of the flower essence is the same. If you bite into a pinyon needle, you will first get a bitter taste that may remind you of your burdens and your emotional bitterness. Yet inside the needle, there is a strong taste of pine without the sourness or bitterness. It's like discovering a powerful essence inside of you that reveals something about your true nature that you haven't felt before. The taste is cleansing and refreshing. The Navajo smeared pitch on a deceased body prior to burial, and the mourners also placed pitch under their eyes or on their foreheads. The Hopi cleansed the bodies and clothes of their deceased in the smoke of the pinyon gum as a purification. Also, the fumes of the pinyon gum clear head colds and earaches. The signature here is the cleansing properties of the tree and its ability to purify negative energy and embrace the earth in times of sorrow or challenge.

Several years ago, I was walking in a juniper-pinyon forest looking for a pinyon tree to take a picture of for this book. This was the fourth time I was to photograph the pinyon, due to my dissatisfaction with the previous photos. I had waited several weeks for the sky to be a deep blue and for the right time in my schedule. I took several shots of different trees and then saw a "perfect pinyon" for a "perfect picture" off in the distance. My eyes rested on this special pinyon as I walked for about fifteen minutes, following its top branches against the clear blue sky. When I approached the tree, a sense of quietness filled me. Underneath the pinyon lay a deceased dog that appeared to have passed to the other world sometime within the previous day. Externally, I could see no injuries. The dog lay peacefully next to the tree. I said a prayer for the dog and thanked both the pinyon tree and the dog for the gifts they gave me. This incident was more than a mere coincidence. I believe that the dog was led to this tree, not only to be nurtured and received by the earth, but also to give back to the earth. The dog's need for cleansing and purifying is shown by its choice to lie beneath the pinyon tree.

- The sap or pitch of the pinyon is sticky, giving it a positive trait of cohesiveness or stick-to-it-iveness and perseverance. Yet it also gives a message that some things that are stuck together may no longer serve us. This signature is about knowing when to stick things out and when to dissolve the stickiness that no longer serves. Learning to know oneself helps develop understanding about what is stuck that is good and what needs to be unstuck.

- The dark-red-colored male conelets correspond with the first or root chakra, which is the base of our life-force center. Connecting with this center helps us let go of needing approval by others and helps us dig deep into our own roots of self-

assurance and stability. The pinkish and purple conelets relate to the fourth (heart) and sixth (brow) chakras, awakening compassion, love, and healing energies in our lives and opening us to spiritual vision and spiritual inspiration. This helps us overcome oversensitivity in how we are affected by others and to focus on living in the present and letting go of regrets.

- The developmental process by which the conelets evolve (taking nearly twenty-six months and three growing seasons) is a significant signature of the pinyon's patience and perseverance. The slow but steady maturation of the tree and the pine nuts teaches us to be patient and persevering in our own lives so that we can bear our fruits at their fullest potency.

Helpful suggestions

Find a comfortable position, then place several drops of the Pinyon essence on your head and rub them in if you wish. Repeat this on your forehead and brow chakra, even around your temples, below your eyes, and around your mouth. Enjoy each moment as part of a process rather than anticipating an outcome. Then place the essence on the outside of your throat, down your neck, and on your heart chakra. Notice how you move and relate to yourself as you engage in this activity. Take your time as you gently rub the essence into each chakra region. Breathe deeply into each area as you rub in the pinyon essence. Place a few drops of the essence on your solar plexus area (right above your navel) and slowly rub it in; do the same on your spleen chakra area (your navel and just below it); and, finally, place some drops on the coccyx area of your root chakra and rub them in.

Then take several drops and place them in your mouth. With your eyes closed, imagine yourself sitting or lying beneath a pinyon tree. Breathe in the fresh scent of the pine. Imagine yourself asking permission from our great earth mother to take a small cluster of pinyon needles with their conelets from the tree. She gives you permission, and you gently break off a small cluster. You take one needle from the cluster and place it on your lap. Then you take the remaining cluster and place it in a clear bowl of pure water. You then place the bowl under a sweeping pinyon branch that lets the sun sift through.

Now you take the needle and place it in your mouth. At first you feel its bitterness. Taking your time, you gently suck on the needle. Slowly, you let your teeth bite gently into the needle and then more deeply inside its center essence. You feel the rush of pine taste flow into your mouth and down your throat. You notice that your nostrils have opened to the pine scent, and your entire being is filled with a refreshing pine energy. You breathe in the taste of pine even more deeply and let it embrace you inside and out.

Taking your time in this experience, allow your journey with pinyon to guide you and just be with it. When you feel completed with this part of your journey, you get up and retrieve the pine-water bowl. You raise the bowl up in the air toward the sky and the pinyon tree, giving thanks and honor to the earth and to Spirit for the gifts you have received. Slowly and consciously, you bring the bowl to your lips as you gently take a sip of the blessed pine water. You feel the soothing, refreshing taste in your mouth and throat. You sit quietly as you notice and experience the sensations and emotions that the pine water gives you.

When you feel complete in your experience of drinking the pinyon water, take the remainder of the water and the pinyon cluster and give it back to the pinyon tree. Thank the tree for the gifts it has shared with you and, in return, place something special that belongs to you under the tree or in her branches.

Slowly open your eyes. Write down your experience in a journal if you wish. Take the gifts that pinyon has given you back into your world.

Affirmations

- "I am free to love myself and others without shame, blame, or guilt."

- "I live patiently in the moment, thanking my Creator for all that I am."

- "I allow the body of the earth to nurture my roots and strengthen my endurance."

case history

Lauren, age thirteen, took the Pinyon essence to help her be more in touch with herself, to help her let go of her shortcomings and old burdens, and to help her stay on task with her homeschooling. She was drawn to the Pinyon essence and made the choice to take it.

Lauren's response to taking the essence is as follows: "I was attracted to the mountains while taking this essence, and it made me very happy at times. I felt in tune with my inner self and found myself daydreaming and somewhat spacey. I felt as if I could see into things, and I felt very feminine and intuitive. It helped me have more insight, feel calmer, and find my inner truths. I felt a refreshing sense of purpose and inner strength."

life's research provers' project findings

Physical Symptoms

Cravings: "Grounding" foods, water, salads

Sensations: "I felt a warming of my heart center and release of the throat center," "the warmth actually spreads throughout the body directly following taking this essence"

Pain: None

Modalities:

    Worse: None reported

    Better: Slept well at night

Head: "I felt a warmth in my head, releasing pressure"

Eyes: None

Face: Opening of the temple regions

Ears: None

Stomach: None

Abdomen: None

Bowel condition: None

Urine: More urination and more fluid intake

Female: More hot flashes

Male: Feel more sensual; "all senses opened up and I feel full of love"

Extremities: None

Back: None

Skin: None

Other: "Gives an energy boost," "releases tension and tiredness," "lots of energy"

Emotional Symptoms

Patterns of Balance: "I felt more inner strength and balance in dealing with personal power issues and in facing challenges," "I felt my inner solar plexus allowing me to speak my power from my heart with clarity and compassion, and with connectedness to the greater whole," "experienced strength and flexibility," "felt secure, safe, and supported," "I was able to hold my own energy while supporting others in the process," "I felt a groundedness and a calmness," "a sense of balance," "I had hurt my foot and the essence was very nurturing emotionally and moved the energy out of the physical and was healing," "the essence helped me take some issues to the inner core of my feelings," "I felt more peaceful and less crisis-oriented," "relates to a sense of being loved by people and cared about," "I felt a general sense of well-being," "helped me to balance kindness," "this essence is excellent for balancing release of stress and allowing time to heal; it gives a sense of warmth, of being in love," "heart opening"

PATTERNS OF IMBALANCE: "anxiety," "a sense of not caring," "impatient"

MENTAL SYMPTOMS

PATTERNS OF BALANCE: "was generally aware of this essence throughout the day and the evening," "felt more flexible mentally and had more mental clarity," "mind was more expansive and grounded," "more intuitive and more creative," "brought up good memories of times with my children and a sense of being lovable," "more balanced mentally," "more creative, but not needing to manifest," "helped me be more grounded, balanced, objective, and aware," "felt security without possession, and protection," "I have been reading more books like *The Celestine Prophecy*, yet those truths I've always known," "I'm more active and interested in catching up," "more mentally active"

PATTERNS OF IMBALANCE: "anxiety," "a sense of not caring"

SPIRITUAL REFLECTIONS

"I feel a sense of great support from the earth and from Spirit when taking this essence; it helps me ground spirituality into the physical and express it in relationship to others; it helped me to be open, connected, and willing to uphold the bigger picture," "I felt more compassionate and willing to be and feel supportive," "felt as if I were waiting," "the essence allows time to just be, without stress or ambitions," "I took time to meditate, contemplate, and align with Spirit," "more active prayer and better discipline," "desire more quiet time," "more meditation," "I have been more attracted to listening to music such as Loreena McKennitt and feminine spirituality while taking this remedy; it made me feel connected," "I feel at peace and very much a part of the universe," "I feel that I have patience to let things unfold without forcing anything"

DREAMS/NIGHTMARES

"The dream images that came to me were vivid, and there were many more than usual. I find I use dream images more than anything else to understand the flower essences; I don't often get physical reactions. In the beginning, the images I had with the Pinyon essence were depressing: from a dark circle and an entangled spider to a moon, a lotus, and a fetus. Moods shifted from dark to light, from oppression to release. A beautiful Indian girl appeared before me. Her face was exquisite. As she looked at me, her eyes began to fill with golden light. My focus shifted to her left eye, and golden tears began to fall. The eye became a beautiful golden sunflower with a dark center, and the girl vanished.... The progression from darkness to light and the radiant yellow light intrigued me. I believe this remedy could be helpful in bringing people out of the darkness into warmth, light, and beauty. I feel this remedy goes very deep."

POMEGRANATE

(Punica granatum)
PRIMARY QUALITY: FRUIT OF LIFE

FAMILY: Pomegranate (Punicaceae)

OTHER NAMES: Apple of Carthage, Grenadier. Latin name derived from *poma granata,* meaning "many-seeded apple." Botanical name also refers to the source of the plant, which was a Roman colony in North Africa named Punicus or Carthage.

WHERE FOUND: Pomegranate is native to Asia, especially Iran, Afghanistan, and the Himalayan slopes. It grows wild on the shores of the Mediterranean and in Arabia, Persia, and Japan, and it is cultivated in the East and West Indies. Pomegranate is cultivated in the western U.S., from the Northwest Coast to Arizona and New Mexico, wherever the climate is sufficiently warm to allow the fruit to ripen. In higher latitudes, it is raised in gardens or hothouses for its beautiful flowers even though it doesn't bear fruit.

ELEVATION: most climates across the North American continent

ENERGY IMPACT (CHAKRA CORRESPONDENCE): first, second, and third chakras

KEY RUBRICS FOR POSITIVE HEALING PATTERNS: abundance, creativity, loving, nurturing, passion, resourcefulness, self-empowerment, sexuality

KEY RUBRICS FOR SYMPTOMS AND PATTERNS OF IMBALANCE: hidden talents, lack of creativity, lack of passion and joy in life, inability to locate resources

OTHER RUBRICS: abundance, adolescence, appreciation, balance, beauty, calm, career, change, clairvoyance, dreams, emotional, female, freedom, fruitful, grounded, heart, home, joyful, kundalini, life force, menopausal, menstrual, mother, optimistic, positive, power, pregnancy, premenstrual, protection, psychic energies, purpose, reproductive, respect, root chakra, solar plexus chakra, spleen chakra, transformation, transition, understanding, underworld, values, wisdom, womb

traditional use

The pomegranate has long been known as an ancient symbol of fertility due to its striking red color and seed arrangement. It is also an ancient design motif. Pomegranate was included in the Egyptian Ebers Papyrus, written in 2000 B.C., and also in the Old Testament (Numbers 13:23). Pomegranate was suspected to be the "forbidden fruit" eaten by Eve in the Garden of Eden, and it was included in the design on the pillars of King Solomon's temple.

In Greek mythology, Persephone was said to have eaten six seeds of a pomegranate after she fell into Hades, the underworld. As a symbol of union, the pomegranate bound her to Pluto, the god of the underworld, in his hidden kingdom for six months from fall to spring (each seed representing one month). Despite this, the symbol of Persephone eating the seeds is also about a birthing period and her return to self. The underworld helped her discover her hidden wisdom, beauty, and power, and allowed her to confront her fears in the darkest moments of her life. In spring, Persephone was free and emerged with the newly found gifts she had given herself.

The medicinal history of pomegranate dates back to Pliny in the first century. The root bark has been used since ancient times to expel worms from the intestinal tract; it has been found most beneficial in cases of tapeworm. In 1804, an East Indian practitioner cured an Englishman of a tapeworm with an infusion of the root bark and used it as a purgative. The bark's active ingredient — liquid alkaloid pelletierine — was discovered in 1878; it was once used in human medicine and is now used in veterinary medicine.

If you bite into the rind of a pomegranate, you will experience its highly astringent nature. About 30 percent of the rind is composed of tannin, a powerful astringent substance. Powdered fruit rind is also used as an astringent, and has been used to treat dysentery, diarrhea, excessive perspiration, and for intermittent fevers, and as a gargle for sore throats. Pomegranate is used in Ayurvedic medicine as a blood purifier to enhance the memory.

Pomegranate fruit is eaten whole, and it is juiced to make delicious drinks and desserts, especially in the Middle East where it has been cultivated for over 5,000 years. Middle Eastern cooks boil the sour pulp to make a pomegranate syrup, which has a distinguished scent and adds flavors to stews and meat dishes. Its sweet juice is also used to make grenadine, a flavoring for cocktails, sherbet, and pickles. The sour East Indian condiment *anardana* is made from the dried seeds of pomegranate and used for stuffings in flavorful breads and pastries. Fabric dyes are also made from the fruits, rind, and bark.

CAUTION: Large doses of the rind or root bark infusion can cause nausea, cramps, and vomiting.

Homeopathic use

The homeopathic remedy *Granatum* is used to get rid of tapeworm with itching of the anus and constant hunger. It is also used to treat persistent vertigo with salivation and nausea, pain in the shoulder so heavy that clothing is intolerable, aching in all the finger joints, and convulsive movements of the extremities.

positive Healing patterns

- Activates the awakening and experience of the kundalini life-force.
- Stirs passion, sexuality, and creative awareness and expression of feminine energy, which nurtures and connects us to the Great Earth Mother; this is helpful for both men and women.
- Teaches us to protect, respect, and honor our vulnerability; to discover

our inner wisdom, beauty, and power in the seemingly darkest moments of our lives; and to make use of these gifts externally by setting healthy boundaries, learning to express our emotions and creativity in safe ways, and feeling free in who we are.

- Attracts an abundance of positive, fruitful inner and outer resources; guides us in personal balance within ourselves, at home, with our family, in our job, and our role within the larger community.

- For women, Pomegranate especially helps us understand how our emotional and mental states affect who we are and how we feel in our physical, sexual, and feminine bodies. It is helpful to women of all ages and in all life cycles — adolescence or premenstrual, menstrual, or menopausal.

- Helps us express a positive nature of joy, optimism, and freedom.

symptoms and patterns of imbalance

Pomegranate may be an appropriate flower essence for those who

- Aren't connected with their creative, sexual, passionate, and feminine nature (men or women)

- Are overly emotional, moody, or mental, especially around premenses, menses, or menopause, or for young teenage girls who generally seem to be "out of whack" emotionally

- Have difficulty finding and nurturing their inner and outer resources, and who feel out of touch or out of balance with their own values and needs; this may relate especially to the struggle between being out in the world with a career or at home with children and family.

features of the original flower-essence water

ODOR: subtle yet sweet
TASTE: slightly sweet, fruity, and delicate; taste lingers at the back of the tongue
SENSATIONS: Tingling and numbing sensation that moves downward. Feels grounded, soothing, and relaxing. Feel warmth in the ovaries that moves upward to abdomen area and continues to move upward to the shoulders.
WATER COLOR: slightly yellow

physical makeup

ROOT, STEM, LEAVES/LEAFLETS, HEIGHT: Pomegranate is a small, deciduous, shrubby tree growing up to 20 feet in height. The trunk's bark is pale brown and is often uneven, and its many slender branches bear spines or thorns at the tips. Leaf buds and young shoots are red, and the bright green leaves are opposite, entire, oblong or lance-shaped, and pointed at the end. They are smooth, thick, and shiny and have short leafstalks. Pomegranate bears fruit about the size of an apple or orange, and its fruit is a globular berry.

The fruit is crowned at the calyx, and it has a thick, reddish yellow, leatherlike peel or rind; it resembles a swollen womb. When the fruit is broken in half, you can see that the brightly colored red, angular seeds are grouped in many compartments or cells. The seeds are fruity, juicy, and very flavorful. The inside rind contains an acidulous pulp that tastes bitter. Pomegranate trees like full sun and lots of water in order to yield plenty of fruit.

FLOWER COLOR: Orange-red to scarlet-red

FLOWERS: The fragrant, showy orange-red to scarlet-red single flowers are somewhat large and emerge at the ends of the young branches. The flowers have five to seven rounded, waxy, wrinkly paperlike petals that grow from the upper part of the tube of the calyx, which is bright red, thick, and fleshy. A somewhat prolific group of yellow stamens with yellow anthers grows from the center of the flower.

BLOOMING PERIOD: April to June

Doctrine of signatures

- The colorful orange-red to scarlet-red flowers, leaf buds, and young shoots, and the red, juicy, flavorful seeds relate primarily to the first or root chakra and second or spleen chakra, which is the seat of the kundalini within the body. This is where our life-promoting energy lies, which influences our circulatory system, our reproductive system, and how our lower extremities operate. The color orange relates to the spleen chakra and is linked to sensation and emotion, which influences creativity. The rounded, feminine appearance of the flower highlights qualities associated with being a woman. The juicy, fruity taste of the fruit, as well as its appearance, stirs passion, sexuality, and creative feminine energy, which nurtures and connects us to the Great Earth Mother. Even the calyx is bright red and fleshy. The astringent nature of the fruit — "the red-juice-dripping, seed-filled pomegranate"[5] distinctly implies the womb and the power, wisdom, and beauty to be discovered by women in their own hidden underworld kingdom. This also relates to the changes within the female body, such as when the blood stops, the process of fertilization, and then when the blood begins a new cycle again.

- The previous signatures may also refer to the intuitive, psychological, and feminine qualities within males. By awakening the "inner feminine," a male can nurture his ability to discover and embody these feminine qualities. The Pomegranate flower essence can also be beneficial for men in the arousal of their passionate and sensual natures.

- The way in which the juicy, red seeds are grouped in compartments yet individual is a signature of their magnetic nature, in which they both attract and give out energy. This magnetic signature represents an abundant gathering of positive and fruitful inner and outer resources, teaching balance in this way.

- The thorns at the tips of the branches and the thick, leatherlike, orangish-reddish rind on the fruit are a signature of protection. They demonstrate a safeguard from being manipulated, taken advantage of, bullied, or eating fruit prematurely or before it is ready and willing. This signature teaches respect and honors vulnerability, healthy boundaries, and safe expression of emotions.

- The smooth, shiny leaves are a signature of the plant's positive nature. The leaves appear luminous, especially on bright sunny days. They express themselves with joy, optimism, and freedom.

- The golden yellow stamens that emerge from the flower's center and the slightly yellow flower-essence water correspond to the third or solar plexus chakra, which is linked to our emotional and mental states and to psychic energies and clairvoyance. The significance of the yellow stamens and the yellow water relates to our ability, especially as women, to understand through experience how certain emotional/mental states can cause who and how we are in our physical, sexual, and feminine bodies. The yellowish rind on the inside of the pomegranate fruit is bitter and

represents an emotional bitterness to watch out for. This signature is another link to being an especially influential remedy for women of all ages and in all life cycles.

Helpful suggestions

Take three to four drops of Pomegranate flower essence, get in a comfortable position, and close your eyes. In your mind, take yourself outdoors and see yourself walking down a path in an autumnal landscape. Feel the wind on your face as it blows the leaves from the trees. The breeze is gentle and refreshing. You feel the crunch of the leaves under your feet, and you can smell the wet earth and the changing of the season. You continue to walk down this familiar path, feeling safe and yet filled with a sense of anticipation.

You come upon a cave and you're mysteriously drawn to enter. As you enter, your senses are heightened and you're pulled deeper inside the cave until you are magically swept down into the core of the underworld. Tasting the darkness, you step forward and follow a small source of light. Standing before you is a cloaked figure. She extends her arms to you, takes you to a ledge in the cave, and invites you to lie down. You allow yourself to trust and follow. You feel the warmth of her hand upon your heart. You begin to breathe slowly, deeply, and with great ease. You feel yourself sink into a place of great peace and soft surrender. Within this space, you hear her telling you that it is safe to let go. Pushing through your fear and with great relief, you begin to release the old. She begins to run her hands gently over your body and asks you to be aware of places where you are holding on. With her help, those places begin to dissolve. She then places her hand upon your womb and you feel an incredible flood of healing and light. You begin to experience a sense of your deepest passion, power, wisdom, and beauty that is the creative feminine. You are filled with the fruits of your own abundance. Gently, she awakens you and leads you back to the mouth of the cave. With much gratitude you embrace her, knowing that you will return. You step back into the sunlight, and with joy and optimism, you greet your life's path.

The following is a poetic journey inspired by the Pomegranate, written by Veronica Vida:

The Stranger

He was back. Once he donated spirit and
sperm only to leave . . . abandon.
The stranger, he was back, claiming blood,
claiming child.
The stranger drew me out, drew me down,
leaving home, leaving innocence.
Abducted into the unknown, the deep
black, my own shadows.
Dripping ruby red blood juice,
pomegranate's own.
First seeds of budding wisdom.
And the journey begins.

Affirmations

- "I flow infinitely and passionately from within, greeting life with joyful abundance."

- "My power is filled with the fruits of my deepest creativity."
- "I embrace my feminine creative self; I open myself to harvesting my inner gifts."

Case History

Magda, age fifty-three, was experiencing financial insecurity. She took the Pomegranate flower essence for a few weeks, and her comments about taking the essence are as follows: "The most striking thing that has happened to me while taking the essence is that I have been more in the flow and have clarity about my life purpose. The financial insecurity I've had has gone away; I've been able to look at and obtain resources from both within and without. I was given an opportunity to look at a new position at a local university that would provide for more security. My clarity was that it was a trap and that it would be off my real purpose, and I was able to say 'no' to this opportunity. As soon as I made this decision, a gift was given to me. An external manifestation of making this choice was that a professional offered to edit for free some videotapes about my Creative Arts Camp. Also, an insurance policy that my mother had taken out a few years before her death became available to me; it had been delayed twice before. Another thing happened while I was taking this essence: a nodular growth appeared on the left side of my forehead and I went to see a dermatologist; due to this incident, I discovered a whole other life insurance policy in my name that I didn't even realize I had. The cost of my surgery to remove the growth was only ten dollars."

lfe's Research provers' project findings

Physical Symptoms

Cravings: Fruit

Sensations: "Energy moved downward, numbing and tingling," "light feeling"

Pain: None

Modalities: Inconsistency in sleep patterns among provers

Head: None

Eyes: None

Face: None

Ears: None

Stomach: Warmth/heat

Abdomen: Warmth in abdomen that rose upward

Bowel condition: None

Urine: None

Female: More hot flashes, more erotic and sexual feelings, more sexual awareness: "I feel I'm experiencing parts of the 'change of life,'" "felt warmth in ovaries"

Male: None

Extremities: Tingling sensation in shoulders

Back: None

Skin: None

Other: More tired than usual

Emotional Symptoms

Patterns of Balance: "felt more positive; I relived past experiences related to love that were traumatic at the time, but now I see them in a more positive light," "I experienced sexual/emotional feelings," "I experienced an inner calming, an inner connectedness, an inner strength, and an inner love — a notion regarding loving everything," "I feel more balanced," "I feel a great change is coming," "I have a feeling of peace," "I anticipate change and transformation"

Patterns of Imbalance: "internalization," "emotionally drained"

Mental Symptoms

Patterns of Balance: "thoughts of a former lover made me think this remedy is related to relationship issues," "better memory for past events in relationships," "I am an artist and this remedy seemed to feed artistic imagery that I will probably resolve in paintings," "reflective that we need periods of transformation (through relationships) in life," "I feel a greater understanding, a sense of doing the right thing," "I am more grounded"

Patterns of Imbalance: "dizziness," "internalizing," "spacey"

Spiritual Reflections

"I marvel at the ability of this flower to produce such powerful imagery — reflecting on the 'power of flowers' and their Creator," "growth takes place through human encounters as a way to encounter Divine experience," "more conscious prayer life and realizing the need for transformation and acceptance of change," "I feel more love," "love everyone and everything"

DREAMS/NIGHTMARES

"I had clear dream images: an eye that turned into a fish blowing bubbles, women, a crown, pentacle, star, spider, fox, and horse. I interpret the eye as representing wisdom, enlightenment, and perception. The fish is the unconscious and images about self-transformation and spirituality. It is a sexual symbol and a Christ symbol. The bubbles refer to possibly a 'bursting bubble,' as in a broken relationship or a new sexual partner. The crown refers to a full awareness of reality. The pentacle to me is about nature, physical life, energy and life. And the fox is a foxy, seductive female beauty. The horse reminded me of power and sex, and the spider is the Spider Woman, full of powerful creativity. This dream seems to deal with becoming conscious and alive and experiencing erotic impulses, personal power, and personal transformation."

PURPLE ROBE

(Nierembergia spp.)
PRIMARY QUALITY: PLENTY

FAMILY: Potato (Solanaceae)
OTHER NAMES: Cup Flower
WHERE FOUND: gardens and greenhouses throughout the U.S.
ELEVATION: most climates in the U.S.
ENERGY IMPACT (CHAKRA CORRESPONDENCE): third and sixth chakras
KEY RUBRICS FOR POSITIVE HEALING PATTERNS: abundance, clairvoyance, expansiveness, insight, vision, wisdom
KEY RUBRICS FOR SYMPTOMS AND PATTERNS OF IMBALANCE: dwelling on lack and being without, inability to see a broader perspective, lack of inspiration and insight
OTHER RUBRICS: abundance, anxiety, awareness, brow chakra, burden, calm, challenged, clarity, collective unconscious, comfort, gentleness, groundedness, inner guidance, inspiration, intuition, meditation, memory, mindfulness, plenty, prolific, psychic, simplicity, solar plexus chakra, spirituality, trust, understanding, warmth

traditional use

Historical use is unknown to author. Today *Nierembergia spp.* is a widely spreading plant that is used as a ground cover. Purple Robe is attractive in flower arrangements and wreaths.

homeopathic use

Unknown to author.

positive healing patterns

- Promotes a sense of abundance and plenty.
- Helps deepen awareness, wisdom, and understanding.
- Helps us regain memory through clairvoyance and vision.
- Offers depth of inner vision, insight, and inspiration.
- Nurtures our inner strength, offering gentleness and ease.

symptoms and patterns of imbalance

Purple Robe may be an appropriate flower essence for those who

- Have an overall feeling of lack and being without
- Are seeking guidance toward higher vision, awareness, and understanding
- Don't trust their intuition and their "higher self"
- Are searching for past memories or healing traumas that require an

in-depth understanding and higher vision of self.

features of the original flower-essence water

ODOR: full, sweet, and pleasant
TASTE: strong, sweet, very soothing and powerful
SENSATIONS: Warm tingling sensations in solar plexus and brow chakra gives a feeling of groundedness. Much warmth and a sense of expansion felt in the brow chakra, with the energy moving upward and out.
WATER COLOR: clear

physical makeup

ROOT, STEM, LEAVES/LEAFLETS, HEIGHT: The stems are smooth, round, flexible, and green, forming many branches toward the top of the plant. Each small branch alternates from its stem and contains tiny, short, alternating leaflets that lead to a cupped flower at the end of the branch. The plant is widely spreading and prolific, and bears abundant flowers. Purple robe can grow up to 2 feet tall and will grow back on its own year after year.
FLOWER COLOR: Deep purple with yellow center
FLOWERS: The deep purple flowers are tubular but flare into a star and bell shape; they are five-petaled. There are two distinct indentations in each petal, and the petals grow approximately 1 inch wide. One firm, thick stamen with a bright yellow anther evolves from the center of the flower, which is also bright yellow. The flowers have a slightly musty smell.
BLOOMING PERIOD: April to October

Doctrine of signatures

- This prolific plant is widely spreading and produces an abundance of flowers. It demonstrates its primary quality of plenty by the way it grows and produces, even though it is a relatively small plant. The structure of the plant is light, delicate, and flexible. The cupped flowers appear delicate although the petals are actually quite strong and pronounced. These signatures give a sense of strength and persistence to grow and spread, yet offer a gentle approach in doing so.

- The deep, rich, purple color of the flower is characteristic of the sixth or brow chakra, which helps bring a sense of purpose, spiritual insight, and wisdom into our lives. The yellow center is indicative of our ability to transmute mental thoughts into higher visions and deeper wisdom. Purple robe says to us, "I am a plant of beauty and simplicity and bring you gifts of abundance. Despite my fullness, I am humble. The small yellow eye in my center is embraced by purple and symbolizes a gift of abundance in your vision, insights, and understanding. I freely give you an abundance of creative depth, vision, and clarity." The yellow eye also represents the third chakra.

- The star shape offers inspiration and illumination, linked to our inner guidance and the ability to trusting the depth of our inner nature and resources.

- The powerful taste of the flower-essence water is warming and gives a feeling of expansion and movement in the brow chakra, as well as a feeling of groundedness.

Helpful suggestions

Create some time to be with yourself and find a quiet, comfortable spot. Take several drops of Purple Robe flower essence and close your eyes if you wish. Go within and find your inner silence. Take a deep breath, hold it gently, and gradually let it go. Repeat. Quietly give thanks and gratitude to your Creator, your family, your friends, and anything that is meaningful to you.

Ask yourself what you can creatively do for or give to another. Your expression of gratitude and willingness to give is a blessing of the abundance that you may receive. You are also giving yourself positive thought-forms that will foster your own inner vision, ideas, and understanding. Helping others is a reflection of the good that may come to you. Your gesture of giving creates abundance and manifestation in your life and raises consciousness for the highest good of all.

tions to manifest that which will abundantly serve my highest good."

case History

Debra, a woman in her late forties, was experiencing a transition in her life that affected her financial situation and also left her with a general feeling of lack (emotionally, mentally, and spiritually). She sought a sense of purpose, an understanding of the meaning of her circumstances, and a willingness to go within to search for guidance and direction.

Taking the Purple Robe flower essence helped Debra to "soften things," and she felt more "comfortable and at ease" with herself and in her situation. "Purple Robe heightened me spiritually. It helped me look at things differently, and I gained a deep personal awareness and understanding of myself and my life path. I felt more inspired, and trusted myself to follow my intuition and wisdom despite the presenting challenges. Purple Robe assisted my ability to focus and to grab hold of my visions, which enabled me to proceed in a new direction with comfort and trust."

Affirmations

- "There is an unlimited supply in my life. I have the choice to create it."
- "I am limitless, boundless, and filled with abundant energy."
- "I creatively weave my thoughts, visions, imagination, and inspira-

LFE's Research provers' project findings

PHYSICAL SYMPTOMS

CRAVINGS: Carrot juice
SENSATIONS: Butterflies in stomach
PAIN: None
MODALITIES: None consistent
HEAD: None

EYES: None

FACE: None

EARS: None

STOMACH: Butterflies in stomach and anticipation

ABDOMEN: None

BOWEL CONDITION: None

URINE: None

FEMALE: Increased hot flashes

MALE: None

EXTREMITIES: None

BACK: None

SKIN: None

OTHER: Clumsiness, more physical vitality

EMOTIONAL SYMPTOMS

PATTERNS OF BALANCE: "I generally felt good," "I felt higher, calmer, and simpler," "more love and understanding," "felt emotionally secure and secure in myself," "old memories came up for me and a reminiscing about the past," "felt at ease, comfortable"

PATTERNS OF IMBALANCE: "avoidance and resistance issues," "anxiety," "burdened," "tendency toward denial," "impatience," "challenged"

MENTAL SYMPTOMS

PATTERNS OF BALANCE: "greater insight and awareness," "boosted my self-esteem," "a readiness to acknowledge myself and move on in positive ways," "a recognition of old patterns and release," "this essence helped me gain deeper insight," "increased memory, more creative, more understanding, more clairvoyant," "while taking this remedy, I am more focused and also am searching and questing deeper," "became more aware of the need for healing past traumas and memories," "gained a new awareness of myself," "this remedy seems to offer healing by increasing awareness"

PATTERNS OF IMBALANCE: "resistance to remembering, and avoidance issues were strong," "I had a resistance to taking this essence," "less clairvoyant, less creative, less intuitive," "denial issues," "memory loss," "doubt and concerns"

SPIRITUAL REFLECTIONS

"experienced a deeper sense of inner understanding," "had many spiritual reflections about how I am and what I am here for," "desire to quest for the truth," "experienced a spiritual memory of my ancestors"

DREAMS/NIGHTMARES

One prover had a series of dream images that included a sphinx in Egypt, an Indian shaman, a golden bull, many Native American faces, a squash, a priest, and a warrior.

Another prover had a dream about her brother going over his mother's will and removing parts of it that he didn't like. Other provers shared some light dreams.

SAGE

(Salvia officinalis purpurescens)
PRIMARY QUALITY: WHOLE-LIFE INTEGRATION

FAMILY: Sage (Labiatae)

OTHER NAMES: Garden Sage, Wild Sage, Meadow Sage. The botanical name *Salvia* comes from the Latin verb *salvere,* which means "to save," "to be in good health," or "to cure." This reflects the vast medicinal reputation of sage in ancient times.

WHERE FOUND: Native to the northern shores of the Mediterranean and to southern Europe. Naturalized in the U.S. for the last three centuries as a garden and wild herbal shrub. Grows best in a warm, dry border but will grow almost anywhere in ordinary sunshine. Can be found as a cultivated plant throughout the U.S. in temperate zones.

ELEVATION: most U.S. climates

ENERGY IMPACT (CHAKRA CORRESPONDENCE): fifth, sixth, and seventh chakras

KEY RUBRICS FOR POSITIVE HEALING PATTERNS: conscientiousness, insight, purification, spiritual inspiration, whole-life balance

KEY RUBRICS FOR SYMPTOMS AND PATTERNS OF IMBALANCE: bitterness, insensitivity, resistance to embracing spirituality in all realms of life

OTHER RUBRICS: aromatic, balance, bitterness, brow chakra, calm, challenge, change, clairvoyance, cleansing, communication, cooling, crown chakra, death/dying, depression, dreams, female, groundedness, imagination, impatience, male, menses, mouth, peaceful, purpose, refreshing, sensitivity, sorrow, sound, spiritual guidance, teeth, throat chakra, understanding, visionary, voice, warming

traditional use

In ancient times and throughout history on many continents, sage was revered for its powers of immortality and longevity, honoring its ability to increase mental capacity. An ancient saying in Asia and Europe was, "How can a man grow old who has sage in his garden?" In the seventeenth century, John Evelyn regarded sage as "a plant indeed with so many and wonderful properties that the assiduous use of it is said to render men immortal." Also in the seven-teenth century, there was a flourishing trade in sage between China and Holland; the Chinese traded three chests of green tea for one chest of sage tea from the Dutch merchants. The Chinese had acquired a taste for sage tea and its medicinal properties of strengthening the digestive system and providing an overall calming effect.

The Romans used sage as a sacred herb, gathered with ceremony. Gerard recommended sage for shakiness, and Dioscorides used an infusion of the leaves and branches to treat diseases of the liver and to cleanse the blood. Culpeper made a hot infusion of sage and recommended it for treating an inflamed throat and hoarseness. He also advised a gargle made of sage, vinegar, and honey. Fresh sage leaves were rubbed on the teeth and gums to cleanse the mouth and strengthen the gums. Pliny used sage to treat snake bites. The juice of sage was used to treat venereal disease and was also recommended for increasing sexual desire.

In the 1800s, Americans used sage externally to cure warts. It was also known to treat epilepsy, insomnia, measles, seasickness, and worms. American Indians used sage externally, mixed with bear grease, as a salve to cure skin sores and as an infusion for baths and rubdowns.

Research performed in 1939 showed that sage has estrogenic properties or hormone precursors that help with irregular menses and menopause. Research has also demonstrated the plant's ability to lower blood sugar levels in diabetics. Sage contains volatile oils, tannins, terpene, camphor, and salvene. One to three drops of sage oil can be used to remove excessive mucus from the respiratory organs, and it is a useful ingredient in lotions or salves to treat rheumatism.

Herbalists of today use sage *(Salvia officinalis)* to treat a variety of conditions, including sore throat, tonsillitis, mouth irritations and sores, sexual debility, hot flashes, irregular menses and menopause, excessive mucous discharges, phlegm, nasal catarrh, excessive secretions of saliva, colds, coughs, diarrhea, digestion problems, dysentery, fevers, flu, sore gums,

headaches, lung congestion, nerve-related problems, night sweats, parasites, liver and kidney complaints, sinus congestion, ulcers, worms, yeast infections, spasms, morning sickness, voice loss, and dandruff. Sage is also used to promote hair growth, return hair to its original color, stop lactation, improve memory, and lower blood sugar levels.

To this day in Bosnia, there are fields upon fields of sage that are harvested for culinary uses. As a culinary herb, sage is lemony, slightly minty, camphor-like, and somewhat bitter. Fresh flowers and young leaves are eaten in salads, and the dried herb is used in a variety of meat and vegetable dishes, soups, and seasonings. Aromatically, sage is an ingredient in perfumes, oils, soaps, and cosmetics. As an ornament, sage makes a colorful and aromatic border in the garden. Cosmetically, infusions of sage have been used to color silver hair. Sage is also used in skin lotions, herbal baths, and aftershaves. Sage also dries well and is used in herbal wreaths, especially culinary wreaths.

Homeopathic use

A mother tincture is made from the fresh leaves and blossom tips and is used to treat cough (tickling), night sweats, and a lung disease called "phthisis."

positive Healing patterns

- Teaches whole-life balance, integrating spiritual principles with practical applications in daily living.

- Helps us demonstrate our spiritual self through our personality self in how we behave in the world.
- Helps us be conscientious about the sounds we make, the words we choose, and the way we communicate with others; guides us toward conscious choice of words and voice tones, and toward speaking with kindness and gentleness.
- Offers spiritual inspiration and visionary guidance.
- Is useful in times of transitions and life-cycle changes by helping us redirect ourselves to higher life purposes and higher ways of living and being.

symptoms and patterns of imbalance

Sage may be an appropriate flower essence for those who:

- Talk about spiritual life and spiritual practices but don't embrace spirituality in their daily lives and with others
- Lack whole-life balance and want to feel more integrated
- Are seeking spiritual inspiration and visionary guidance (this is a suggested essence to take on a vision quest)
- Are experiencing a life transition or a lifestyle change, and are seeking their higher purpose in life
- Are spiritual philosophizers or teachers, yet are insensitive about

their choice of words, voice tones, and general ways of communicating that turn other people off
- Lack the ability to access spiritual vision, intuition, and guidance
- Have physical conditions such as light sensitivity, frontal sinus infections, inability to focus, or mental confusion.

features of the original flower-essence water

ODOR: slightly spicy and somewhat minty; refreshing and aromatic

TASTE: refreshing, cooling, and aromatic; somewhat bitter with a hint of mint

SENSATIONS: Feel a smooth coolness in the back of the throat and a slight tingling of cool energy from the throat to the third eye and out the top of the head. Gives a refreshing feeling. My three-year-old daughter said, "It makes me feel good. That's good water, Mom."

WATER COLOR: clear

physical makeup

ROOT, STEM, LEAVES/LEAFLETS, HEIGHT: Sage is a hardy semievergreen subshrub with a somewhat shallow root system. The wiry stem is square and woody and is covered with fine hairs. It grows from 12 to 30 inches tall. The soft, velvety, gray-green leaves are thick and hairy and grow in opposites up to 2 inches long. The underside of the leaves is smooth and veiny with a pronounced center vein. The topside of the leaves is covered with a network of

small intricate veins that appear pebbly
and puckery and look like the small
bumps on a tongue. The leaves are oblong
and long-stalked, with round-toothed
margins. All parts of the plant are highly
aromatic, refreshing, spicy, and somewhat
pungent. They have an astringent taste
due to the volatile oil in the tissues; they
taste bitter, cool then warm, and have a
drying effect. Tiny dark-brown seeds
appear in an oval nutlet at the base of each
flower after flowering. The seeds should
not be consumed.

FLOWER COLOR: Violet-purple-blue with
white streaks

FLOWERS: The flowers blossom in whorls
along the stem, with four to eight at each
axil. They generally are a violet-purple or
bluish color, although less commonly
there are white and pink flowers. The
flowers are about $^1/_2$ to $^3/_4$ inch long.
They are deep-throated and two-lipped,
with the upper lip either straight or
arched, and they look like an open
mouth with lips and tongue. They also
appear spurlike, with the fuzzy base of
the calyx being bell-shaped and male, and
the flower opening being more female,
like a gateway. Two white streaks appear
at the front of the mouth, or the lower
lip, and a whitish color emerges from the
center opening of the flower. There is a
tiny ring of hairs on the inside. Stamens
emerge from the center of the flower with
purple anthers. The soft sepal looks like a
five-pointed cup that gently holds the
flower.

BLOOMING PERIOD: June through July

Doctrine of signatures

- The network of intricate, pebbly
  veins on the leaves resemble the
  small bumps on a tongue. The soft,
  velvety, hairy leaves, smaller than
  but similar to mullein leaves, call to
  mind the soft hairs lining the
  mucous membranes. The deep-
  throated two-lipped flowers look
  like an open mouth with lips and
  tongue. These signatures significantly relate to the mouth and
  throat. If you put a leaf in your
  mouth and breathe in, you will feel
  a cooling sensation in your throat
  and then a warming feeling. It also
  has a drying effect. It's no wonder
  this plant is used to treat mouth
  sores and irritations, tonsillitis,
  voice loss, excessive mucous discharges, phlegm, nasal catarrh, and
  excessive secretions of saliva. These
  signatures, as well as the hint of
  bluish color in the flowers, also
  relate to the throat chakra and the
  mode of expression through communication of voice and sound.
- The violet-purplish color of the
  flower corresponds to the brow
  chakra, which is linked to the pituitary gland, the endocrine system,
  and the corpus callosum that
  unites and balances the two hemispheres of the brain. The male and
  female symbolism of the flower also
  suggests balance. The brow chakra
  serves as a visionary or guide, opening us to clearer and broader

perceptions, imagination, inspiration, and spiritual understanding and insights. This signature opens us to see beyond our ordinary vision, helping us connect with our own spiritual essence.

- The pungent, bitter taste of the plant is a signature of how deeply affected we can be by our own bitterness, which causes personal setbacks, lack of direction, the inability to manifest, and, most importantly, a lack of spiritual guidance and spiritual inspiration. Yet the refreshing, soothing flower essence drink — even with a slight hint of bitterness — along with our intention can help redirect us to our higher purpose.

- The white streaks in the flower are associated with the seventh chakra and imply purification, stabilization, and cleansing of the entire energy system. They serve as a boost to the process of healing associated with each individual when taking this flower essence.

Helpful suggestions

Take a few drops of the Sage essence and pack a light backpack, making sure you include your Sage flower-essence bottle in the pack. Choose an outdoor area or nature area you would like to explore more. If you are not able to physically do this exercise, then do a visualization.

When you arrive outdoors, breathe in and smell the fresh air, observe the sky, and take in your surroundings. Follow the lines of the horizon and notice the colors around you. Listen to your inner voice. Feel the sensations of your feet as you walk on the earth and feel the earth below your feet. If you can, walk for at least half an hour before you stop to rest. If you are a yoga or martial arts practitioner or have other forms of conscious exercise, you may want to engage in that exercise before you sit down to rest. Find a comfortable spot to sit.

Take several more drops of the Sage flower essence. Again, notice where you're sitting and look around you. Look above and look below. Place your hands on the ground and feel the earth. Think of a favorite song or chant, and sing it while your hands continue to touch the earth. Feel the sensations inside your throat as you sing. As you stop briefly for a breath, breathe into your heart and continue to sing. Next time you stop for a breath, breathe into your solar plexus and continue to sing. Repeat this exercise with your abdomen, then your spleen chakra, and then your base. Extend your breathing to the earth and imagine yourself breathing into and from the earth. When you are ready, quiet your voice and sit in silence. Continue to breathe into and from the earth as long as you want. Close your eyes and just be.

When you are ready, slowly open your eyes and observe how you feel. If you want, write down your experience and any inspirations or insights you gained. Take your inner journey with you as you return home and hold it as long as you can. Remind yourself of this journey and this time with yourself, especially as you are taking the Sage essence.

Affirmations

- "I open my inner doorway and step inside the core of my being."
- "My voice is a vessel of sound, speaking my truth all around."
- "I allow the light of my body to guide and fill me."

Case History

Mateo, age thirty-five, is an entrepreneur and world traveler. He took the Sage flower essence with the following intention: "My intention is to take the essence and sit quietly and merge into Oneness with this purple-flowered essence of earth — to feel the easy flow of spiritual wisdoms grounding themselves into my being through daily life as my work emerges effortlessly in writing, speaking, and teaching. I vow to observe and write in my journal daily all the inspirations flowing through me."

Mateo took the Sage flower essence regularly. He found that this essence created deep sensations in his throat and kept him from feeling hunger, yet he still felt strong. He also experienced a significant grounding energy that helped him to integrate his spirituality into his physical world. Mateo shared a dream he had while taking the Sage flower essence: "I met a Sage man who took me walking through a lush landscape that eventually led upward. As we climbed up the huge moss-covered rocks, deeply verdant canopies of trees and tropical shrubbery cascaded alongside the largest waterfall I've ever seen. So electric was the air shooting straight out from the waterfall that my body tingled with excitement as I watched in amazement this very old, bearded man glide ahead of me. We reached the top to view an exquisite panorama from a sheer cliff that dropped to the ocean. Deep blues and greens were layered from sky to ocean. The Sage man said he was taking me to the Masters. I breathed deeply as he took me into this magnificence."

LFE's Research Provers' Project Findings

PHYSICAL SYMPTOMS

CRAVINGS: Steak

SENSATIONS: Surge of energy

PAIN: Teeth hurt into my head

MODALITIES: Not enough provers to make a valid study

HEAD: Headache

EYES: None

FACE: None

EARS: None

STOMACH: None

ABDOMEN: None

BOWEL CONDITION: None

URINE: None

FEMALE: Started my moon cycle early; hot flashes and a surge of energy

MALE: Lack of sexual energy

EXTREMITIES: None

BACK: None

SKIN: None

OTHER: None

EMOTIONAL SYMPTOMS

PATTERNS OF BALANCE: "after being incredibly depressed, I felt a peaceful and calming sigh of relief," "emotionally helped me to stay with some personal stuff and be with it," "helped me to detach myself from my 'trips,'" "I felt deeply sensitive while taking this essence," "once you make it through the storm, an incredible calm comes"

PATTERNS OF IMBALANCE: "impatience," "irritation in interacting with others," "anger," "experienced an incredible depression"

MENTAL SYMPTOMS

PATTERNS OF BALANCE: "I was more able to clearly see myself and other people, too; this was depressing at first, but I was able to get through it," "seeing my behavior and how I am was a good challenge," "my mental activity was strong and reflective," "more clairvoyant"

PATTERNS OF IMBALANCE: "the clairvoyance I experienced depressed me," "lots of waking up and thinking about things"

SPIRITUAL REFLECTIONS

"I felt a challenge to love and live love," "I felt a difference in who I am and how I fit into my world"

DREAMS/NIGHTMARES

Provers stated that dream activity increased. One prover stated that she had "huge epic dreams." Another prover had a dream of an old memory.

SAGUARO

(Cereus giganteus)
PRIMARY QUALITY: THE GUARDIAN

FAMILY: Cactus (Cactaceae)
OTHER NAMES: Sahuaro, Giant Cactus
WHERE FOUND: in the Sonoran Desert along rocky slopes and flats
ELEVATION: 600' to 3,600'
ENERGY IMPACT (CHAKRA CORRESPONDENCE): first, third, and seventh chakras
KEY RUBRICS FOR POSITIVE HEALING PATTERNS: endurance, honoring sacred space, perseverance, protection, purpose, stamina, wisdom
KEY RUBRICS FOR SYMPTOMS AND PATTERNS OF IMBALANCE: disrespect, lack of dignity, impatience, restlessness, feelings of unprotection, lack of purpose in life
OTHER RUBRICS: abundance, ambition, ancient, authority, awareness, consciousness, creativity, crown chakra, dreams, energize, expansion, giving up, guardian, insight, irritability, light, maturity, meditation, memory, nervous system, nighttime, passion, patience, prayer, radiance, reserves, root chakra, silence, solar plexus chakra, spine, spirituality, strength, understanding

Traditional Use

The saguaro has had many uses for early Native Americans of central and southwestern Arizona for centuries. The Hohokam Indians, who inhabited the region until about A.D. 1200 allowed saguaro wine to ferment to vinegar (acetic acid) and used it to engrave sea shells centuries before Europeans began using a similar etching technique. These people, as well as the Tohono O'Odham (the "desert people") who came after them, dislodged the fruit from the high branches with pieces of saguaro ribs tied together. The syrup, yams, fruit wine, and flour made from the seed sustained them through the hot summer months when little else was available. The O' Odham credit the saguaro with saving them from starvation before they began to farm. The placentas of newborns were often buried at the base of the saguaro to request of Spirit a long life for the baby.

Woodpeckers often peck holes in the saguaro. This causes the damaged saguaro to line the hole with scar tissue, creating a bootlike void that owls, hawks, and other desert birds use for shelter. This shelter protects the birds from the heat of the day because its inside temperature is thirty degrees cooler than the outside temperature. In the winter season, the sunlight radiates into the nest and keeps it warm.

The roots and the boot-shaped nests were used as containers by the Indians. The wooden ribs of dead saguaros were used to make roofs, shelters, fences, hiking sticks, knickknacks, and simple furniture, as well as to line graves. In earlier times, the Indians gathered their families and walked to the harvest grounds to collect saguaro fruit. The process could take up to three weeks. The women would gather the fruit and make syrup, leaving the empty fruit husk inside-out to encourage rain. The men would hunt for food and gather wood for the fire, then ferment the syrup into a low-alcoholic-content wine. The wine was then drunk in a ritual rainmaking ceremony of thanksgiving; drinking the wine was symbolic of the earth drinking or absorbing the rain. The elders faced the four sacred directions one by one, drinking the wine and praying for rain. Today, Indian families still harvest the saguaro fruit — but they usually make the round trip in only one day, driving a pickup truck.

The saguaro fruit eventually fall on the ground, attracting a variety of wildlife such as javelina, rabbits, birds, and ants.

Today there is a large market for saguaros among collectors and landscapers. They are considered prized additions to many a yard.

Homeopathic use

Unknown to author.

positive Healing patterns

- Helps us to persevere in times of struggle, to open our awareness through our own developmental process and that of our children, to become mature people who act wisely when we are given authority,

and to learn to pace ourselves and to build up our own reserves for times of need.

- Teaches us to build a strong nation of people who stand by their truths, who guard against negative ways of being and living, who protect their children and their environment, and who live with dignity; also shows us strength, insight, and wisdom through humbleness.

- Gives us an ancient connection and an ability to tap into our infinite storage bank of information that will help us evolve into our own spirituality; helps us emerge toward our higher wisdom and awareness, even in the darkness, and to find strength in our inner selves.

- Channels light, energy, and consciousness throughout all the chakras and in all parts of the body.

- Stirs passion, sensuality, creativity, and positive abundance at all levels; promotes the magic needed to energize and produce positive resources and reserves from within and outside of ourselves.

- Encourages us to find our inner silence, to honor that which is sacred, and to take time during the day for prayer, meditation, and devotion.

symptoms and patterns of imbalance

Saguaro may be an appropriate flower essence for those who

- Lack flexibility in their outlook toward life and who tend to be impatient, restless, and irritable
- Give up easily and don't live up to their abilities and talents
- Hold themselves back from expanding in consciousness, exploring their internal depths, and identifying their values and belief systems
- Prevent access to higher spiritual awareness and knowledge.

features of the original flower-essence water

ODOR: strong, powerful, and fruity
TASTE: strong, powerful, fruity, and smooth
SENSATIONS: gives a feeling of total relaxation and calmness
WATER COLOR: yellowish green, somewhat sea-green

physical makeup

ROOT, STEM, LEAVES/LEAFLETS, HEIGHT: The largest cactus in the United States, saguaros average 30 feet in height, and some grow to 50 feet. They are about $2\frac{1}{2}$ feet in diameter and can weigh up to nine tons! The Saguaro's green trunklike stem is characterized by columns with twelve to thirty prominent ribs. Saguaros branch out from the primary trunk as they grow older, forming branches or arms as large as 20 inches in diameter and creating a variety of humanlike shapes. This spiny, leafless cactus has many organs called "areoles"; fifteen to thirty whitish gray (slightly pinkish) 3-inch spines emerge from each areole. The saguaro grows at a slow, steady pace and has a long lifetime — up to two hundred years. The Saguaro grows only $\frac{1}{2}$ inch tall the first year, and stands at about 6 inches when it is nine years old. It takes nearly fifteen years for the saguaro to reach 1 foot. When it grows to about 8 feet in height, the first flowers begin to blossom. In forty to fifty years, the saguaro may grow to 10 feet in height, and then it takes seventy-five to one hundred years for it to reach 20 feet tall. At about this age, the saguaro begins to form its branches. The young saguaros are very vulnerable to the desert heat; they need another plant such as a creosote bush, paloverde tree, or older saguaros to nurture, shade, and protect them. Tiny holes in the saguaro's outer surface open during the nighttime, which help the cactus to breathe. The saguaro has a shallow root system that spreads out over a 50-foot radius. Following a good rain, the roots bring in the water and cause the plant's accordion-like folds and spongy stem tissue to become larger. Saguaros that have reached full growth may absorb up to 200 gallons of water in a single rainstorm. During the dry season, the saguaro gradually becomes slender again. Mature saguaros yield at least 100 fruits per season, which ripen and split open in July. The fruit is egg-shaped and about 3 inches long and $1\frac{3}{4}$ inches around. Each fruit's scarlet lining and succulent deep-red pulp average 2,000 tiny black seeds. A single saguaro produces several million seeds during the course of its life.
FLOWER COLOR: Creamy white
FLOWERS: The creamy white flowers are

waxy, smooth, soft, and very heavenly. They sometimes appear as a white halo or crown in terminal clusters on the saguaro's branches and main trunk. Each flower is about 3 inches in diameter and has a layered effect. The outer part is artichoke-like and prickly, while the inner petals are soft and smooth. Numerous yellow stamens with yellow anthers emerge from the center of the flower. One long, thick, pale-yellow pistil resembles a tiny long arm and a hand with many fingers. The flower buds open only once, beginning at nighttime and staying open during the latter part of the next day. The flowers have a strong, sweet, melonlike fragrance that lures bees and many insects in the daytime, and moths and bats during the night.

BLOOMING PERIOD: May through June

Doctrine of signatures

- The saguaro's amazing endurance, stamina, patience, steady rate of growth, and longevity are a signature that represents great perseverance, maturity, and a sense of authority with wisdom. The saguaro's ability to soak up water and nurture itself in spite of the demands of a hot desert climate is also a signature of the plant's ability to persevere as well as to build up reserves for times of need. These signatures resemble an ancient ability that each of us has inside ourselves, if we so choose, to persevere in times of struggle, to open our awareness through our own developmental process and that of our children, to become mature people who act wisely when we are given authority, and to learn to pace ourselves and build up our own reserves as a safety net.

- If you see one saguaro, you will see many saguaros. They grow in large communities scattered throughout the desert. Their presence is one of protection, likemindedness, silence, and humbleness with dignity. They are the guardians of the desert and, due to their height and size, they appear to oversee and protect their environment. Yet saguaros have a humble presence in spite of their great strength and size. Their presence speaks of surrender, dignity, higher truths, and awareness. These signatures represent our own need for a strong nation of people who stand by their truths, who guard against negative ways of being and living, and who protect their children and their environment. The art of being humble also shows great strength, insight, and wisdom. Saguaro teaches us to find our own inner silence within the Silence.

- The saguaro's towering posture and gigantic spine resemble the human spine and the nervous system. The saguaro is characterized by columns with twelve to thirty prominent ribs. The human body's spine is a column of bones and cartilage that extends from the seat of the skull to the pelvis, protecting the spinal cord and sustaining the head and the trunk. The entire spinal column protects and surrounds the spinal cord, which is a column of nerve tracts moving from the brain. Peripheral nerves shoot off from the main branch or spinal cord to every part of the body, and their roots move through the vertebrae. The signature of the saguaro's spine represents its ability to channel light, energy, and consciousness throughout all the chakras and in all parts of the body.

- The creamy white saguaro flowers relate to the seventh chakra or crown chakra. They are soft, light, radiant, heavenly, and sweet. The areoles of the saguaro allow the flowers to grow and emerge from the plant's tremendous body. The flowers give us an ancient connection and ability to tap into our infinite storage bank of information that will help us evolve into our own spirituality. The flowers remind us of the devotion and silence needed every day to help us become our purpose and live our lives fully. The yellow stamens are associated with the higher wisdom and intellect of the third chakra as related to the seventh chakra. The flowers bud only once, beginning at nighttime and staying open during part of the next day. This signature helps us gain access to our higher

wisdom and awareness, even in the darkness, and to find strength in our inner selves.

- The succulent deep-red fruit, like that of the pomegranate, stirs passion, sensuality, creativity, and positive abundance at all levels. The magic of this special fruit is indicative of the mystery of the saguaro and of life, and of the ability to energize and produce positive resources and reserves from within and outside of ourselves.

- The unique yellowish sea-green color of the water indicates the saguaro's fascinating relationship with the earth and her changes. It also relates to the fourth chakra. Along with the red fruit (first chakra) and creamy white flower (seventh chakra), the fourth chakra is the center and marriage of the three upper and the three lower chakras. These unique signatures show the saguaro's balanced nature and its creative force of energy and power.

Helpful suggestions

Take three or four drops of Saguaro flower essence and find a comfortable position. Imagine that you are walking on a Sonoran desert trail, weaving through arroyos, ascending gracefully to a desert mesa. You feel guided to leave the trail. You're searching for your higher purpose, for strength and power. You are drawn to a distant ridge on the edge of the mesa. As you begin to approach the ridge, you can feel the thermal activity, a rising current of hot air. You see a cluster of mature saguaros that guide you to them, graced with paloverde and mesquite trees and other desert shrubs. You find yourself standing in the center of the saguaro's circle, and there you feel the power and nurturing embrace of the mysterious desert giant. You prepare for a ceremony with this majestic plant.

In the ceremony, you gently leave behind your mortal thoughts and feelings, fears and doubts, and you feel protected as you enter into the sacredness of the Sonoran mystery. As a warrior, you feel the shield of protection offered by the saguaro's towering presence. Within this protection, you are ready to cross the threshold of their sacred space. As you begin to enter ceremony, still centered in the circle of saguaros, you listen to the inner silence of the desert. Then you hear the wind rustling through the shrubs, and you hear the distant cry of a bird of prey. Through breath and senses, body, mind, soul, and earth become one. Feeling one with the saguaro, you feel rooted and balanced. The consciousness of this balance rises up your spine like the towering plant, awakening and stimulating each sacred center from the root to the crown, opening, flowering, and receiving the light, warmth, and radiance of the sun. Through this expansion, you feel a quickening of the nervous system to its purpose, wisdom, and unity with Spirit. You give thanks to Spirit for your journey and the channel of Light you feel throughout your being.

Affirmations

- "I am guided by the wisdom and understanding of the Ancient Ones."
- "I protect, honor, and respect all that is sacred and that all are sacred."
- "I am patient and enduring, strong yet humble."

Case History

Ellen, a woman in her mid-forties took the Saguaro flower essence because she was attracted to the plant. Within twenty-four hours, she realized that she felt "heavy-hearted." To her, this meant that she had some energetic obstacles to work through that needed to lift. Ellen also was aware of her emotional state, which seemed impatient, restless, and somewhat irritable. She found herself drawn toward spending some inner quiet time with herself. She went into her bedroom and did a meditation in which she sets up a matrix of energetic support systems. She felt a yearning to quest for deeper insight into her financial situation and ways to access abundance. She also did some energy work on herself.

Ellen felt the "heavy-hearted" energy lift, and she regained a sense of calm. She also felt strong and positive, with a willingness to be more patient and enduring in her life situation. She realized that she felt a desire for passion and creativity, and she sensed the need for understanding her greater spiritual purpose in life. One of Ellen's visions is to be able to protect the natural environment of the sixty-eight-acre pristine land where she lives and to prevent this land from being taken over by development firms. She feels she is a guardian for this land and a protector of this natural and precious environment. Saguaro flower essence is helping her stay with her vision and her higher purpose, and is directing her to be steadfast and to act in practical and positive ways toward her goals.

LFE's Research provers' project Findings

PHYSICAL SYMPTOMS

CRAVINGS: Water

SENSATIONS: None

PAIN: None

MODALITIES:
  WORSE: None reported
  BETTER: Slept well at night

HEAD: None

EYES: None

FACE: None

EARS: None

STOMACH: None

ABDOMEN: None

BOWEL CONDITION: None

URINE: None

FEMALE: None

MALE: None

EXTREMITIES: None

BACK: None

SKIN: None

OTHER: "I felt physically strong, energetic, and motivated."

EMOTIONAL SYMPTOMS

PATTERNS OF BALANCE: "I felt happy but also concerned, and felt this was a serious essence relating to my life's path somehow," "a lot of emotions were felt — happy, sad, melancholy — and I felt motivated to get a new start in my life and to bring back some balance," "I experienced an elimination of old ways and unhealthy behaviors," "I felt strong, positive, and creative," "it brought up certain uncomfortable emotions, which then led to calm," "it gave me strength," "this essence helped me to create harmony"

PATTERNS OF IMBALANCE: "I experienced agitation and a feeling of obstacles that had to be dealt with in the outside world and with myself internally — like a flurry of activity; the outer circumstances pushed the emotional/mental revolution of it," "provoked a healing crisis, which seemed worse at first but then calm," "overactivity of pressure and responsibilities to handle," "irritability and impatience," "restlessness," "felt burdened and challenged"

MENTAL SYMPTOMS

PATTERNS OF BALANCE: "this essence helped me make choices to get my life back into some order, purpose, and balance," "I thought about my life and my world," "this helped me get a boost toward putting things into perspective," "this essence heightened my understanding, intuition, memory, and creativity," "I had a clear sense of things," "it helped me think about making plans to resolve certain issues," "this essence brought a greater awareness and deeper insight," "I was more aware of my environment"

PATTERNS OF IMBALANCE: "irritability,"

"lack of patience," "restlessness," "overactive mind"

SPIRITUAL REFLECTIONS

"I enjoyed more time with myself during this essence," "this essence helped me focus on my spiritual growth," "I reflected on my inner spiritual self; I felt this was a gentle essence, but it was also strong at times," "this essence gave me the silence to see," "this essence brought obstacles to the surface to be seen and dealt with"

DREAMS/NIGHTMARES

"I had dreams that reminded me to get back on my spiritual path, which I've been neglecting. I have thought about my new surroundings and how it's been difficult to set up good energy for myself to meditate in, and my dreams were gentle reminders that it will turn out okay."

"I had a dream that I was at a friend's house outside in some sort of a mudslide, and I couldn't get up this mudhill to her house. I kept sliding down to the bottom of the hill. My friend suggested that I go down to the far, smaller end of the hill and try again. I did this and was able to make it to the top of that small, short end of the hill. I knew this meant for me to start over with the Development classes that are going to begin in the later part of this year. I knew I would need to take "baby steps" again. My father, who has passed on, was also in this dream, giving me support and encouragement just by letting me see him. I felt happy when I woke and knew this was an important dream to learn from. I also had a dream about my grandmother, and I rarely have dreams or any contact involving my father or my grandmother."

"I had a deeper sense of my dream pictures (like trying to bring up the subconscious)."

SCARLET PENSTEMON

(Penstemon barbatus)
PRIMARY QUALITY: COURAGE

FAMILY: Snapdragon or Figwort (Scrophulariaceae)
OTHER NAMES: Golden-Beard Penstemon, Beardlip Penstemon, Red Penstemon, Southwestern Penstemon, Hummingbird Flowers. *Penstemon* means "five stamens." The botanical name is derived from the Latin word *barbatus* or *barba,* meaning "beard."
WHERE FOUND: roadsides, oak and conifer forests from southern Colorado and Utah to central Mexico
ELEVATION: 4,000' to 10,000'
ENERGY IMPACT (CHAKRA CORRESPONDENCE): first, second, third, and fifth chakras
KEY RUBRICS FOR POSITIVE HEALING PATTERNS: creativity, confidence, self-expression, masculine sexuality, passion, intimacy
KEY RUBRICS FOR SYMPTOMS AND PATTERNS OF IMBALANCE: agitation, anger, depression, lack of courage and faith, lack of confidence
OTHER RUBRICS: acceptance, breakthrough, challenges, change, comfort, emotion, expression, face, freedom, gentleness, healing, love, mouth, nurturing, passion, positive, purpose, reproductive, risks, root chakra, sensation, sensitivity, serenity, solar plexus chakra, spleen chakra, strength, surrender, throat chakra, vitality, voice, wisdom

Traditional Use

There are over 250 species of penstemon native to North America in a variety of colors. Native Americans used the leaves to make a poultice for the skin; to treat swellings, gun, and arrow wounds; and as a wash to treat eye problems. They also drank a tea made of penstemon to treat constipation, stomachache, internal injuries, bronchitis, kidney problems, and whooping cough. It is also used by the Navajo as a common medicine for treating fractured or broken bones in sheep. The fresh leaves, mixed with sweet almond, apricot kernel, or olive oil can be made into a salve as a skin dressing to treat irritations of the outer skin, anus, and lips.

Homeopathic Use

Unknown to author.

Positive Healing Patterns

- Gives us the courage, faith, vitality, and strength to face life's challenges, and the courage to allow ourselves to grow.
- Helps us have the courage and the creativity to take needed risks.

- Serves as a remedy — for men in particular, although it is also helpful for women — to have the courage to make positive changes; to let go of old patterns (especially sexual patterns); to have the courage to be sensitive in the way they feel, think, and act; to have the courage to be vulnerable to love and to be loving; to have the courage to be soft and nurturing; and to have the courage to share their fire and sweet nectar in a gentle and passionate way.
- Helps us to rebuild our faith and to let go when we need to.
- Promotes the courage to be creative in expression of voice, speech, and actions.

symptoms and patterns of imbalance

Scarlet penstemon may be an appropriate flower essence for those who

- Lack courage and confidence in themselves, especially when faced with life's setbacks
- Lack courage and creativity in self-expression, and who act out their feelings of agitation, irritability, and emotional upsets in insensitive ways
- Lack the courage (men in particular) to make positive changes, to be sensitive in the way they think, feel, and act, and to be gentle, nurturing, and passionate

- Have difficulty letting go and need to rebuild their faith and courage.

features of the original flower-essence water

ODOR: slightly pungent yet slightly sweet
TASTE: slightly pungent, then sweet; very full
SENSATIONS: warm tingling in the back of the throat and down to the root chakra
WATER COLOR: clear

physical makeup

ROOT, STEM, LEAVES/LEAFLETS, HEIGHT: Scarlet penstemon's narrow grayish green leaves arise in pairs from the stem and have smooth margins. They are long and grasslike and grow up to 5 inches long. The plant forms a clump of slender stems growing upward and ending with numerous drooping flowers growing from the stems on short stalks.

FLOWER COLOR: Bright red or scarlet red
FLOWERS: The flower petals form a narrow tube that is distinctly two-lipped and grows about $1^1/_2$ inches long. The lower lip bends downward and back with a beard of long yellowish hairs dangling from its lip. The upper lip has what looks like two tiny teeth that project forward. Scarlet penstemon is one of nearly fifty flowers in the Southwest, and one of nearly forty species of penstemon in western North America, that are pollinated by hummingbirds. Hummingbirds are attracted by the red flowers, and they can hover to sip the sweet

nectar. Bees on the other hand can't see red and there is no place for bees or butterflies to perch to sip the nectar.

BLOOMING PERIOD: June to October

Doctrine of signatures

- The scarlet color of the flower relates to the root or first chakra, which is linked to the reproductive system, activities of the testicles and ovaries, and the circulatory system. This is our center for life-promoting energy and is also connected to our "roots" and where we came from and how we respond to who we are at the very core of our being. The second or spleen chakra is also addressed here due to the orange-red appearance of the flower. This chakra relates to creativity, emotion, and sensation. These two colors together give a signature of the flower's courage, vitality, faith, and strength.

- The funny little face on this flower is unique. The upper lip with its tiny "teeth" and the lower lip with its golden bearded tongue certainly contribute a unique signature to scarlet penstemon; this signature is related to the throat chakra. The golden-yellow tongue corresponds to the third or solar plexus chakra and, as it hangs toward the ground, it gives a sense of having the courage to release emotions and old emotional patterns whether spoken or unspoken. The taste of the

flower-essence water, which is at first pungent and then sweet, is symbolic of facing or releasing the old in order to receive the new.

- The flower faces downward as an expression of surrender. The flower's long, narrow tube contains sweet nectar deep inside, which requires a strong and courageous intention to go deep within to find it. Once the nectar is found, its sweet taste is comforting and nurturing. When I first journeyed with the scarlet penstemon, the plant reminded me of the Serenity Prayer: "God grant me the serenity to accept the things I cannot change, the courage to change the things I can, and the wisdom to know the difference." The message of the journey went on to say: "Accept life's painful challenges as lessons to rebuild your faith, and have the courage and strength to take the next step. Seek your inner guidance and find the courage to go deep inside yourself. Have the courage to take a sip of your sweet nectar, giving you even more courage, strength, and wisdom. It takes courage and the willingness to take risks in order to follow your life's path. And it takes even more courage to face life's setbacks, and the wisdom to trust and to be patient in your process."

- The soft elastic petals of the flower, its tubular phallic appearance, and the scarlet-red-to-orange colors are a signature of male sexuality and simply being a male. Along with the above signatures, it encourages men to have the courage to make positive changes, the courage to let go of old patterns, the courage to heighten their sensitivity in the way they feel, think, and act, the courage to be vulnerable to love and to be loving, the courage to be soft and nurturing, the courage to share their fire and sweet nectar in a gentle and passionate way.

- The soft grayish green pastel color of the leaves, along with their smoothness and the way they grow in pairs, brings balance and calm within the fire.
- The warming sensation of the flower-essence water is also indicative of the lower chakras.

Helpful suggestions

Take several drops of the Scarlet Penstemon flower essence, then stand up and droop your head and arms downward. Slowly move your body from side to side with your head hanging down. Stick out your tongue, letting it hang between your lips, and make it vibrate. Take a deep breath down into your root chakra and slowly breathe it out as you continue to droop. Then take a deep breath and breathe into your spleen chakra and slowly let it go. Then take another deep breath and this time breathe into your solar plexus chakra right above your navel. Continue to let your head and tongue hang as

you breathe out. Check to see how you are feeling. Are there any sounds you'd like to express?

Make any sounds, songs, voices, or words that will help you release. Do this for as long as you'd like or until you feel your release has completed itself.

Now allow yourself to gently drop to the floor and lie on your back. Stretch out your legs and rest your arms at your sides. Take in a deep breath from your solar plexus and slowly release it. Repeat at least two more times. Now breathe in deeply into your spleen chakra and slowly release it and repeat this a few more times. Next breathe deeply into your genitals and then slowly let the breath release. Repeat this several times. Now imagine yourself poking your head inside the two-lipped scarlet penstemon. Stretch your head as far as you can deep inside the tubular flower. Stick out your tongue and reach for the nectar. Stretch a little farther and reach out again. Don't settle for less. Have the courage to stick your head even farther inside and gently stretch your tongue to taste the sweet nectar of the flower. Take in the nectar. You made it! Notice how you feel. Take in as much nectar as you wish, then slowly back your head out from the flower's head. Thank the scarlet penstemon for its sweet nectar and for the courage you gained from sticking your head and tongue deep inside. Thank yourself for having the courage to do this exercise!

Affirmations

- "God grant me the serenity to accept the things I cannot change, the courage to change the things I can, and the wisdom to know the difference." (The Serenity Prayer)

- "I have the courage to let go of the old and the courage to bring in the new."
- "I have the courage to go deep inside myself, to be vulnerable to love, and to be loving."

case History

Mary came to me in her early thirties for a flower-essence consultation, explaining that as the second child in her family, she "was the glue that held the family together." She felt that as a child she lacked the courage and confidence to speak up for herself, and that today as an adult those patterns were still prevalent. She described herself as "lacking faith and trust" and "wanting the courage and strength to allow herself personal growth." She asked for a remedy that would help her stabilize her root chakra and help her "let go more," giving her the courage to be herself.

After I gave Mary Scarlet Penstemon and a personal consultation, she went out for lunch by herself and then went to the Holy Chapel in Sedona, located in a setting of gorgeous red rocks. She later told me that, at the church, she released a lot of sadness and felt she made an emotional purge. She said it took a lot of courage for her to first allow herself to feel unwanted emotional wounds, and then to let them go. When she returned home and continued taking the essence,

she felt she had more courage to be her own person.

In October of 1994 my stepson Adam, who was thirteen years old then, was going through a difficult time in relation to his identity, peer pressure, drugs, school, parents who divorced when he was eight years old, and the continued bridging of a new family. I asked him if he would be interested in taking a flower essence. I tried to find some symptoms that would relate to a particular flower. He and I had a discussion about Leadership Day, which occurred at school, and Adam said he was bored at school — that "there's nothing to learn." When trying to help me find a remedy, he wanted me to know that he didn't like it when we asked him questions, he wanted more privacy, he didn't think he should have boundaries or anyone telling him what to do, and that he didn't think he "should have to share."

I got out some flower essences that I thought might be appropriate, and we read the description for each one. I felt he needed to make the choice and that it wouldn't be nearly as effective for me to make it for him. When we reached the description for Scarlet Penstemon, I read the Serenity Prayer out loud to him and talked about Scarlet Penstemon in terms of having the courage to find himself and to say no. This flower essence stirred him more than the previous seven.

Adam took the essence religiously for about four days, and then he just finished off the bottle on the last day. There certainly was more work involved than taking a flower essence for Adam, but his comment in taking Scarlet Penstemon was that "it gave me more courage with my friends and helped me to talk more." I have found it useful to let kids choose which flower essences they are drawn to, and I believe that Spirit works in special ways.

lfe's Research provers' project findings

PHYSICAL SYMPTOMS

CRAVINGS: None

SENSATIONS: None

PAIN: None

MODALITIES: No consistent reports

HEAD: None

EYES: None

FACE: None

EARS: None

STOMACH: None

ABDOMEN: None

BOWEL CONDITION: None

URINE: None

FEMALE: None

MALE: None

EXTREMITIES: None

BACK: Lower backaches

SKIN: None

EMOTIONAL SYMPTOMS

PATTERNS OF BALANCE: "this remedy may help someone 'stand up for their rights' or may bring up issues concerning that which may cause irritation, emotionally or mentally, and having to confront those feelings or thoughts, so possibly 'courage' might also apply," "brings balance," "self-relief," "brought up the need for more personal time," "brought up the feeling for

me to comfort myself and nurture what I've been neglecting," "I felt a calming from this essence, a welcome relief," "I had a calming, nurturing relief, and a 'let go' type of feeling"

PATTERNS OF IMBALANCE: "slight irritation," "I have been down, detached, and feel like I attract the constant challenge"

MENTAL SYMPTOMS

PATTERNS OF BALANCE: "I generally felt good and was happy to know I was getting back on track with my life. I feel like I have more understanding and knowing," "I did less thinking — just sort of let go," "this essence helped me to think less and feel more," "I think this essence would be good for someone going through or coming out of a depression or down time in their life"

PATTERNS OF IMBALANCE: "aggravated," "spaced out," "confused," "questioning"

SPIRITUAL REFLECTIONS

"I felt the desire to let go and just realize I'm doing the best I can to help myself and my situation and that now I need to be patient and continue to strive to renew or to continue down my spiritual path," "I had a desire to learn more or to experience spiritually," "I was helped to go within to find answers and that they aren't necessarily outside of myself"

DREAMS/NIGHTMARES

Dreams were clear, but none specifically recorded.

STRAWBERRY HEDGEHOG

(Echinocereus engelmannii)
PRIMARY QUALITY: PASSION

FAMILY: Cactus (Cactaceae)

OTHER NAMES: Strawberry Cactus, Hedgehog Cactus, Engelmann Hedgehog, Engelmann's Cactus, Torch Cactus, Strawberry Echinocereus. The botanical name *Echinocereus engelmannii* was given in honor of George Engelmann, a botanist and doctor from Germany who came to the United States in 1832 at the age of twenty-three. He gradually succeeded in an obstetric practice in St. Louis while maintaining an interest in plant life and botany. Many botanical explorers sent specimens for him to identify, and he has long been remembered for his botanical work with the cactus family. The "strawberry" part of the plant's common name comes from the dark red mahogany-colored fruits that are juicy and rich in sugar and may be eaten like strawberries. "Hedgehog" refers to the plant's stems, which are rounded like a hedgehog.

WHERE FOUND: low-moisture and well-drained soils, rocky flats, sandy desert areas, and hillsides in Arizona and California deserts

ELEVATION: sea level to 5,000'

ENERGY IMPACT (CHAKRA CORRESPONDENCE): first, third, and fourth chakras

KEY RUBRICS FOR POSITIVE HEALING PATTERNS: compassion, love, intimacy, sexuality, self-worth

KEY RUBRICS FOR SYMPTOMS AND PATTERNS OF IMBALANCE: aggression, insecurity, insensitivity, inhibition, shut-down sexuality

OTHER RUBRICS: balance, creativity, expression, fear, female, femininity, freedom, giving, heart chakra, kundalini, male, mother, nurturing, passion, procreation, protection, receiving, relationship, reproduction, respect, root chakra, security, sensitivity, sensuality, solar plexus chakra, spleen chakra, trust

Traditional use

The Strawberry Hedgehog cactus is a survival plant of the desert. Although it reduces in size in the summer heat, it recovers in size and moisture with the downfall of rain. Thorns can be removed by cutting off the outer skin from the cactus while the stem is still rooted. Placing the thorns back into the ground allows them to propagate. The inner cactus flesh can then be used for sunburns, bites, stings, open wounds, cuts, abrasions, and even to treat earaches. The flesh, as a food, can be eaten raw in hot weather and either cooked or roasted in cold weather. Although the texture is slimy, it is a good emergency food in the desert. The Pima Indians regarded the fruit as a delicacy, and the fruits are important in the diets of birds and rodents.

Homeopathic use

Unknown to author.

positive Healing patterns

- Promotes relationship and sexual openness based on trust, security, protection, intimacy, and expressing love with a partner freely and passionately.
- Increases our sensitivity, creativity, appreciation, and awareness of ourselves and our partner.
- Gives a strong balance of male and female roles in positive ways.
- Assists those who want to experience the kundalini life-force during sexual interactions.
- Promotes heart-centered energy that opens us up to love, compassion, and passion.

symptoms and patterns of imbalance

Strawberry Hedgehog may be an appropriate flower essence for those who

- Feel closed down, insecure, inhibited, or blocked sexually and emotionally and lack self-worth and appreciation of self, especially women
- Fear yielding, giving, or receiving
- Are insensitive of their partner's needs
- Want more sexual excitement and satisfaction
- Are obsessively sexual and aggressive, and desire immediate sexual gratification without a whole-body experience
- Are in need of healing and loving their mothers, especially for women.

features of the original flower-essence water

Odor: roselike, subtle, and soft
Taste: very pleasant and roselike with a full yet light taste that stays in the mouth
Sensations: Obvious light tingling in the vagina; feel the lips of the vagina open as if to receive and give energy; also feel a warm tingling in the heart chakra.
Water Color: clear

physical makeup

Root, Stem, Leaves/Leaflets, Height: Grows in open clumps that form a loose or thick cluster up to 3 inches wide and 20 inches long, looking like spine-covered cucumbers standing on end. They are green and cylindrical, and grow up to 3 inches in diameter. The straight spines are usually yellow, although they can vary in color from white or gold to pinkish to black, and they tend to point downward. There are ten to fourteen protruding ribs on each stem with areoles (small open spaces) set about $^1/_2$ inch apart. Each areole consists of eight to twelve $^1/_2$-inch-long radial spines, and up to six central spines that can be up to 3 inches long. The plant's ribs appear tough, yet they are very delicate and are protected by the spines.
Flower Color: Magenta
Flowers: The deep magenta flower makes an opening in the skin of the cactus right above the areoles (the small open spaces), where two to six central spines come together along the plant's ribs. The flowers carry a very sweet fragrance. They are delicate, transparent, and elastic. The

cup-shaped flowers are up to 3 inches wide. The inner petals are more intense in their magenta color, and the outer petals are a softer pink. There are dozens of soft, airy, lemon-yellow stamens that grow close in the center and around the pistil, then spread out in a circle inside the base of the flower. Inside the very center is a profound green pistil that is firm yet soft and looks like a miniature tree with nine to eleven small fingerlike segments. The sepal is thorny with alternating whitish long and short spines. The flowers bloom for several consecutive days, attracting bees and beetles to their abundant pollen and sweet nectar. The blooms are followed by green spiny fruit, which becomes red when ripe and grows up to $^1/_4$ inch long and 1 inch in diameter. The ripe, succulent fruit is juicy and rich in sugar, and may be eaten like strawberries.

BLOOMING PERIOD: March to April

Doctrine of signatures

- It is amazing that a beautiful, sensual, soft flower can emerge from a cucumber-like organ that is covered with needles. The cylindrical stem of the cactus is actually very delicate, and the needles provide protection. This signature in and of itself is certainly symbolic of both the male and female, and gives a strong balance of male and female roles in positive ways. The needed protection of the spines or needles indicates sensitivity toward each other. Even the flower is able to find its place to emerge from the

skin of the stem at a cluster of spines, protected yet free to express itself. The stem (resembling the male organ) is able to receive the flower's sweet nectar from within the skin, even with the spines all around. And the stem is able to give to the flower so that the flower can emerge from the stem's sustenance. What a fascinating signature!

- As if the above signature weren't enough, we're going to take this a few steps farther. The deep magenta petals are more intense on the inside of the flower, like the deeper, brighter reddish colors inside the vagina, especially when a woman is sexually excited and passionate. The womb is protected, and the vagina opens up like a flower in its peak blossom! The strawberry hedgehog's flowers are elastic, giving a feeling of stretching. Yes, this is true. The petals are strong, yet yielding and gentle. The outer petals are a softer pink like the vulva and its surrounding area. This signature certainly points to female sensuality and passion. Another added attraction to this signature is the male-looking pistil in the center of the flower. The pistil is firm yet soft, and emerges right from the very center of the flower as yet another gift from Mother Nature. Also, it's another indication of the balance of giving and receiving sexual energy.

- The magenta flower and the red, juicy fruit correspond with the first or root chakra, the seat of the kundalini life-force and sexual energy within our bodies. It's linked to the reproductive system, and influences the functions of the testicles and ovaries. It stems from who we are and is related to our self-worth and our appreciation of self so that we can open up and experience our sexuality at its fullest. This signature relates to the experience of kundalini, sexuality, and creativity in a highly evolved and positive way. A more challenging aspect would be for those who are obsessively sexual, aggressive, insensitive, and only desire immediate gratification without a whole-body experience. The softer pink outer petals represent the fourth or heart chakra, which gives the ability to transmute and open the sexual energy into a hot-pink, passionate love. My friend Eileen refers to this as "being in love with the act of living in the moment." These signatures relate to more than just sexual passion and expression. They also relate to the heart-centered energy that opens us to love and to the nurturing we may need so that we can love. The femininity of the flower relates to the female as the mother and also represents the healing of our love toward our mothers and ourselves.

- The red, juicy, succulent fruits also represent sensuality and sweet passion.
- The soft lemon-yellow stamens that emerge profusely from the center of the flower's cup correspond to our third or solar plexus chakra and the emotions we feel in relation to ourselves, our sexuality, and our passion.

Helpful suggestions

Take some alone time for yourself and set up a supportive environment for this experience. You may want to light some candles and incense or arrange an altar with things that are special to you and have an intimate meaning that demonstrate the ways you appreciate yourself. Enjoy the time you spend doing this, and use your imagination creatively. Take a champagne glass or a special goblet and fill it halfway with pure water. Then add about four to six drops of the Strawberry Hedgehog flower essence, and place the glass or goblet on your altar (or nearby). If you have a deep magenta cloth or veil of any kind, place it where you will be lying down to do this exercise (on your bed, a futon, or a comfortable spot on the floor). If you don't have a magenta cloth, you can visualize having one as part of this exercise.

First, sit by your altar on your magenta cloth, or just sit comfortably wherever you choose. Drink a few sips from your special glass and take five or ten minutes to sit in silence and reflect on what you appreciate about yourself. Then lie down on your magenta cloth and wrap it around you. Close your eyes and visualize the magenta color radiating from the base of your spine to your coccyx to your rectum and below and around to your genitals. Breathe the color into each area and feel its warmth. Then bring the magenta color below and around your genitals. If you are a woman, take the color and the warmth deep inside to your uterus; slowly take several long, deep breaths, breathing the warmth and color deep into your womb. If you are a man, take the magenta color into your genitals and imagine it radiating outward from there. For both genders, gradually let the color and the warmth flow from inside to outside your genital area and again breathe it in. Feel your genitals open to receiving this radiant light and the warmth it brings.

Let the magenta color and the warm feeling flow upward through your abdomen to your solar plexus and up to your heart chakra. Breathe in the deep magenta color and feel its warmth. With the magenta color on the inside, visualize a soft glowing pink encircling the magenta around your heart chakra. Feel your heart open and allow the radiance of the colors to enter deep inside. Breathe warmth into this area and continue to visualize these colors in and around your heart as long as you wish, feeling the warmth they provide. Imagine your whole body surrounded by deep magenta, with soft glowing pink encircling your auric field. Lie there as long as you'd like, taking in the warm, loving energy these colors provide. Holding this energy, slowly open your eyes and sit up when you're ready. Take a few more sips of your drink and feel its sensations. Sit in silence and let your next step be guided by Spirit.

Affirmations

- "I am an abundant resource, giving love and receiving love."

- "I allow the creative, sensual petals of my personality to burst forth and to receive, give, and share in life's celebration."
- "I unconditionally allow myself to passionately receive and express the pleasures of blissful love."

Case History

Terri, in her late thirties, came for a flower-essence consultation, and here is her story about taking the Strawberry Hedgehog flower essence: "Before taking the Strawberry Hedgehog, I felt as though I had lost touch with a part of myself. I couldn't quite put my finger on it. I felt homely and plain. I had lost some of my desire for closeness and intimacy with my husband. I knew this was not because I wasn't attracted to him physically or emotionally. There seemed to be a wall within myself that I couldn't break through.

"I began taking the Strawberry Hedgehog flower essence and concentrated on what that wall might be. Within a short time, I began to realize that I had suppressed my femininity. I began to rejoice in my own feelings and all that being a woman truly means. I was able to see myself from a different point of view. I felt myself soften. I felt more attractive and enjoyed being close to my husband again. I could allow myself to be pampered without feeling a loss of my independence. My desire for intimacy and for sex increased as I allowed myself to feel good about being me. Also, my sexual fulfillment and gratification intensified. With the use of Strawberry Hedgehog, I was able to rediscover my feminine side and let down my protective wall without feeling vulnerable. Instead of the weakness that I feared, I became stronger and more able to relate to others in a healthy way."

LfE's Research provers' project findings

Physical Symptoms

Cravings: None
Sensations: None
Pain: Lower back
Modalities: None consistently reported
Head: None
Eyes: None
Face: None
Ears: None
Stomach: None
Abdomen: None
Bowel condition: None
Urine: None
Female: Less frequent hot flashes; I have more energy than before; increased sex drive
Male: None reported
Extremities: None
Back: Lower back pain
Skin: None
Other: None

Emotional Symptoms

Patterns of Balance: "I felt more grounded and more in control," "I felt the need to be spending more time with my mother, which I did; I love and respect her very much, and she's a strong influence in my life. We spent most of our time together while I took this essence. I don't know if this essence is related to 'female' or 'mother,' but it sure felt like it to me," "I feel grounded and confident about myself while thinking about relationships in my life," "I am thankful to have these people in my life," "I felt appreciative of who I am and thankful for people who are positive and influential in my life," "I am reminded that I still need to nurture and appreciate myself," "felt more calm and a new sense of peace," "I feel more loving," "I wanted more intimacy"

Patterns of Imbalance: "I feel like a basketball or tennis ball being bounced all over my emotions"

Mental Symptoms

Patterns of Balance: "I put things more in perspective and in a more rational way," "I noticed I spent some time thinking about the relationships in my life (mother, sister, boyfriend, best friends, etc.)"

Patterns of Imbalance: None reported

Spiritual Reflections

"I feel stronger and more grounded than usual," "I had subtle reminders of my spirituality and loving guardians in my life"

Dreams/Nightmares

Dreams were inconsistent and not emphasized with this essence.

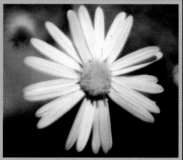

Aster (Desert Aster)
(Machaeranthera tephrodes)

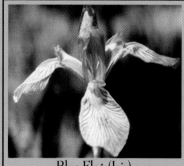

Blue Flag (Iris)
(Iris missouriensis)

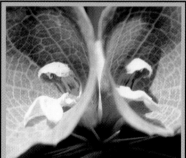

Bells-of-Ireland
(Moluccella laevis)

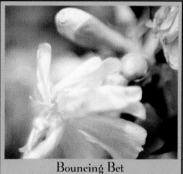

Bouncing Bet
(Saponaria officinalis)

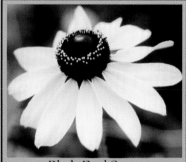

Black-Eyed Susan
(Rudbeckia hirta)

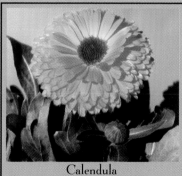

Calendula
(Calendula officinalis)

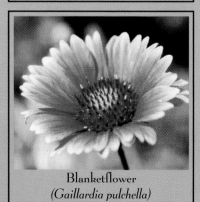

Blanketflower
(Gaillardia pulchella)

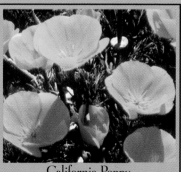

California Poppy
(Eschscholzia californica)

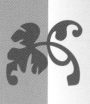

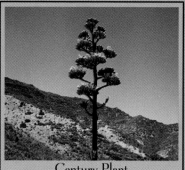

Century Plant
(Agave parryi)

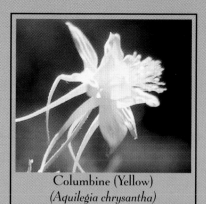

Columbine (Yellow)
(Aquilegia chrysantha)

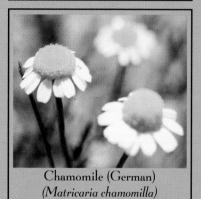

Chamomile (German)
(Matricaria chamomilla)

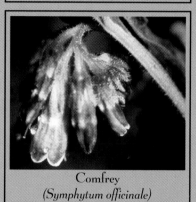

Comfrey
(Symphytum officinale)

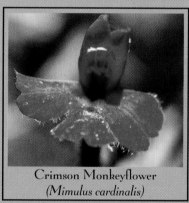

Chicory
(Cichorium intybus)

Crimson Monkeyflower
(Mimulus cardinalis)

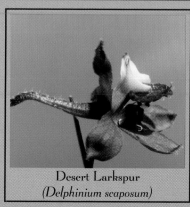

Cliff Rose
(Cowania mexicana)

Desert Larkspur
(Delphinium scaposum)

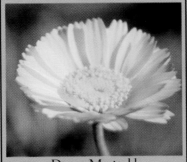

Desert Marigold
(Baileya multiradiata)

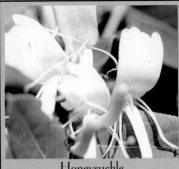

Honeysuckle
(Lonicera japonica 'Halliana')

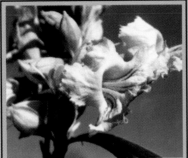

Desert Willow
(Chilopsis linearis)

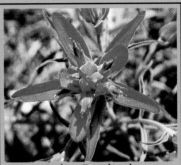

Indian Paintbrush
(Castilleja chromosa)

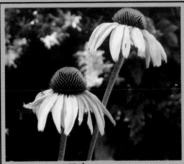

Echinacea
(Echinacea angustifolia)

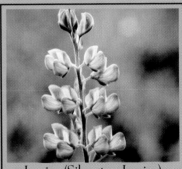

Lupine (Silverstem Lupine)
(Lupinus argentus)

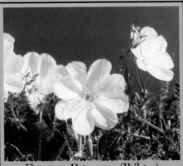

Evening Primrose (White)
(Oenothera caespitosa)

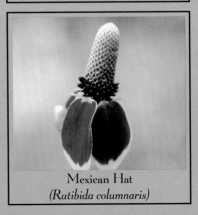

Mexican Hat
(Ratibida columnaris)

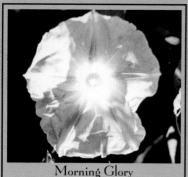

Morning Glory
(Ipomoea purpurea)

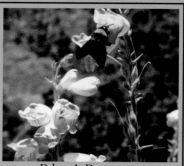

Palmer's Penstemon
(Penstemon palmeri)

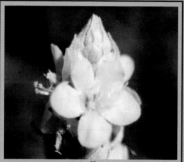

Mullein
(Verbascum thapsus)

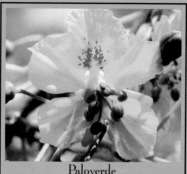

Paloverde
(Cercidium floridum)

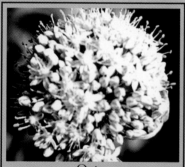

Onion
(Allium cepa)

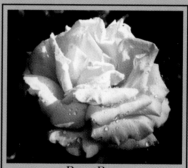

Peace Rose
(Rosa peace)

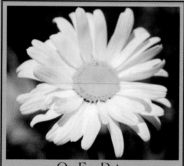

Ox-Eye Daisy
(Chrysanthemum leucanthemum)

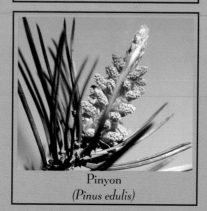

Pinyon
(Pinus edulis)

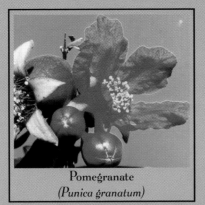

Pomegranate
(Punica granatum)

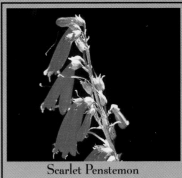

Scarlet Penstemon
(Penstemon barbatus)

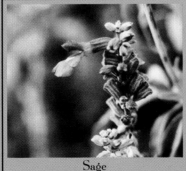

Purple Robe
(Nierembergia spp.)

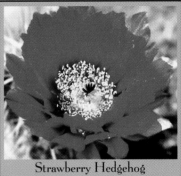

Strawberry Hedgehog
(Echinocereus engelmannii)

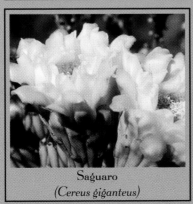

Sage
(Salvia officinalis purpurescens)

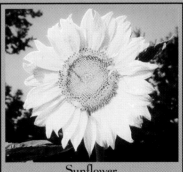

Sunflower
(Helianthus annuus)

Saguaro
(Cereus giganteus)

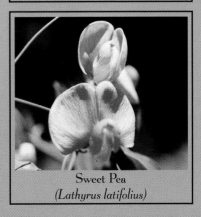

Sweet Pea
(Lathyrus latifolius)

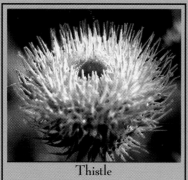

Thistle
(Cirsium neomexicanum)

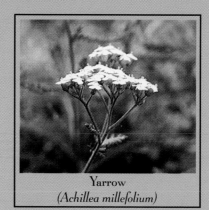

Yarrow
(Achillea millefolium)

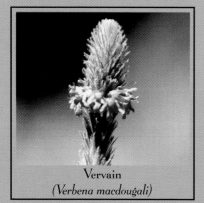

Vervain
(Verbena macdougali)

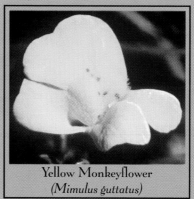

Yellow Monkeyflower
(Mimulus guttatus)

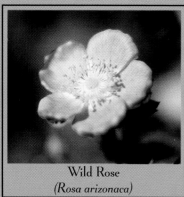

Wild Rose
(Rosa arizonaca)

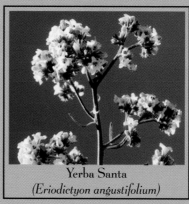

Yerba Santa
(Eriodictyon angustifolium)

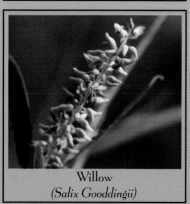

Willow
(Salix Gooddingii)

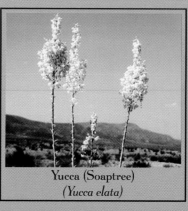

Yucca (Soaptree)
(Yucca elata)

SUNfLOWER

(Helianthus annuus)
PRIMARY QUALITY: FOUNTAIN OF YOUTH

FAMILY: Sunflower or Daisy (Compositae)

OTHER NAMES: Sunflower, Tall Sunflower, Giant Sunflower, or Big Sunflower. The botanical name *Helianthus* comes from *anthos,* meaning "flower" and *helios,* meaning "sun." Its golden-rayed flowers resemble the sun.

WHERE FOUND: Native to Central America and widespread in North America, the Mediterranean, Eastern Europe, and the former Soviet Union. Over sixty species of the sunflower can be found in every state in the U.S. and southern Canada, especially along washes and roadsides.

ELEVATION: 100' to 7,000'

ENERGY IMPACT (CHAKRA CORRESPONDENCE): third chakra

KEY RUBRICS FOR POSITIVE HEALING PATTERNS: cheerfulness, determination, direction, expansion, playfulness, vision, warmth, wisdom

KEY RUBRICS FOR SYMPTOMS AND PATTERNS OF IMBALANCE: anger, despair, exhaustion, fear, guilt, hopelessness, panic, pessimism, lack of goals or direction, unworthiness

OTHER RUBRICS: aggressiveness, appreciation, assertion, awareness, balance, blame, brow, celebration, centeredness, certainty, clarity, communication, compassion, confidence, conscious, courage, creativity, critical, defensiveness, ego, encouragement, faith, focus, freedom, fun, happiness, innocence, insight, intellect, joy, leadership, life force, light, liveliness, masculine, observation, optimism, personal power, pleasure, positive, protection, purpose, radiance, rebirth, relaxed, renewal, self-empowerment, self-honor, solar plexus chakra, spirituality, stability, sun, transformation, will, world peace, yang, youthfulness

Traditional use

The sunflower is believed to have originated in Peru, where the sun-worshipping Incas wore headdresses of the flower and adorned their temples with flowers wrought in gold in honor of their god. Aztec sun priestesses also adorned themselves with sunflowers and gold jewelry with sunflower emblems. Sunflower was cultivated some 3,000 years ago by the American Indians, and archaeologists also found seeds in clay containers made at about that same time. The sunflower has always been respected as a symbol of the sun.

Native Americans found many uses for the plant, including soap, snares and arrows, flutes, flour, cereal, cornmeal, mush, breads, soups, oil, and dyes. They boiled the flower heads to obtain seed oil to grease their hair, and they extracted the seeds to make a purple and black dye for clothes and baskets. The flower was boiled to make a yellow dye. The Pueblo Indian women decorated their dresses with sunflowers during corn dances. Sunflowers were worn in women's hair, and woven in a circle and placed on the men's hats for the harvest dance.

Medicinally, sunflower root was used to treat snakebite, rheumatism, and inflammation, and the stem juice was used to clean cuts and wounds. Early Russians made a liniment for rheumatism and used decoctions and teas to treat jaundice, diarrhea, malaria, and heart, kidney, and bladder ailments. The Chinese have cultivated sunflowers for centuries, and they use them to make acupuncture moxa, delicate silks, and thick ropes. The sixteenth-century Spaniards cultivated the sunflower as a decorative plant, and the Dutch used it to reclaim marshy land because of its great capacity to absorb water from the soil.

The sunflower is an extremely useful plant; all parts of it can be used. The seed kernel can be eaten and is rich in vitamins such as B1, B2, D, and niacin, as well as calcium, iron, fluoride, magnesium, sodium, phosphorus, potassium, sulfur, vegetable fats, and proteins. Hot drinks can be made from the hulls. Stems are ground into fodder and used in paper-making and textile production, and are smoked as a tobacco substitute.

The pith (stem tissue) is one of the few substances known for its light weight and has become common in scientific laboratories. An infusion of the pith stalk can be used as an eyewash and to treat cases of sore, inflamed eyes. The dried stem becomes very sturdy and makes a good source of fuel. The flower is eaten in salads or steamed. Medicinally, sunflower seeds are used as an expectorant and a diuretic to treat coughs, colds, sore throats, pulmonary problems, and bronchitis. The leaves and/or flowers are used to treat heart difficulties, malaria, and fevers. Sunflower oil has become popular to eat and cook with; it makes a pale yellow oil, high in unsaturated fats. Sunflower oil is recommended over butter because of its low saturated-fat content. The oil is also fed in products to sheep, cattle, and poultry. The oil can also be used in liniments, ointments, and medical compounds.

Ornamentally, sunflower offers a windbreak, a splash of garden color, and a natural birdfeeder. It is often planted for its beauty as well as its prolific and tasty seeds.

The sunflower has become a well-known decorative symbol, and is popular as a design on clothes, tablecloths, window curtains, fabrics, towels and washcloths, bedspreads, jewelry, and more.

Homeopathic use

A sunflower homeopathic remedy (*Helianthus annus*) is used to treat intermittent fever, catarrh, nasal hemorrhage, thick scabs in the nose, rheumatic pain in the left knee, vomiting, mouth dryness and congestion, and spleen. This remedy is indicated if a patient's stools are black, and symptoms are usually irritated by heat and soothed by vomiting.

positive Healing patterns

- Gives us the ability to think and reason, to gather the strength and power from deep within our roots, to find purpose and desire in life, and to empower ourselves.
- Strengthens our higher will and our ability to follow the Light and to allow spiritual wisdom and vision to flow through our thoughts.
- Gives us the ability to assert ourselves physically in the world with positive determination, optimism, and direction.
- Helps us find balance in our lives and provides us with warmth and compassion as we lovingly embrace ourselves, others, and our life's purpose.
- Nurtures and restores our youth and innocence, fun and play, liveliness and pleasure, bringing the child within each of us alive and directing us toward creative action and thought, joy and humor.
- Connects us with the source of the sun, its love and its power. Helps us take on the radiant energy the sun provides within each of us; lets our "sun shine" by expressing ourselves creatively in the world.

symptoms and patterns of imbalance

Sunflower may be an appropriate flower essence for those who

- Have emotions that cloud their mental judgment, lacking the mental power to be positive, optimistic, and creative; this cloudiness may include fear, panic, hopelessness, despair, guilt, unworthiness, uncertainty, worry, anger, hatred, nostalgia, and lack of courage
- Lack the intention and the Higher Will to follow through with ideas and practical solutions in life
- Tend to become bogged down with what others think, and lack a feeling of recognition and self-esteem
- Have become depleted and withdrawn — who feel they have lost their power, purpose, and Higher Will to be creatively expressive
- Are out of touch with their child self, youth and innocence, pleasure and liveliness, fun and play, and feel lost in the darkness of the self
- Are overly confident and assertive (male or female), and misuse their power within themselves, with others, and in the world at large
- Lack strength, warmth, and compassion from others that is necessary for a healthy ego (children or adults).

features of the original flower-essence water

ODOR: strong and musty
TASTE: light and airy
SENSATIONS: tingling down to the feet, giving a feeling of groundedness and vital energy, then tingling up through the chakras giving a great sense of mental clarity, lightness, and energy
WATER COLOR: yellow

physical Makeup

ROOT, STEM, LEAVES/LEAFLETS, HEIGHT:
The sunflower's root system is far-reaching
and deep, drawing out trace minerals not
always present in topsoil. The outer stem
is rough, hairy, stout, and sturdy. The
inner stem is fibrous and light. The sunflower's rough, hairy leaves are large with
coarse, irregularly toothed edges. The
many leaves vary from opposite to alternate along the stems, and are triangular or
somewhat heart-shaped. They are mid-
green in color with three prominent veins,
growing up to 12 inches long. The entire
sunflower plant generally ranges from 3 to
12 feet in height.

FLOWER COLOR: Golden-yellow with
yellowish/purplish or brownish disk

FLOWERS: The sunflower's head is golden
yellow and daisy-like in appearance, with a
center disk that is yellow-purplish or
brownish. The disk is encircled by brilliant
ray flowers extending outward. The disk
flowers are fertile and composed of small
tubular flowers without petals that ripen
into seeds. The seed head forms a dazzling
geometric circle pattern. The outer shell of
the seed is flat, and oval, thinly covered,
and gray with brown and white stripes.
The shell is about $1/2$ inch long. Seed ker-
nels are light gray, flat, and oval. The seeds
are rich in vitamins and nutrients, and very
tasty. The sunflower's nutritional qualities
are said to be related to the plant's ability as
a heliotrope, which refers to the flower
head's astonishing trait of following and
facing the sun from morning to night.

BLOOMING PERIOD: May to October

Doctrine of signatures

- The deep root system of the sunflower is far-reaching, giving it the
ability to draw out trace minerals
that may not be found in the topsoil. The root system also absorbs
water from the soil, and it is
believed to open pathways in the
soil that allow natural warmth from
the sun to pass through. The flower
head's ability to follow the sun
throughout the day is also a signature of the plant's amazing talents.
Along with the vitamins and other
nutrients found in sunflower seeds,
these signatures symbolize the
wealth of nutrients the plant has to
offer us and its incredible relationship with the sun.

- The golden-yellow color and the
shape of the sunflower's round
flower head, along with the golden-
yellowish, purplish disk, is also
symbolic of the sun. As with the
century plant, these colors that are
characteristic of the sun represent
the fire of life, the will. Also like
the century plant, the stalk is sturdy
and tall and gives a feeling of great
strength, endurance, and a desire to
reach toward the sun's natural
power and light. No wonder the
ancient ones honored the sun
with adornments of the sunflower.
These signatures relate to the third
chakra, will, purpose, power, self-
empowerment, and self-honor. This
is the energy center that gives us

the ability to think and reason, to gather the strength and power from deep within our roots, to find purpose and desire in life, and to empower ourselves with who we are. The third chakra helps us strengthen our mind and pursue a state of positive faith, self-direction, courage, and stability. This chakra is complemented by the violet-purple ray of the sixth chakra (like the purple disk of the sunflower), which strengthens our ability to receive higher inspiration, to follow the Light, and to allow spiritual wisdom and vision to flow through us and guide our thoughts.

- The third chakra or solar plexus center is sun energy. It is associated with the left side of the brain and its activities, representing the male or yang energy. The sun is also known to represent the male. In relation to the signatures already mentioned, the male energy within each of us — whether we are male or female — with the assistance of the sunflower, gives us the ability to assert ourselves in the world with positive determination, optimism, and direction. It helps us find balance in our lives, and provides us with warmth (from the sun) and compassion as we lovingly embrace ourselves and our life's purpose, and as we embrace others. The solar plexus and the sun also represent the direction south in Native American traditions. The south is about youth and innocence, fun and play, liveliness, pleasure, and creativity. It is about nurturing our will with all of these things, and connecting with the source of the sun, its love, and its power. Even the flower-essence water is yellow.

- The sunflower's large disk represents an eye. The eye of this plant is open wide and offers a journey of seeing and believing. In some cases, the eye is brownish and dark. The leaves and stems are coarse and hairy. In times of misery, emotional pain, suffering, and feeling "stuck," like the black-eyed Susan this plant will restore youth and liveliness, bring the child within each of us alive, and direct us toward creative action and thought. The sunflower guides us to follow the sun — the light — just as its youthful head turns toward the light.

Helpful suggestions

Take several drops of the Sunflower essence and get into a standing position. Close your eyes and stand with your feet about 6 to 8 inches apart. Imagine your feet and toes reaching deep inside the earth, going deeper and deeper and deeper. The deeper your feet go into the earth, the more energy you feel in your body. Finally your feet begin to feel a wetness as they reach water. They absorb the water and other nutrients, sending these nutrients up through your ankles, legs, thighs, buttock, genitals, abdomen, stomach, arms, hands, fingers, chest, heart, throat, face, and to the top of your head. You spread your arms outward with your hands open, and stretch your arms upward as if reaching for the sun. Tilt your head back and feel the warmth of the sun on your face as you slowly move your head from one side to another, as if following the radiance, light, and warmth of the sun. Take in this warmth and feel it shine through your head and face.

Maintaining the warmth on your head and face, bring the warmth back down through your throat, heart, chest, fingers, hands, arms, stomach, abdomen, genitals, buttock, legs, ankles, and all the way to your feet and toes that are reaching deep into the earth. Feel the connection of the warmth from the top of your head and on your face all the way down to your toes stretching deep into the earth. Allow your body to be a channel of this warmth, penetrating light, and radiance throughout your energy channels.

Affirmations

- "I am renewed in radiance and light, compassion and warmth."
- "I allow my personal power to shine from deep within my roots and outward toward the sun."
- "I joyfully celebrate my fountain of life and living."
- "I embrace the power and light of the sun."

case History

Dean was a forty-seven-year-old man who had been highly optimistic about completing a major project he had been working on for nearly nine months. He was faced with many obstacles and challenges in this project, and in the past few weeks he had found that self-doubt, self-criticism, depletion of energy, withdrawal, uncertainty, and a lack of recognition for his efforts were beginning to take over his mind and his overall energy output.

Dean prayerfully took the Sunflower essence one evening, realizing that he needed to make a shift to help him follow through with his life's purpose. When he awoke the next day, he found that he had regained some faith and determination, had released some grumpiness, and experienced the day with more joy and humor than he had felt for days. That evening, he didn't take the Sunflower essence and awoke the following day feeling depleted, realizing that he had lost his youthful energy and outlook on life. So again he took the Sunflower essence, and within minutes he felt his energy level change to a brighter and more positive nature. By taking the Sunflower essence consistently and with prayer and intention for several days, Dean was back on track again, feeling determined and positive about aligning himself with his higher will and his life direction, and regaining the ability to act on his intention.

LFE's Research provers' project findings

PHYSICAL SYMPTOMS

CRAVINGS: None

SENSATIONS: None

PAIN: None

MODALITIES: None

HEAD: None

EYES: None

FACE: None

EARS: None

STOMACH: None

ABDOMEN: None

BOWEL CONDITION: More bowel movements

URINE: None

FEMALE: None

MALE: None

EXTREMITIES: None

BACK: None

SKIN: None

OTHER: More physical vitality

EMOTIONAL SYMPTOMS

PATTERNS OF BALANCE: "I was able to take other people's emotional negativity lightly," "it helped me protect my feelings," "helped me to not take others' emotions and actions personally," "I felt more relaxed, centered, and certain," "I felt optimistic and positive," "I felt a sense of encouragement and certainty about positive outcomes," "this essence contrasted positive over negative," "I found myself feeling encouraged," "I felt more confident and cheerful," "I felt freedom with this essence," "I felt like laughing"

PATTERNS OF IMBALANCE: "defensiveness," "I was aware of needing to be careful about my fears," "my ego needed to stand out of the way," "it brought up aggressiveness, blaming, criticalness, and anger that needed to be worked with," "misunderstanding"

MENTAL SYMPTOMS

PATTERNS OF BALANCE: "I was more aware mentally of how people reacted to my words and actions," "I was more left-brained," "more clairvoyant," "more aware of the sensitivities of others," "I was more focused and determined," "I had more mental clarity and was able to watch a process unfold," "I think this essence would help people be more positive in a critical situation," "I was more observant"

PATTERNS OF IMBALANCE: "overly mental; trying to think things out and forcing things to happen"

SPIRITUAL REFLECTIONS

"I experienced spiritual growth in a way of being able to help others in sorting out problems and an awareness or encouragement that this is possible," "I felt that my prayers were being answered and that light was shedding on a particular situation"

DREAMS/NIGHTMARES

One prover shared a dream filled with images. No other dreams were reported.

SWEET PEA

(Lathyrus latifolius)
PRIMARY QUALITY: GROWING CHILD

FAMILY: Pea (Fabaceae, Leguminosae)
OTHER NAMES: Common Sweet Pea, Hardy Sweet Pea
WHERE FOUND: in gardens and greenhouses, on bank covers, trailing over rocks, on trellises or fences, and naturalized throughout the U.S.
ELEVATION: most U.S. climates
ENERGY IMPACT (CHAKRA CORRESPONDENCE): fourth chakra
KEY RUBRICS FOR POSITIVE HEALING PATTERNS: belonging, compassion, confidence, love, protection, social integration
KEY RUBRICS FOR SYMPTOMS AND PATTERNS OF IMBALANCE: desertion, fear, insecurity, lack of confidence, loneliness, feeling unloved and unprotected
OTHER RUBRICS: adolescence, appreciation, awareness, calm, centeredness, change, children, community, creativity, emotional pain or suffering, feminine, gentleness, groundedness, growing up, healing, heart chakra, inner child, insight, inspiration, nervousness, perseverance, puberty, purification, responsibility, right-brained, social integration, spirituality, transformation, transition, uncertainty, worry

traditional use

Father Cupani, a Sicilian priest, gave sweet pea seeds from his monastery garden to a schoolmaster in London, England. These seeds are reputed to be the ancestors of all the common sweet peas known today in our gardens, greenhouses, and naturalized settings. There are hundreds of varieties of sweet peas that vary in colors, petal shapes, and fragrance. The traditional use, however, is unknown to the author

homeopathic use

Unknown to author.

positive healing patterns

- Promotes protection, security, self-confidence, and self-acceptance.
- Helps us to be gentle and compassionate and to love ourselves and others unconditionally.
- Guides and nurtures us to be with those who offer positive support and who honor our personal growth.
- Helps us radiate our creative life-force energy and power, and to affirm our personal freedom through positive integration with the world at large.

symptoms and patterns of imbalance

Sweet pea may be an appropriate flower essence for those who

- Are insecure, lack confidence, or feel unprotected
- Are impatient and unloving toward themselves and others
- Need help finding positive people in their lives who will offer support and compassion, not codependence
- Lack nurturing, or who have or have had abusive or addictive child-hoods.

features of the original flower-essence water

ODOR: sweet and light
TASTE: very subtly sweet
SENSATIONS: quiet, soothing, and gentle-feeling
WATER COLOR: clear

physical makeup

ROOT, STEM, LEAVES/LEAFLETS, HEIGHT: *Lathyrus latifolius* is a perennial vine with smooth pastel-green stems and leaves that consist of a pair of narrow leaflets and a terminal branched tendril or leafless organ that attaches and twines around some other body so that the plant can climb. It likes sun and thrives in good soil; its climbing vines need support such as a trellis or fence to grow on. *Lathyrus latifolius* will live a long time and doesn't like to be disturbed. The blooming season can be extended by cutting the blooms often to prevent seed formation.

FLOWER COLOR: Pink (Other colors this plant produces are lavender, reddish purple, and white.)

FLOWERS: Each flower consists of one broad, roundish petal that is upright (shaped like a hood), two smaller side petals that resemble wings, and two lower petals that form together. The way the petals fold and display themselves offer the flower's character of protection. The stamens have golden yellow anthers, and the sepal has five parts. The fragrance of the flower is sweet and light.

BLOOMING PERIOD: May to October

doctrine of signatures

- The broad, hood-shaped petal represents protection, as if a child is sitting with a hood or cap over its head. Inside the hood, the child feels safe, calm, secure. The two smaller side petals that resemble wings indicate freedom, and the two folding lower petals also offer the flower's character of protection and security.
- The climbing feature of the sweet pea, whereby the vines need a support structure to grow on, is similar to the growth of a child, the child's gradual growth process, and the support needed to grow in a positive way. A child who finds secure

footholds by which to gain confidence and emotional security is better able to find himself or herself integrating with the world at large.

- The pink color of this sweet pea corresponds to the fourth or heart chakra and our ability to gain the willpower and creativity needed to be strong in who we are. Balance in the heart chakra helps us radiate our creative life-force energy and power. It teaches us to love ourselves and others unconditionally.

- The soft, gentle beauty and nature of sweet pea is a reminder of the gentleness and compassion needed to raise a child — or to relate with our own inner child. The flower-essence smell and taste also reinforce the sweetness and gentleness of the plant's character.

Helpful suggestions

Take some time to be with yourself. Get comfortable, take several drops of Sweet Pea flower essence, and close your eyes. Take a few minutes to breathe, relax, and find that deep space within that allows you to be truly connected and in touch with who you are and how you're feeling in the moment.

Imagine yourself sitting under a large pink hood with your arms wrapped around your legs. You are surrounded by the color pink everywhere. You see pink with your eyes closed and with your eyes open. Breathe in the soft pink color and let your breath flow through your throat

and upward to your brow and out the top of your head. When your breath reaches the top of your head, hold the breath for a few seconds then slowly release it. Take in another breath, and this time let the breath flow downward all the way through your throat, heart, solar plexus, spleen, genitals, and to your feet. When you reach your feet, hold the breath for a few seconds, then visualize releasing the breath out through your feet. Repeat the breathing exercise a few more times. Then slowly unfold your arms from around your legs, open your eyes, stand up, and stretch. Remember to be gentle with yourself and to take time out to nurture and honor yourself and your growth.

Affirmations

- "I appreciate and love who I am, acknowledging my pleasures and my pains."
- "I take responsibility for integrating and participating in the world at large."
- "I make choices in my life that give me security and personal growth."

Case History

Shandor, age three, wasn't fitting in well with the other children at his preschool. (For the first part of his story, see Case History for Onion.) He demonstrated a lack of positive social integration, and he began to hit other children as a way of relating. Shandor was feeling threatened by the other children because his mother was the preschool teacher. He sought attention by acting out. Beneath the surface, Shandor seemed worried, upset, and insecure. He was given Sweet Pea flower essence, and within just a few days his mother commented that he was becoming friendlier and less defensive with his peers. She also said that he seemed more "accepting of himself, which made it easier for others to accept him." Within a week, Shandor showed noticeably more emotional security and social integration.

LFE's Research provers' project findings

PHYSICAL SYMPTOMS

CRAVINGS: None

SENSATIONS: Nervous tension

PAIN: None

MODALITIES: Documentation not consistent

HEAD: Ease of mental pressure and fatigue

EYES: None

FACE: None

EARS: None

STOMACH: Nervous upset, restless

ABDOMEN: None

BOWEL CONDITION: None

URINE: None

FEMALE: None

MALE: None

EXTREMITIES: None

BACK: None

SKIN: None

OTHER: "Had lots of energy, felt good with this essence," "had a slight increase of physical energy"

EMOTIONAL SYMPTOMS

PATTERNS OF BALANCE: "I had an easy feeling with this essence; it helped me attain a little peace and ease; it felt very feminine," "this essence helped relieve tension and a feeling of struggling," " I felt more at ease and calm," "I felt more optimistic about life and also more creative"

PATTERNS OF IMBALANCE: "felt confused about situations in my life," "I felt the need to hide my feelings and pretend I was happy," "I felt I lost control to remain relaxed and calm," "felt sadness," "I think I felt the opposite effects of this essence; if someone was naturally not grounded, unhappy, or confused then this essence could help"

MENTAL SYMPTOMS

PATTERNS OF BALANCE: "experienced relief of mental stress," "I felt at peace and more calm mentally," "this essence helped me to be more optimistic," "helped me to think clearer," images came to my mind: many images of women, an Indian woman, a woman with a mask, a woman sitting on a chair, and a woman with a dove," "this essence has helped me experience the transformation of worry into work, which has been very positive; it also helped me with the connection between suffering and its expression through my artwork," "I felt more creative"

PATTERNS OF IMBALANCE: "more mental confusion and mental tension," "spent more time in the worry world"

SPIRITUAL REFLECTIONS

"It helped me to ease turbulent spiritual growth struggle," "I wanted to take time out for myself during the day," "I experienced a spiritual unfoldment that included rebirthing, transformation, beauty, and deep growth," "this essence helped me reflect on the spiritual growth that is possible through the transforming effect of pain and suffering," "it also helped me recognize the potential for wholeness in every human being"

DREAMS/NIGHTMARES

One prover had two separate nightmares. She also had an uplifting dream with many images that included a dog, a fish, an egg, and a flower.

THISTLE

(Cirsium neomexicanum)
PRIMARY QUALITY: BALANCE

FAMILY: Sunflower (Compositae)
OTHER NAMES: New Mexico Thistle, Bullthistle; *cirsium* is an ancient Greek word for "thistle."
WHERE FOUND: Foothills, desert mesas, and plains in Arizona and New Mexico westward to the eastern borders of the Mojave Desert. Many other species of thistles can be found throughout the United States and in many European countries.
ELEVATION: 1,000' to 6,500'
ENERGY IMPACT (CHAKRA CORRESPONDENCE): fourth, sixth, and seventh chakras
KEY RUBRICS FOR POSITIVE HEALING PATTERNS: calm, centeredness, confidence, clarity, inspiration, union, vision
KEY RUBRICS FOR SYMPTOMS AND PATTERNS OF IMBALANCE: anxiety, fear, lack of confidence, nervousness, tension, lack of inspiration and vision
OTHER RUBRICS: balance, brow chakra, crown chakra, dreams, extreme tendencies, heart chakra, protection, purpose, spiritual, wisdom

Traditional use

There are at least seventeen species of thistle in the Southwest, and numerous species throughout the United States, Europe, and Asia. The thistle has an extensive history, which includes the "Blessed Thistle's" virtues as described in Turner's *Herbal* in 1568. Culpeper, Pliny, Dioscorides, and Gerard studied various species of thistle and recommended using them for treating conditions such as nervous complaints, rickets, hair loss, pleurisy, toothaches, ringworm, and itching. When crushed to remove the prickles, the leaves of all thistles are a good source of nutrients for cattle and horses. The Chinese make thistle teas and decoctions as a treatment for appendicitis, internal bleeding, and inflammations.

Native Americans ate the roots of the New Mexico thistle raw, boiled, or roasted. These thistles make good emergency food, as they are easy to identify and they grow abundantly. By taking a sharp knife and holding the plant upside-down, the prickly leaves can be cut from bottom to top. The stems can then be peeled and are generally sweet and juicy. Flower buds picked at the immature stage can also be eaten raw or steamed and dipped in lemon butter; they taste similar to artichoke hearts (artichokes are thistles, too). Native Americans also steep the entire thistle plant to drink as a tea to prevent conception.

Thistle infusions can be used as a tonic, astringent, and diuretic. They are known to treat stomach conditions, fevers, diarrhea, dysentery, skin eruptions and ulcers, and poison ivy rash.

Homeopathic use
Unknown to author.

Positive Healing patterns
- Helps us see, understand, and experience the balance between hard and soft, inner and outer, light and dark, sweet and bitter. Reminds us to look at our tendencies to overdo or underdo.
- Shows us our own rough edges and helps us capture our beauty and sweetness from deep within.
- Helps us find our center, where the balance and union of the upper and lower chakras meet.
- Offers protection, wisdom, and spiritual insight, allowing Light to enter our bodies.
- Grounds Spirit with matter.

symptoms and patterns of imbalance
Thistle may be an appropriate flower essence for those who

- Have extreme tendencies and need to find balance within themselves
- Are nervous about a particular situation, such as stage fright, and need help finding their center from within
- Are consciously working toward balance in their lives — especially with the chakra system — for wholeness and union with self
- Lack spiritual insight and are seeking the Light.

features of the original flower-essence water
Odor: pleasantly mild lavender-like smell
Taste: slightly bitter
Sensations: Tingling sensation and energy enter in feet and move upward through the body and out the top of the head.
Water Color: clear

physical makeup
Root, Stem, Leaves/Leaflets, Height: New Mexico thistle, from which this flower essence is made, is a hearty plant with spiny stems and dark green leaves that alternate along the stems. The center of the stem is often sweet and juicy, and the immature buds can be eaten raw or steamed, much like artichokes. The prickly leaves are spiny, coarsely pinnately lobed, and edged with many spines. The leaves thin out toward the top and they grow up to 7 inches long. The plant bears seeds with many bristles. The plant itself grows from 2 to 6 feet tall.
Flower Color: Pinkish purple and white
Flowers: The flower head is composed of a soft array of delicate, stringy spines that emerge from the center and make a round,

plush lavender circle. Midway inside the circle, the lavender spines become white, with tiny white tips that reach toward the sky. The center of the flower is filled with soft, bright pinkish lavender tips on shorter lavender spines. The flower disk is about 2 inches wide. The disk is encircled with long, spine-tipped bracts, and the outer thornlike bracts point down toward the earth. When the flower is full in blossom, if you try to remove the flower head from its thorny throne, you will discover that the spines are soft and silky.

Blooming Period: March to September

Doctrine of Signatures

- The thistle's spiny stems and prickly leaves appear rough, edgy, thorny, and abrupt, as if in need of protection. Yet inside the stem lies a sweet juice, and underneath its surface emerges a soft and delicate flower. Perhaps this is a reflection of what each of us, as human beings, truly are. The thorns and roughness show us our own edges — the edges to work with in order to capture our own beauty and sweetness from deep within. The edges and thorns also help us when we are in need of protection, yet this plant demonstrates a balance of soft and hard, inner and outer, light and dark, sweet and bitter. It reminds us to look at our tendencies to overdo or underdo and teaches balance and the ability to find our center.

- The soft, stringy spines that emerge from the flower head resemble tiny nerve fibers; this is a signature of the flower's ability to help us carry information from the lower chakras to the upper chakras, and vice versa. It is also a signature of the softness that lies within each of us.

- The soft and subtle pinkish, lavender, and white colors of the thistle represent the fourth, sixth, and seventh chakras. The fourth or heart chakra is our center, located between the three upper and three lower chakras. At this center, the Spirit/Vision/Light/Wisdom/Communication from above unites and balances with the matter/survival/procreation/knowledge/personality from below. The signature of balance is again shown here. When the heart center is in balance, it radiates a creative force of energy and power. The sixth chakra is the visionary chakra, which gives us wisdom and spiritual insight. It allows light to enter our third eye, which is the vibrational point where the darkness from the center of the earth comes together with the light from the center of the sun. The signature of balance is again demonstrated. The seventh chakra aligns us with our spiritual essence and an intrinsic knowing that is linked to our higher consciousness.

- The flower-essence odor is pleasantly sweet, yet the flower-essence taste is mildly bitter. This is another example of bringing opposites together to create balance.

Helpful suggestions

Take the Thistle flower essence when you can consciously focus on creating the balance you are seeking in your life or in your personality. Thistle can assist you in softening your character if needed, or in protecting yourself in circumstances where you need to bear those thorny edges. Thistle will help you achieve the balance in your being that you are striving for. With a conscious intention, ask yourself in what ways the parts of you need to come together to form balance and union.

Lie down in a comfortable position and take several drops of Thistle flower essence; hold them in your mouth. Slowly let the drops enter the back of your throat before you swallow. As you swallow, imagine the drops sliding down your throat and into your heart chakra. Next, visualize the long, spiny, soft, delicate flower tips stroking the top of your chest where your heart chakra lies. Take a deep breath and breathe into the slow strokes of the flower. Feel the flower's softness and gentleness.

Now imagine the tender strokes spiraling in a circle around your heart chakra. Continue to breathe into the feeling of the flower's strokes. Slowly breathe in and out.

Imagine the strokes of the flower spiraling within your heart chakra and now extending down to your stomach and up to your throat. Breathe into that feeling that still takes you into the center of the heart chakra but now extends to your throat and stomach chakras. Feel the gentle sensation of the thistle flower spiraling around those areas. Now imagine the strokes getting bigger, extending and spiraling down to your spleen and root chakras, all the way down to your feet, and back up to your brow and crown chakras all the way to the top of your head. Visualize yourself in the center of the spiral and relax into the gentle strokes encircling and spiraling around you and on you.

Slowly let the spiraling get smaller and smaller until you feel the strokes only on your heart chakra again. Breathe into the center of your heart chakra, and as you hold your breath in the center, imagine a soft lavender and white light entering that space. Gradually release your breath. Continue breathing and bringing the light into the center until you are ready stop.

Affirmations

- "Darkness will ultimately be lost in the light of transforming love."
- "As I breathe deep into my heart, I feel balanced and at peace with myself."
- "I allow the rough edges of my personality to be softened from deep within."
- "I take time to be with myself and to nurture the union of my opposite natures."

Case History

Andrea was appearing for the first time as a belly dancer. It also was the first public performance for the troupe she was in. Andrea was very nervous for herself and for the troupe. Several other women who had solo numbers were also nervous. Andrea described the nervousness as a "mixed bag," filled with anxiety, anticipation, and optimism, yet lacking confidence. She felt out of sorts and out of balance with herself.

Andrea happened to have a bottle of Thistle flower essence in her purse, which she discovered in the dressing room. She took some and passed it around to the other women. Andrea says that within a few minutes she and her friends found their center; they felt in sync, at ease, and in balance within themselves and each other. It helped them visualize how they wanted to perform — and their performance was awesome.

LFE's Research provers' project findings

PHYSICAL SYMPTOMS

CRAVINGS: More thirsty
SENSATIONS: None
PAIN: None
MODALITIES: No consistent comments
HEAD: None
EYES: None
FACE: None
EARS: None
STOMACH: None
ABDOMEN: None
BOWEL CONDITION: More frequent bowel movements
URINE: None
FEMALE: None

MALE: None
EXTREMITIES: None
BACK: None
SKIN: None
OTHER: Most provers commented that they were more physically active with this remedy. One prover was more tired than usual and had unusual sleep patterns.

EMOTIONAL SYMPTOMS

PATTERNS OF BALANCE: "I felt more emotionally steady, not major 'lows' or 'highs,'" "I felt detached from my emotional patterns and experienced them as an observer," "felt more emotionally stable," "felt more grounded," "this essence helped me connect with the earth and nature and enhanced my creativity," "I felt protected, safe, calm, and centered," "felt more motivated," "had good, positive emotional feelings," "this remedy helped me get back on track with my goals; I had good feelings taking the remedy," "I felt motivated and confident"

PATTERNS OF IMBALANCE: "anxiety, restlessness, and impatience"

MENTAL SYMPTOMS

PATTERNS OF BALANCE: "I am more alert than usual to subtle signs that I normally don't respond to," "I had an increase of mental imagery," "this remedy made me think about how most growth takes place when life is darkest," "I feel this remedy is to help find the transformational potential in each of us," "had more clairvoyance and a greater vision by taking this remedy," "was more analytical," "I had very little spaciness, and had more of a determined feeling, thinking and looking to the future and making decisions for change," "helped me to focus," "I think this essence would be helpful for those needing to make choices and detaching themselves from outside influences; it would be useful in grounding energy while integrating spiritual influences into the body or the person's reality," "I gave more attention to my future goals and changes that I'm working toward," "I made a very conscious effort in putting my mental energy to work for me," "I had more positive mental activity and visualized myself in a new job," "more mental clarity," "positive communication skills," "this essence gave me a boost and initiative to stay focused with my goals"

PATTERNS OF IMBALANCE: "anxiety, fear, despair," "worry and negative thoughtforms"

SPIRITUAL REFLECTIONS

"I had a definite feeling about the power of love and goodness over darkness," "I experienced various images, such as a heart, a rose, a butterfly, and a bat, that seemed to interplay between darkness and light, truth and love; that left me reflecting about the meaning of this remedy," "I wanted more quiet time," "I realized that life is full of balancing energies such as dark and light, good and evil," "the remedy helped me appreciate the power of beauty," "I felt very grounded, but at the same time I was frequently contemplating spiritual aspects of my reality," "I felt more of a desire to make deeper connections and have more discipline with my practices, such as meditation, prayer, and connecting with nature"

DREAMS/NIGHTMARES

Most provers indicated that they had an increase in dream memory.

One prover shared a dream in which "a rose appeared with a heart at the center, which changed from dark to light and shimmering." Another prover shared an image she had when she closed her eyes to go to sleep: She vividly saw her back porch surrounded by paradise trees (a type of tree that grows in Arizona). The porch seemed lighted, as if a porch light was on.

VERVAIN

(Verbena macdougali)
PRIMARY QUALITY: REACH FOR THE STARS

FAMILY: Verbena or Vervain (Verbenaceae)

OTHER NAMES: New Mexico Vervain, Spike Verbena, Tall Verbena, Blue Vervain, Macdougal Verbena. Derived from the Latin word *verbenae* and named for Dr. David Trembly Macdougal (1865–1958), a plant physiologist with the Carnegie Institute and an authority on desert vegetation.

WHERE FOUND: most common in Arizona and the southern Rockies, in valleys, roadsides, mountain meadows, and open flats

ELEVATION: 6,000' to 8,000'

ENERGY IMPACT (CHAKRA CORRESPONDENCE): sixth and seventh chakras

BACH FLOWER REMEDY: *Verbena officinalis* is used to treat those who are strongly opinionated with tendencies to preach or teach and philosophize. They are easily provoked by injustices, and when taken to the edge have tendencies to be overly enthusiastic, argumentative, and overbearing.

KEY RUBRICS FOR POSITIVE HEALING PATTERNS: accomplishment, direction, insight, inspiration, leadership, motivation, purpose, uplift

KEY RUBRICS FOR SYMPTOMS AND PATTERNS OF IMBALANCE: complicated thoughts, being judgmental, lack of motivation, nervous exhaustion, being opinionated, rigidity, tending to be overstressed

OTHER RUBRICS: achievement, balance, brow chakra, crown chakra, elegance, extreme, goals, grace, groundedness, heart, idealism, integration, integrity, moderation, nervousness, relaxation, relief, simplicity, spiritual, stress, strive, tension, uplifting, vision

traditional use

The genus *Verbena* is referred to as "holy bough," and vervain is known as "the enchanter's plant." It has been associated with mysticism and magic for centuries. The Romans placed vervain plants on their altars, and the ancient Egyptians devoted the plant to the goddess Isis. The Druids of Celtic Britain used vervain to purify the water used in sacred rituals; the word *vervain* is believed to be of Celtic origin, meaning "a stone-expeller." It was used to treat urinary stones and gravel. Vervain is also associated with Christ's crucifixion; according to myth, it stopped the bleeding from Christ's wounds. In medieval days, necklaces of vervain were worn as lucky charms for protection from headaches and snakebites. Known as the "herb of Venus," vervain was also used

the complete book of flower essences

in love potions and lucky charms. In seventeenth-century England, Culpeper used vervain to treat "pain in the secret parts."

Today vervain has multiple medicinal uses: sedative, mild tranquilizer, diaphoretic, emetic, diuretic, bitter tonic, and antispasmodic. It is used to treat the onset of a cold, especially if accompanied by upper respiratory inflammation. Vervain induces sweating, and it relaxes and settles the stomach. It eases nervous tension, depression, insomnia, headaches, jaundice, and stomach, bowel, and menstrual cramps. A salve made of vervain leaves is used to treat sprains, deep bruises, and muscle tension. Drinking a tea will assist in reabsorption of blood from ruptured tissues. A decoction of leaves and flowers can also be added to bathwater as an enchanting way to relieve tension.

The Navajo and other Native American tribes used vervain petals as a source of blue pollen to replace larkspur when unavailable, and they used the crushed petals ceremonially like corn pollen. The Navajo also used vervain as a medicine in their Water Way, Life Way, and Plume Way ceremonies.

Homeopathic use

Mother tincture is prepared from the entire fresh plant. It is used to treat disorders of the nervous system, such as nervous depression, nervous exhaustion, insomnia, and epilepsy and other spasms. It raises the absorption of blood and relieves pain in bruises. It is also used as a remedy to treat various skin irritations, such as from poison oak.

positive Healing patterns

- Encourages direction, leadership with open-mindedness, encouragement, and a sense of crowning achievement. Promotes an inner excitement to "reach for the stars."
- Gives the insight and perspective to see ahead and to strive for accomplishments not yet present.
- Helps bring an organizational framework to goal-setting and lifestyle that promotes simplicity, moderation, elegance, grace, integrity, and integration.
- Helps us remain relaxed, peaceful, and grounded while striving for goals and ideals or in relating to others.
- Allows us stay open and tolerant with others, letting others make their own choices.

symptoms and patterns of imbalance

Vervain may be an appropriate flower essence for those who

- Tend to be overcomplicated, overjudgmental, overopinionated, argumentative, and rigid, and take extreme measures to make their point from a place of personal (ego) will
- Lack direction and motivation, along with a lack of desire or an inability to see the whole picture
- Tend to be over-idealistic and are not down-to-earth
- Act overenthusiastically and lack

physical, emotional, and mental strength, especially due to stress and nervous exhaustion.

Features of the original flower-essence water

Odor: subtle and slightly bitter
Taste: full, pleasant, soft, and slightly sweet; doesn't taste like it smells
Sensations: Slightly warming and calming; tingling from toes to head; gives a feeling of balance, integration, and focus.
Water Color: clear

Physical makeup

Root, Stem, Leaves/Leaflets, Height: The strong, thick, square stem is sticky and composed of many layers. The stem is hairy all around. The branching stems arise from spreading roots. Dark green lance-shaped, mintlike leaves are widely spaced and grow in opposites. The leaves are up to 4 inches long, with larger leaves at the base and smaller leaves toward the top. The prominently veined leaves are prickly yet fuzzy, and are irregularly toothed. The entire plant has a slight bitter smell. Its average height is 2 to 3 feet.
Flower Color: Lavender to purple
Flowers: The flowers grow on a long, erect spike. Forming a ring around the spike, the flowers first open at the bottom of the spike and then appear to progress up the spike as the season progresses. Seed pods appear below and flower buds appear above. The singular, tiny flower is composed of five petals or lobes, with three petals bending downward and two petals bending upward. The center of each tiny flower (about $1/4$ inch wide) is whitish yellow and star-shaped. The flowers have a slightly bitter smell.
Blooming Period: June through September

Doctrine of signatures

- The formation of the spike and the ring of flowers progressing upward signifies integrity, direction, leadership, inspiration, and a sense of crowning achievement (seventh chakra). This also represents the plant's ability to see ahead and to strive for accomplishments not yet present. It also demonstrates the plant's openness and its capacity for calmness and a higher perspective for the good of all.

- The lavender/purple color relates to the sixth chakra and signifies spiritual vision, peacefulness, inspiration, and purpose.

- The tiny star shape in the center of the flower also symbolizes an upward direction, as if encouraging us to "reach for the stars" and to stay open and receptive to the good of all.

- The organizational structure of this plant as a whole — especially the neat appearance of the spiraling spikes along with each circle of flowers and each layer that makes up the stem — represents simplicity, moderation, elegance, and integration without overcomplication or extreme measures.

- The leaves growing in opposites represent balance, and the soft hairiness of the leaves and stem represent nerve endings and the plant's ability to relieve stress and tension. Along the wiry stems are knots that resemble a ladder, hinting of the tension that increases or escalates when a feeling of peacefulness is absent.
- The spreading roots and the sturdy branching stems symbolize the plant's ability to remain grounded while striving for ideals and goals, as represented by the spiraling spike.

Helpful suggestions

Take several drops of Vervain flower essence. If you can, go outside at night and look at the stars. If weather permits, sit outside and do this exercise, or just imagine yourself in this simple visualization. Find a comfortable spot and locate one star to gaze at. If you have a pair of binoculars, take several moments to look through them. Imagine what it would feel like to be a bright star shining in the night sky. Ask yourself what your true life goals are and in what ways you would like to achieve personal fruition.

What could you do to help yourself achieve a long-awaited goal? How could you achieve this goal while staying down-to-earth and being responsible for daily activities? How could you simplify your life while striving for and staying focused on your goal(s)? Gaze into the star. Listen to its messages. Do this exercise at least three nights in a row, and then as often as possible throughout a month. Only act harmoniously without pushing, and avoid trying to make things happen.

You also may want to take the essence prior to sleep. Observe how you feel when you wake up. Observe your thoughts and inner dialogue. Stay in touch with this plant and see how it affects you. Look at its photo. What can you gain from it? Go on a plant journey throughout the month and see where it takes you.

Affirmations

- "I honor each step and cycle that I experience and learn from as I move toward my vision and goals."
- "My commitment to myself today is to engage in an activity that releases stress and tension."
- "I live for simplicity, balance, moderation, and peace of mind, body, and soul."

Case History

Jill, age forty-one and an occupational therapist, was experiencing a loss of direction in relation to her life goals. Due to the geographical area where she lived, she had been traveling many miles to make home visits to work with her clients. Jill's job also required her to spend at least one night per week out of town, which was not preferable to her and her husband. She found that she was becoming self-critical and self-judgmental about having taken on this lifestyle. She felt shut down in her heart and lungs, and she yearned to simplify her lifestyle.

Jill was with me when I made the Vervain flower essence. She journeyed with the plant and drank its water. She immediately felt calmed by the pleasant, soft, sweet taste of the Vervain flower-essence water. She felt that the plant helped her get in touch with her true goals in life and helped her shift her focus in the direction she wanted to take. Jill made a vow that day to return home and establish an action plan to help her find a different job to be more conducive to her lifestyle. It took nearly six months for Jill to make these changes, and now she has a different job that is closer to home. She thanks the Vervain flower essence for its role in her changes.

LFE's Research Provers' Project Findings

PHYSICAL SYMPTOMS

CRAVINGS: None

SENSATIONS: "The first time I took the essence I got hot and prickly from the top of my ears to the top of my scalp"

PAIN: None

MODALITIES: Some provers had better sleep, while some did not

HEAD: Headaches

EYES: None

FACE: None

EARS: Ears ringing

STOMACH: None

ABDOMEN: None

BOWEL CONDITION: None

URINE: None

FEMALE: None

MALE: None

EXTREMITIES: None

BACK: None

SKIN: None

OTHER: "I first experienced total fatigue, followed by pleasant dreams and restfulness." Two provers said that this essence made them feel tired.

EMOTIONAL SYMPTOMS

PATTERNS OF BALANCE: "felt tension at first, then calm," "felt protected," "had more faith," "felt strength," "balance"

PATTERNS OF IMBALANCE: "tension," "irritability," "anxiety," "wanted to be alone," "tired of other people's problems," "burdened," "blameful"

MENTAL SYMPTOMS

PATTERNS OF BALANCE: "I have reality checks more often," "this remedy helped me to be more clairvoyant, intuitive, and creative in my mind," "more mindful"

PATTERNS OF IMBALANCE: "tension," "blameful toward others," "irritable"

SPIRITUAL REFLECTIONS

"I am more aware of the struggle between light and dark forces, and I firmly believe that the Light wins out," "I am more firmly fixed in my attitude of faith and embracing the goodness," "I deeply believe in the power of love, prayer, and healing"

DREAMS/NIGHTMARES

Two provers commented that they remembered their dreams more than usual, and that they saw colors and beautiful images in their dreams.

WILD ROSE

(Rosa arizonaca)

PRIMARY QUALITY: LOVE

FAMILY: Rose (Rosaceae)

OTHER NAMES: Arizona Rose. The name "rose" comes from an ancient root *wrod*, the modern translation of which is *vard*, an Old English word meaning "thornbush."

WHERE FOUND: ponderosa forests and shady streamsides

ELEVATION: 4,000' to 9,000'

ENERGY IMPACT (CHAKRA CORRESPONDENCE): third and fourth chakras

BACH FLOWER REMEDY: *Rosa canina* is one of Dr. Edward Bach's thirty-eight flower remedies. Wild rose is for the "apathetic" — "those who without apparently sufficient reason become resigned to all that happens, and just glide through life, take it as it is, without any effort to improve things and find some joy."[6]

KEY RUBRICS FOR POSITIVE HEALING PATTERNS: beauty, compassion, devotion, freedom, protection, vitality

KEY RUBRICS FOR SYMPTOMS AND PATTERNS OF IMBALANCE: apathy, avoidance, depression, dissociation, disinterest, grief, weariness

OTHER RUBRICS: aliveness, anxiety, appreciation, brokenheartedness, celebration, cheerfulness, creativity, displaced, dreams, gratefulness, healing, heart chakra, joy, love, misery, motivation, pain, passion, release, resignation, solar plexus chakra, sorrow, suffering, surrender, vibrancy

traditional use

The rose began its long European history in Greece, where its legend goes back to the Greek historian Herodotus. Its cultivation then spread to southern Italy, and from there to Persia and China. For over 3,000 years the rose has been the "queen of flowers." People of all lands have honored and cherished the rose. Cleopatra enticed Mark Anthony knee-deep in rose petals on her palace floor to gain his affections. The Romans crowned bridal couples with roses, and Roman banquets were decorated with rose centerpieces. Roses were a sacred flower to Aphrodite, the Greek goddess of love and beauty. Even as early as the tenth century, rose water (made by placing rose petals in water) was prepared as a purification.

The Muslim conqueror Saladin had the Omar mosque purified in rose water upon entering Jerusalem in 1187. In the sixteenth century, an essential oil called an "attar" or "otto" was prepared from rose petals; its production has been a prominent industry in France ever since. The rose became known as the "gift of the angels" due to its safe, soothing healing qualities. Rose water became popular for cooking, and is an ingredient in a candy called "Turkish delight." Wine prepared from rose petals was made in ancient Persia, and rose petals have historically been used in jams, vinegar, and pies, and as a garnish.

American Indians gathered the wild rose for ornaments and for medicinal uses. Young braves picked wild roses for their brides. Wooden needles from the rose bush were used for leatherwork. They used rose petals with bear grease to treat mouth sores, and they made a rose powder to treat fever sores and blisters. Sore eyes were treated with rose rainwater (rose petals in rainwater), and the inner bark of the rose root was used to treat boils. Indians also cooked the seeds and ate them to relieve muscular pains. The leaves were made into a poultice and used to soothe insect stings.

Most parts of the Rose plant can be made into a wash to cleanse cuts, wounds, and infections and the petals can be used as a bandage. Medicinally, rosehips are recommended in a tea as a source of vitamin B-complex and vitamins A, E, C and rutin, and as a mild laxative and diuretic. Rose hips tea is also said to expel kidney stones. The petals offer a flavor to medicines in the form of a syrup and have been used in tonics and gargles to treat catarrhs, sore throats, mouth sores, and stomach problems. Flowers steeped in hot water are a good treatment for diarrhea and gallstones. The flowers also relieve nervousness. Rose petals have been used to ease uterine cramps and labor pains, and to soothe the mother after childbirth. Roses are considered cooling and are used for soothing the mind in Ayurvedic medicine.

The petals are also common in potpourris. One of the most popular, best-loved fragrances is that of the rose. Its soothing aroma is associated with love and femininity and is found in perfumes, bath oils, soaps, hair tonics, skin lotions, ointments, creams, and air fresheners. One of the most costly oils is made from damask roses, which are cultivated in Bulgaria. Chewing on the fresh petals offers a pleasant taste, and placing rose petals in a tub of butter or margarine for a few days makes a delightful spread.

Homeopathic use

Unknown to author.

Positive Healing patterns

- Promotes a vibrancy, a feeling of wanting to do something.
- Helps us go beyond our miseries to face the deepest pains, especially those associated with "heartaches," in order to release them and move forward in life.
- Offers devotion and love toward life and living.
- Helps us find our passion for being alive.

symptoms and patterns of imbalance

Wild Rose may be an appropriate flower essence for those who

- Show disinterest or indifference in themselves and their life circumstances
- Feel they live in misery, whose heart is closed down, and who may have limiting conditions such as a terminal illness, a permanent disability, or the loss of a loved one
- Have chosen to live among the thorns and do nothing about it
- Are weary, lack vitality, and lack love and joy in living.

features of the original flower-essence water

Odor: especially sweet
Taste: especially sweet
Sensations: Soothes the throat and very pleasant to drink. Is quieting and soft.
Water Color: clear

physical makeup

Root, Stem, Leaves/Leaflets, Height: This rosebush grows from 1 to 3 feet high. The stems are brownish in color and many-branched. Its thorns are up to $^1/_4$ inch long and they are hooked. The bright green leaves are made up of three to nine toothed leaflets that are somewhat oval and range from $^3/_4$ inch to $2^1/_2$ inches long.

Flower Color: Pink

Flowers: The flower carries a sweet rose fragrance and has five wavy petals. The petals grow up to $2^1/_4$ inches wide. A clump of many yellow stamens with yellow anthers give a "loose" appearance as they emerge from the inside. The fleshy, rounded, orangish red hip is small, dry, and hard, and a one-seeded berry-like fruit follows.

Blooming Period: June through August

doctrine of signatures

- The wild rose bush has many branching stems that are covered with prickly thorns. I have walked in the wilderness and studied many wild rose bushes. The rose always seems to be protected amidst the thorns. When reaching for the rose, one must take great care to not get pricked by a thorn. This has always reminded me to have a clear intention and to pay attention when I pick a rose flower or when I'm near a rosebush. There have been times when I have gently pulled aside branches so that the flowers have more room to breathe. And although the flower seems to say "Leave me alone," at first, it also seems relieved to have received some attention and to have more space to grow in. The thorns are the plant's expression of protection; they represent our need to protect ourselves from life's blows, our pains, our challenges, and our suffering. The flower's destiny is to live among the thorns. As people, we will always have our challenges, pains, and suffering. The question is whether to accept that there can be anything else in the midst of these pains. Some people like living in their own misery and indifference as a form of protection: "Nothing can get better, so there's no need to hope for anything that might not happen." Yet the flower itself holds a vibrancy, an energy that says, "It's time to get up and go."

- The pink color of the flower corresponds to the heart or fourth chakra, the center that awakens our compassion, our love, our joy for life, and the way we love ourselves. It relates to loving emotions such as grieving the loss of a loved one, feeling a lack of love in life and for one's self, and perhaps feeling self-pity and despair with no interest in change one's circumstances.

- The clump of yellow stamens relates to the third or solar plexus chakra, which is associated with psychosomatic diseases caused by feelings that can break down and lead to apathy, dissociation from others, disinterest, indifference, lack of motivation, and lack of positive change.

- The wild rose bush represents a signature of abundance and growth, freedom and beauty. It demonstrates the power of our emotions and thoughts, once stuck among the thorns, to find a new freedom toward personal growth and change, and a true desire to make the best of living.

Helpful suggestions

Take several drops of Wild Rose flower essence and close your eyes. It may be helpful to take this essence at bedtime if you can make time to be alone. Visualize yourself walking along a wilderness trail in a ponderosa forest. You come to a clearing, and you see several wild rose bushes in full bloom before you. You feel a sense of excitement as you approach the bushes. You notice that the stems and leaves seem to be going in all directions, and they are somewhat scattered in appearance. As you step closer, you can see the prickly thorns on the stems and you carefully keep your distance from them. Your eyes are attracted to the simple yet beautiful flower that emerges from the thorny stems. You ask Spirit for permission to pick a flower. With permission, you find a flower that calls out to you. Mindful of the thorns, you slowly reach your hand into the rosebush and carefully separate the base of the flower from its stem. Carefully, you step away from the rosebush with the flower.

Now find a soft spot on the ground in which to sit. Place the flower gently in the palm of your hand. Look it over. You will see five broad pink petals with yellow stamens in the center. Study the flower's features. Notice how simple it appears.

Notice how beautiful its simplicity is. As you sit holding the flower, imagine yourself living in a bed of thorny stems. In what way have you accepted the thorns or pains in your life? In what way have you adjusted to living in your miseries? Is there no sense of hope?

Bring the flower to your nose and smell its sweet fragrance. Place the flower on your heart. Imagine yourself being picked up amidst the thorns or pains, being held in the palm of someone's hand, then placed next to that person's heart. See a soft pink glow all around you. Imagine how it would feel to be picked up and held. Imagine how it would feel to be embraced so lovingly. Bring the wild rose to your lips. Gently kiss the flower. Absorb the flower's sweet fragrance. Let the fragrance surround you. Let the fragrance and flower energize you. Feel how it feels to become alive again! Experience your devotion to yourself as a blossoming flower. Hold the power of this journey within. Hold the power of your devotion within.

Take the flower and step toward the rosebush. Tenderly place the flower at the base of the bush and thank the wild rose for helping you regain a new desire to live. Walk back into the forest and thank Mother Nature for all of her gifts. Take your journey into your dreams. Write down your experience when you wake up and hold the energy of the wild rose during your time with it. You can always come back whenever you desire.

Affirmations

- "I celebrate life with all its joys and sorrows."
- "I release my deepest heartaches and devote myself to love."
- "I begin this day in love, and live in love all day long."

Case History

I had given Wild Rose flower essence to R. M., age forty-seven, to help her deal with her depression and apathy. She told me a story about a situation she found herself in a few months later.

R. M. had offered to take care of someone's poodle while the owner went out of town. The poodle was high-strung and nervous. After five days of having the poodle, the poodle hadn't eaten and had hardly drunk any water. It stayed in its bed most of the time. R. M. worried that the dog would have kidney failure, and she didn't know what to do. Then she remembered her bottle of Wild Rose essence. She put four drops in a dropper bottle and filled it with water. Then she nearly forced the drops down the dog's throat. Ten minutes later, the dog was up and drinking water. He started playing with a dog biscuit and proceeded to eat it. R. M. was very relieved that the Wild Rose essence helped the dog, and the dog seemed happy to have regained its desire to live. R. M. had no more problems with the dog, and the owner was happy to know that R. M. took such good care of her dog.

Lfe's Research provers' project findings

PHYSICAL SYMPTOMS

CRAVINGS: Chinese food

SENSATIONS: "felt a releasing in my heart," "heart palpitations," "muscles tensed and then relaxed," "felt stoned"

PAIN: None

MODALITIES: Lack of consistency

HEAD: Relieved pressure in head

EYES: None

FACE: None

EARS: None

STOMACH: Nausea

ABDOMEN: None

BOWEL CONDITION: None

URINE: None

FEMALE: None

MALE: None

EXTREMITIES: "felt feet and legs open as if experienced a release and open to receive," "arms twitched then calmed"

BACK: None

SKIN: None

EMOTIONAL SYMPTOMS

PATTERNS OF BALANCE: "I felt very motivated to finish projects, and there was more energy available for this," "I felt hope, happiness, and a bright outlook," "I felt more peaceful and happy," "I got along with my daughter much better because I was more peaceful and centered," "this essence increased my creativity and creative drive," "was able to live in the flow," "seems good for the holidays when there's a lot to be done and you need to get back in the flow," "I was very adamant about bringing issues to the surface," "I was anxious to discuss my emotions with my boyfriend who didn't feel like it; I was concerned with getting things out in the open and didn't settle for anything else," "wanted to bring things out in the open to be faced and dealt with," "I felt joy, happiness, freedom, and lightheartedness," "I felt grateful for family connections," "I felt happy and optimistic," "I released some sadness," "I felt my heart opening," "felt grounded," "I felt soothed, calmed, and serene," "I experienced my heart release"

PATTERNS OF IMBALANCE: "I didn't feel like myself when taking this essence; I felt kind of displaced," "felt anxious," "irritable," "felt scattered"

MENTAL SYMPTOMS

PATTERNS OF BALANCE: "my mind was clear," "experienced some joyful memories," "have more mental clarity," "helped me be more creative in my artwork," "I think this essence is for those who take life for granted," "felt relaxed and at peace," "felt quieter," "I was more alert"

PATTERNS OF IMBALANCE: "anxiousness," "sometimes I felt my mind was playing tricks on me and I had to say to myself, 'Wait, slow down; what's going on here?'" "felt scattered"

SPIRITUAL REFLECTIONS

"Aware of my spirituality, more on a feeling level," "I felt a joy of balancing in this life, growth through sadness, liberation and light out of darkness and sorrow," "I have more faith," "I experienced spiritual joy and compassion," "I feel fortunate in spite of stresses; I made a change to appreciate my life with all its ups and downs"

DREAMS/NIGHTMARES

Dreams were more lucid, and provers remembered them better than usual.

WILLOW

(Salix Gooddingii)

PRIMARY QUALITY: FORGIVENESS

FAMILY: Willow (Salicaceae)

OTHER NAMES: Goodding Willow, Western Black Willow, Dudley Willow

WHERE FOUND: along banks and streams in the western U.S.

ELEVATION: below 7,000'

ENERGY IMPACT (CHAKRA CORRESPONDENCE): fourth and seventh chakras

BACH FLOWER REMEDY: Bach used *Salix vitellina* to treat those who felt injustice and who were resentful or bitter. The positive aspect of Willow is optimism without bitterness.

KEY RUBRICS FOR POSITIVE HEALING PATTERNS: clarity, compassion, flexibility, letting go, patience, understanding

KEY RUBRICS FOR SYMPTOMS AND PATTERNS OF IMBALANCE: blame, confusion, criticism, emotional bitterness, impatience, injust acts, resentment, resistance, rigidity, vengefulness

OTHER RUBRICS: appreciation, awareness, breakthrough, calm, change, consciousness, crown chakra, expansion, flow, forgiveness, grace, heart chakra, peace, relief, resistance, resolution, security, victim, vulnerable, water, wisdom

Traditional use

There are many species of willow. It is difficult to identify some species due to the variation of leaves and the cross-breeding of different species. Due to the complexity and numbers of willow trees, this section speaks to the general history and uses of a variety of willows.

The willow has a fascinating history of uses and symbology. It was considered to be a symbol of death and/or immortality by several cultures. The Chinese viewed it as a symbol of immortality because a new tree can be grown from a small branch. The willow was sacred to the Greek and Roman goddesses Circe, Hecate, and Persephone, all of whom are Mother Goddess death aspects. The plant has also been seen as a symbol of mourning in the form of the weeping willow. Ancient Greeks wore willow leaves around the neck after a heartbreaking love affair.

Dioscorides prescribed willow for pain and inflammation, and the historically far-removed Hottentots used a willow concoction as a remedy for rheumatic fever. The American Indians used the willow similarly and passed along this information to the white settlers. They also used branches as poles for tipis and to build sweat lodges. Willow was fed to livestock as fodder; mixed with cotton and fur, the down of some types of willow was made into stockings. Basket makers have used the plant shoots to make sturdy baskets, and the resilient wood was used at one time to make tool handles and fences. Willow is currently used in making artificial limbs.

Today, willow branches are still commonly used to make sweat lodges, especially in the southwestern U.S., and they provide the structure for hoop weavings and dream catchers. They are known for their flexibility and strength.

Medicinally, willow bark has been used for centuries for its cooling actions to reduce pain and inflammation as well as to lower fevers. In the 1820s, the active ingredient salicin was isolated. In the late 1800s, a German chemist by the name of Felix Hoffman was looking for some relief for his father's arthritis. He formulated a drug now widely known as aspirin from salicin. Salicin extracted from the bark of the willow was also used as a substitute for quinine. Salicin is an active ingredient used to treat arthritis and rheumatism. Also, by steeping willow bark and twigs in water, you can make a bitter drink to relieve pains and chills.

Various willows have numerous other medicinal uses. They are used to make eye drops, as an astringent, as a sex depressant, for restoration of the stomach and liver, and to treat hay fever, chills, dandruff, diarrhea, earache, flu, heartburn, headache, impotence, chronic inflammation and infection,

muscle soreness, night sweats, rheumatism, worms, dysentery, and disability of the digestive organs. Willow's antispasmodic qualities have been used to treat whooping cough and asthma. The willow herb has wonderful antiseptic qualities and can be used to treat infected wounds, ulcerations, or eczema. This makes it a useful first-aid herb for hikers to be familiar with.

Cosmetically, whole willow is found in face creams, detergents, lotions, and herbal baths due to its astringent properties. As an ornamental plant, willow is valued for its beauty. Willows offer practical landscaping solutions, especially in marshy areas and to stabilize stream banks.

homeopathic use

Salix nigra, or Black Willow, is a homeopathic remedy that regenerates the organs of both sexes, treats hysteria and nervousness, restrains genital irritability, and tempers sexual passion. It is used to treat conditions such as red and swollen face, sore and bloodshot eyes, nervousness before and after menses, painful menstruation, excessive menstrual discharge, pain associated with movement of the testicles, and back pain across sacral and lumbar areas.

positive healing patterns

- Helps us take our personal matters to their root cause, encouraging us to understand ourselves and any bitterness, resentment, or roughness that we may feel.
- Teaches us to be flexible in the ways

we approach life and all living things, and to move with the ebb and flow of life's wisdom and grace.

- Helps prevent ourselves from being worn out by the bitterness of others so that our own bitterness does not seep in.
- Gives us the ability to seek and gain higher spiritual evolution and awareness in spite of our challenges. Helps us understand ourselves as a system of energy, guiding us to be mindful of the situations we find ourselves in and to expand our conscious awareness of our biological heritage.
- Helps us find compassion within ourselves, open our hearts toward others, and act accordingly.

symptoms and patterns of imbalance

Willow may be an appropriate flower essence for those who

- Feel resentment and emotional bitterness, especially related to unjust situations or people; symptoms of sleeplessness, restlessness, and impatience may develop
- Lash out blamefully, criticize others in a vengeful manner, and have closed hearts
- Lack flexibility in how they approach life and carry grudges against others
- Feel victimized in an unjust world
- Are patient, understanding, and

compassionate as long as they possibly can be in challenging situations until they are set off by people who are petty, who stretch boundaries, who take them to the edge where they snap when such injustices become blatant and unnerving, then impatience, restlessness, and bitterness seep in.

features of the original flower-essence water

Odor: very fragrant, "green," and spicy

Taste: bitter, strong, spicy; very potent and cooling

Sensations: Opens the nostrils and clears a tightness in the solar plexus. There is a slight tingling in the brow and crown areas. Can feel the crown chakra open and lift.

Water Color: clear

physical makeup

Root, Stem, Leaves/Leaflets, Height: This willow species has a deep root system that helps stop stream erosion. The grayish bark is thick and rough, with deep indentations that have narrow ridges. The trunk can grow up to 30 inches in diameter, and usually has many branches growing from it. The branches are gray, thicker, and rougher toward the bottom, but light, slender, smoother, and yellowish toward the top. In fact, they are so light that they bend and sway gracefully in the wind. The shiny leaves are bright green or lime green, narrow, lanceolate, finely toothed, and long-pointed. The curved leaves are longer and larger toward the bottom of the stem and shorter and smaller toward the top of the stem. The leaves have one central vein and can grow up to 5 inches long and $3/_4$ inch wide.

FLOWER COLOR: Green/white

FLOWERS: The flowers grow in a small clustered spike that consists of tiny, unisexual, petalless flowers called "catkins." The tiny closed flowers alternate along the stem and are followed by white cottony seeds that bud open. The catkins are light and delicate, and grow up to $3^1/_2$ inches long.

BLOOMING PERIOD: March through May

Doctrine of Signatures

• A significant signature of the willow is the strong, unique, bitter taste in the leaves and in the flower-essence water. The bitterness that the leaves and flower essence leaves in your mouth is similar to the bad feeling of bitterness toward an experience or person in your life. Emotional bitterness may cause resentment, biting criticism, slashing or snapping out, and a feeling of vengefulness. It may also feed on the feeling of being a victim in an unjust world. When injustice is experienced, an emotional bitterness toward life may be carried over into other situations and relationships. The lesson of this signature is that we need to be cautious about how bitterness thrives within each of us.

Rather than falling into victim consciousness or vengeful consciousness, we need to find a way to gather the power to come into our heart to let go of the bitterness and resentment. The acts of injustice done by others will sooner or later come back around to them, and these injustices will be taken care of in a natural way that is much bigger than us.

• The willow tree likes dampness and commonly grows along rivers and streams. Growing near water represents deep emotions which, if not allowed to flow with the waters, are kept inside where unhappiness, resentment, and bitterness can grow. The willow's deep root system holds the soil and stops streambank erosion. When the creek or stream rises, the willow holds the soil together to keep it from being eaten or worn away. This signature also relates to the one previously mentioned: When we are able to "keep it together," we can prevent ourselves from being worn out by the bitterness of others so that our own bitterness does not seep in. The positive willow will give a person the needed inner strength (related, again, to holding the soil together) to flow with the water or emotions and to release whatever bitterness, feelings of despair, or resentment a person is holding onto.

• The thick, rough ridges of the lower

bark also symbolize our own rough emotional edges and our ability to deal with barriers in life that may appear to hold us back and drain our energy. Yet these barriers help us grow in our own inner strength. The upper branches are smooth, graceful, and flexible. They dance and move with the wind — with the ebb and flow of life's wisdom and grace. This signature relates to our ability to be flexible in the way we approach life and all living beings. Willow also demonstrates flexibility and the flow of life in the way it grows along water and is nurtured by water. If you try to force the branches to bend, they may snap; when they are moistened in water, they gain even more strength, endurance, and ability to stretch and bend.

- The green tiny catkin flowers are petalless. They gently and humbly hang along the stem. They represent the fourth chakra, the heart. The opening of our hearts helps us let go of resentments and emotional wounds, past hurts, suffering, and bitterness. Slowly, tiny white cottony seeds emerge from the opening bud and expand into a soft cotton down covering the catkin, becoming exposed to the light. This signature relates to the seventh chakra, the expansion of consciousness, and the ability to seek and gain higher spiritual awareness in

spite of our challenges. The passage from the closed, bitter, limiting catkin to the white cottony seed-bud opening is symbolic of reaching a broader understanding with ourselves and the Divine Power that is bigger than, yet inclusive of, the physical world and our experiences in it.

Helpful suggestions

Take several drops of the Willow flower essence. Play some of your favorite soft music if you'd like. Stand up in an area where you have the space to move freely. Close your eyes. Take a deep breath in and slowly exhale. Repeat. Imagine you are a willow tree that grows along the river. Overhead, you hear the flapping of wings from a pair of mallard ducks. Upstream you hear the trickling flow of the nearby waters. Take another breath and slowly breathe out. Feel the rustling of the wind through your branches (arms). Slowly move one arm and allow it to hang, bend, and move. Sway your arm gracefully above your head, from side to side. Now move the other arm and do the same thing. Next take a step with one foot and allow your whole body to bend and sway, moving your head, neck, shoulders, arms, torso, stomach, buttocks, thighs, and legs. Imagine the water flowing throughout your being. Sway from side to side, and then from front to back. Feel the energy moving in your body. Feel your strength. Feel your grace. Feel your body bend. Notice anywhere that you feel soreness or pain. Gently let your body move through the pain. Breathe into the soreness and then breathe it out, allowing your body to gracefully release any discomforts. Continue to move as you wish and let your movements be guided by your intuition. When you are ready to stop, gradually let your body finish moving where it wants to. Stand still and feel the energy of your body/mind temple. Take in another breath and slowly let it out. While holding this energy, lie down and rest.

Affirmations

- "I bend with life's opportunities."
- "I allow the waters of life to flow and weave throughout my body/mind/soul, bestowing agility, flexibility, and a deep level of forgiveness."
- "As I am generous and forgiving of myself and others, all resentments are released."

Case History

Leah, a woman in her early forties, took the Willow flower essence because of some resentment she was feeling about her husband's relationship with himself and his health condition. She and her husband were planning to relocate due to his health, which meant she would be giving up her income and her security.

Leah described her experience by saying, "I believe the essence has helped me deal with my fears, resentment, and stuckness. This has been a struggle for many

years and is a high trust issue for me. It got me to see that there was an underlying bitterness that I was not conscious of. The affirmations helped me heal this part of myself. I feel very positive about this essence and I believe it affected me very deeply. I feel more flexible, less bitter, and less fearful."

LFE's Research Provers' Project Findings

Physical Symptoms

Cravings: None

Sensations: None

Pain: None

Modalities: None reported

Head: None

Eyes: None

Face: None

Ears: None

Stomach: None

Abdomen: None

Bowel condition: None

Urine: None

Female: Increase in sexual feelings

Male: No male provers

Extremities: None

Back: None

Skin: None

Other: More energy

Emotional Symptoms

Patterns of Balance: "I felt a breakthrough of sorts — a sense of relief, calmness, clarity, and hope," "I found this essence rejuvenating," "loneliness," "able to let go and move on," "had more strength," "felt more peaceful," "felt more love pouring in on a global level," "am more patient," "felt very feminine"

PATTERNS OF IMBALANCE: "I have had feelings of emotional imbalance and confusion," "I am having difficulty letting go of what was the past and who I need to be for myself in the moment," "I have some resistance to change," "felt fear, which was probably related to a medical diagnosis," "my heart was in a state of chaos regarding security issues," "I felt more vulnerable," "I feel a strong need for security"

MENTAL SYMPTOMS

PATTERNS OF BALANCE: "this flower essence helped me realize that I need to continue to clear old habits and beliefs before I can be involved in a partnership," "was more understanding and patient," "the remedy brought on more awareness," "my beliefs about security in relationships were illuminated," "brought resolution," "I got a distinct awareness that I should lighten up and move through past hurts but am not sure how to do it," "I was able to have more mental clarity in the face of intense emotions," "this essence gave me more insight and clarity," "heightened my awareness," "this essence was very calming," "I took this essence on my mother's

birthday, which was a happy time for me," "gave me feelings of independence," "this essence helped me be a little less serious about things"

PATTERNS OF IMBALANCE: "this essence showed me ways I needed to change and also my resistance in doing so," "had more mind chatter and loss of focus," "worry that led to confusion"

SPIRITUAL REFLECTIONS

"I had an increased awareness and ability to see myself clearly as a first step toward change," "this essence helped me be patient with my spiritual growth," "I felt surrounded by love and peace," "I gained a sense of the reality of physical mortality and the true purpose of disease," "I felt influenced spiritually, but can't say how; I felt I was being helped by this essence because it arrived at the same time my physical/medical crisis occurred"

DREAMS/NIGHTMARES

"I dreamed of a plant completely submerged in water, and I was worried about it drowning. Then I saw that it was flowering with white flowers, and I knew it would be all right."

YARROW

(Achillea millefolium)

PRIMARY QUALITY: PROTECTION

FAMILY: Sunflower (Compositae)

OTHER NAMES: Common Milfoil, Chiliophyllon, Soldier's Woundwort, Carpenter's Weed, Noble Yarrow, Old Man's Pepper, Ambrosia, Supercilium veneris, Ballusticum, Centifolia, Sideritis, Thousandleaf, Cammock, Millefeuille, Nosebleed, Sneezewort, Devil's Nettle, *Herbe aux charpentiers, Garbenkraut, Jungfernaugen, Tausendblatt,* and *Blutstillkraut.* Named for Achilles, the Greek hero of Homer's *Illiad,* who is credited with finding the medicinal qualities of this genus. The species name is derived from the Latin word *millefolium, mille* meaning "thousand" and *folium* meaning "leaves."

WHERE FOUND: Native to Europe, Asia, and North America. Grows along roadsides and abandoned areas, pastures, fields, embankments, and in pine-forest clearings. Yarrow plants like the full sun and acclimate to a variety of soils.

ELEVATION: 5,500' to 11,500'

ENERGY IMPACT (CHAKRA CORRESPONDENCE): seventh chakra

KEY RUBRICS FOR POSITIVE HEALING PATTERNS: cleansing, energy, insight, prevention, shield, inspiration

KEY RUBRICS FOR SYMPTOMS AND PATTERNS OF IMBALANCE: anxiety, exhaustion, over-responsibility, run down, "wounded warrior, wounded healer"

OTHER RUBRICS: apprehensive, burnout, clarity, consciousness, crown chakra, detachment, freedom, grounded, harmony, light, mind, nervousness, positive, protection, rejuvenated, release, stagnation, strength, stress, surrender, tension, tired, unprotected, uplifting, vulnerable

traditional use

Yarrow pollen found on fossils in Neanderthal burial caves indicate that the plant's history of human use dates back 60,000 years.

Divining sticks made of fifty dried yarrow stalks were used by the ancient Chinese in association with the *Yarrow Stalk Oracle,* more commonly known as the *I Ching* or the *Book of Changes.* Some 3,000 years ago, the Greeks used yarrow in the Trojan wars, and the Greek hero Achilles is said to have staunched the bleeding of wounded soldiers with yarrow. Yarrow's reputation as a woundwort remedy continued through the American Civil War. Yarrow also had a reputation for being a magic herb and was included in the Saxon amulets for protection. It was put under the pillow for bringing a dream vision to the sleeper about his or her true love.

At least forty-six Native American tribes used yarrow leaves externally to treat burns, skin rashes, bruises, cuts, and wounds, and to reduce swellings and ease rheumatic joints. They also drank yarrow leaves and flowers in a tea for spiritual guidance and to treat an overall run-down feeling, as well as for conditions such as internal bleeding, fevers, and indigestion. The nostrils were packed with the fresh yarrow leaves to stop nosebleeds, and yarrow was used to help people recover from a coma.

In the first century A.D., Dioscorides spread yarrow on ulcers to prohibit inflammation. In the 1500s, Gerard recommended yarrow to alleviate pain and swelling of the "private parts." In the seventeenth century, Culpeper used yarrow on wounds. Yarrow was also a common remedy to the Shakers, who used it to treat hemorrhages, flatulence, and indigestion, and as a general tonic. Also known as "carpenter's weed," yarrow's delicate, lacy, saw-toothed leaves look like a saw. The bruised leaves were also used as an astringent. Yarrow induces sweating, and hot yarrow tea is a traditional home remedy for a cold, fever, and flu.

Yarrow was included in the U.S. Pharmacopoeia from 1836 to 1882. It was still in the pharmacopoeias of Austria, Hungary, Poland, and Switzerland in 1982. In the 1950s, an alkaloid was discovered in yarrow that helps make blood clot faster. Some varieties of *millefolium* contain a volatile oil called azulene that acts as an anti-inflammatory. In the 1960s, research

showed that yarrow contains flavonoids (effective as an antispasmodic) and salicylic acid derivatives (like aspirin); this may explain yarrow's ability to treat fevers and relieve pain.

"Nosebleed" is a country name given to yarrow because of its effectiveness in stopping bleeding. British herbalist Maude Grieve says that yarrow can also cause nosebleeds to relieve a headache. Due to the plant's reputation for stopping or inducing bleeding, it is a recommended women's remedy to help bring on suppressed or irregular menses, to reduce excessive bleeding, or to help break up stagnant blood in the reproductive tract. It is also effective for treating inflammation of the ovaries, prolapse of the uterus, or vaginal discharge, and for ease in menopause. Herbalist Maria Treben advises women of all ages, from age thirteen to ninety, to have a cup of yarrow tea from time to time. Women with uterine fibroids can benefit from a yarrow sitz bath to help stir up and remove blood. Yarrow is helpful in treating blood blisters and is known today to be used by American Indians to treat cancer, as indicated by massive blood infections.

Yarrow also has a powerful effect on the stomach and intestines, and activates sluggish digestion. Gardeners add a yarrow leaf or two to compost to stimulate fermentation and help the compost "digest"; yarrow works similarly in the large intestine, aiding the process of healthy digestion and fermentation. Thus yarrow is a good remedy for bloating, flatulence, gurgling or burping, and yeast infection. In a classroom lecture, herbalist

Matthew Wood says that yarrow "stimulates the mucous membranes, removing heat and inflammation, dampness and pathological flora." Yarrow is also recommended for hemorrhoids associated with bright red bleeding and hemorrhage from the stomach, intestines, and urethra. Yarrow also regulates the function of the liver.

Yarrow is also used today to treat arthritis, bladder infections, bronchitis, cancer, constipation, jaundice, leukemia, liver congestion, bleeding lungs, lymphatic problems, rheumatism, scurvy, skin problems, thyroid imbalances, ulcers, tumors, spleen and stomach problems, menses, and burns. Yarrow is also a highly useful remedy in the treatment of colds, influenzas, measles, chickenpox, smallpox, high blood sugar, fevers, and inflammation of the mucous membranes, especially associated with the respiratory tract. Richard Katz and Patricia Kaminski of the Flower Essence Society use a Yarrow flower essence for people undergoing radiation therapy to energetically protect them from radiation burns and sensitivity toward radiation. They also use the flower essence for psychic protection.

According to Matthew Wood, herbalist Victor Rangel recommends yarrow for healing "cuts to the bone." This phrase indicates both the physical abilities of yarrow to heal (bleeding, cuts, and bones) and its use for people who may feel emotionally "cut to the bone." Herbalist Matthew Wood describes yarrow as the remedy for the "wounded warrior and the wounded healer": "People with the 'wounded warrior personality' tend to be strong and courageous. They are the ones who run around putting fires out, but they may get 'cut to the bone.' Most of the patients I have seen Achillea help had a somewhat noble, warriorly carriage."[7]

Drinking an infusion of yarrow flowers will expel phlegm in the upper respiratory tract, or yarrow can be applied externally as a wash to treat eczema. A dark blue essential oil is extracted by steam distillation of yarrow flowers and is used as an anti-inflammatory to treat conditions such as inflamed joints or rubbed onto the chest to treat colds and influenza. The oil is also antiallergenic and antispasmodic.

Yarrow is one of many groups of plants described as "medicine twigs" or Life Medicine by the Navajo, who use the plant in various ceremonial ways.

Yarrow is also used as an ornamental, in skin lotions, and as a source of yellow dye. Young, finely chopped yarrow leaves can be added to salads and eaten as a garnish.

CAUTION: Yarrow contains a substance called thujone, which can cause abortion in pregnant women who drink too much of the tea (two to three cups per day).

Homeopathic Use

Yarrow (Millefolium) is a homeopathic remedy prepared from the leaves and flowers. It is used to treat various types of hemorrhages with bright red blood, incarcerated hernia, smallpox (with pain in the pit of the stomach), falls from a great height, and bloody mucus. Conditions may include dizziness, a feeling of forgetfulness, cutting pain from the eyes to the root of the nose, bloody urine, hemorrhaging bright red blood (bowels, lungs or uterus), hemorrhoids (bleeding), or a cough with bloody expectoration.

positive healing patterns

- Offers an energy shield to protect one from feeling drained by others or by one's environment (including electromagnetic radiation).
- Helps us to seek the Light within ourselves, which keeps us strong and helps us thrive energetically in spite of our tendencies toward weakness or reactivity.
- Provides natural protection and guidance to live according to our Highest Good by capturing a glimpse of the Light and allowing us to glow in that Light.
- Promotes cleansing of our thoughts and helps us release toxic buildup and stagnation at all levels throughout our being. Relieves tensions and nervousness, and allows us to become conscious, centered people in the way we live and act in the world.

symptoms and patterns of imbalance

Yarrow may be an appropriate flower essence for those who

- Feel vulnerable, run-down, and stressed out
- Tend to react from within their own weaknesses
- Demonstrate the personality of the "wounded warrior, wounded healer" (See Traditional Use), especially those who are exposed to the public daily or who provide healing for others, such as teachers, lawyers, store clerks, and healers; who have job burnout, are overworked, and feel an overload of responsibility
- Feel unprotected and unsafe (especially children).

features of the original flower-essence water

ODOR: fresh, strong, pungent "green"
TASTE: cool, refreshing, and menthol-like; smooth, bittersweet, and astringent
SENSATIONS: Soothed throat, pressure lifted from top of head, warmth in the solar plexus, felt calm and grounded.
WATER COLOR: clear

physical makeup

ROOT, STEM, LEAVES/LEAFLETS, HEIGHT: Yarrow is a thriving plant with creeping underground roots that allow the plant to spread quickly and to nurture large colonies. Its pale green, stout, slender, rough, finely hairy stem is hollow and branches near the top. It grows from 1 foot to 18 inches in height. Yarrow's slightly woolly, grayish green, finely dissected leaves are narrow, deeply cut (swordlike), fernlike, lacy, and feathery. The upper leaves clasp the stem at the base and the lower leaves are stalked, alternating upward toward the branched flower heads. Leaves grow up to 6 inches long and are highly aromatic, giving off a spicy, earthy odor that continues after drying. The tiny seeds are flat and tear-shaped, grayish brown in color.

FLOWER COLOR: White or bone-white

FLOWERS: The small daisy-like ray and disk flowers bloom in flat-topped clusters at different places along the stem, frequently forming additional clusters toward the top. They sometimes appear slightly pinkish. The tiny disk florets are usually composed of five white ray petals and five tiny stamens with pale yellow anthers. The pollen is soft orange in color. When you breathe in the flower scent lightly, it is sweet. Breathing in the full scent, the flower has a powerful earthy, woody, pungent odor.

BLOOMING PERIOD: June through September

Doctrine of signatures

- The most obvious of yarrow's signatures is the feathery, lacy, saw-toothed leaves. The signature of the leaves points to the plant's ability as a woundwort remedy and all the physical conditions that relate to cuts, burns, wounds, blood, and inflammatory conditions. The flowers also have a lacy appearance and are usually bone-white in color, or sometimes pinkish. This signature

also suggests bones and blood. But the same signatures also demonstrate the plant's vulnerability despite its incredible ability to thrive and to heal. In both cases, these signatures are described by herbalist Matthew Wood as the "wounded warrior, wounded healer." Through the plant's signatures, we are also shown the need to protect ourselves (especially when we feel "cut to the bone") from the energies and forces of others and our environment.

- Yarrow's tough and nurturing underground root system is also symbolic of the yarrow-type person who is tough, strong, and courageous. This signature also demonstrates the person who spends his or her energy on everyone else, and who needs to take time out to protect and nurture him- or herself.

- Yarrow's strong scent, volatile oils, and bitter qualities make a statement of the healing powers of this plant. Although yarrow heals us strongly on the physical level in many ways, it also makes an impression on who we inherently are. The whitish flower heads are indicative of the seventh chakra, which governs both our conscious and unconscious thoughts. Yarrow promotes cleansing of all our thoughts and helps us release toxic buildup, stagnation, and tension at all levels throughout our being. It helps us relieve tension and nerves, thus allowing ourselves to become conscious, centered people in the way we live and act in the world.

Helpful suggestions

Take several drops of the Yarrow flower essence and lie down in a comfortable position. Close your eyes and imagine yourself walking up a mountain path. The path is somewhat steep, and you begin to feel you are running out of breath. You pause and take a moment to catch your breath and rest. Then you continue along your journey up the mountain path. As you near the top of the mountain, you see an open meadow and you experience a pleasant anticipation. You walk into the open meadow and see three grandmother alligator juniper trees in the near distance (alligator junipers have rough bark that resembles alligator skin). You are drawn to the incredible energy of the trees and you walk toward them. As you get closer to the trees, you notice an enticing colony of dainty little white-headed flowers that appear to be dancing in their own merriment. Feel a tingling of excitement move through your body and all the way up to the top of your head. You finally reach your destination and find yourself in the center of the three alligator juniper trees, surrounded by the precious yarrow colony. Find a cozy spot on the grassy ground between the yarrow flowers and lie down, looking up into the yarrow's feathery leaves and its bone-white lacy flowers. You catch a glimpse of sunlight in your eyes and, feeling tired, you close your eyes. Feeling nurtured and protected by the yarrow plants and the juniper trees, you allow yourself to go to sleep and enter the dream world. Enjoy your journey.

Affirmations

- "I take personal space to gather my strength and regain my energy."
- "I wrap myself up in my protective cocoon."
- "I lovingly detach myself from other people's problems."
- "My inner Light glows within me and surrounds me."

Case History

Sharon, a woman in her late forties, led a busy life as a senior editor in a publishing firm on the East Coast. She had been feeling "very tired and burned out." Not only was her job high-stress, but Sharon's boss had an unpredictable temper that left her feeling "on edge" whenever he was around. In addition to her demanding job, she commuted nearly every weekend from Maryland to New York to visit her mother, who was ill. Sharon had also divorced about a year before and moved to her own apartment. That same year, she discovered that her son had AIDS. Sharon was feeling listless and said, "I'm pushing myself too much and I hope nothing is wrong with me. The wise part inside me says it's natural to feel tired and take time to rest."

Taking the Yarrow flower essence was an amazingly immediate energetic boost to Sharon. She responded quickly to the essence and felt an energetic shift inside herself that helped her make wiser choices in dealing more effectively with her job and her life situations. Overall, she felt a "clearing of energy" and a "protected circle of Light" surrounding her.

Another case history is a story about a little kitten who came into a new home. The kitten was withdrawn and frightened, and had a loss of appetite. He did not play, and he wanted to be held as much as possible. He clung to his owner, Marjorie, and wouldn't let her go; he constantly meowed due to his emotional distress. Marjorie put Yarrow flower essence in his bowl of water. Within twenty-four hours, the kitten "perked up." His appetite increased, he became active with the other cat in the house, and he made more contact with other people.

LFE's Research provers' project findings

PHYSICAL SYMPTOMS

CRAVINGS: None

SENSATIONS: Tingling in legs and feet

PAIN: None

MODALITIES: None

HEAD: None

EYES: None

FACE: None

EARS: None

STOMACH: None

ABDOMEN: None

BOWEL CONDITION: Better bowel movements, softer and increased frequency

URINE: None

FEMALE: None

MALE: None

EXTREMITIES: None

BACK: Pain in lower back

SKIN: Red, dry rash in a circle about as big as a quarter; dry skin

OTHER: Most provers felt a general energy boost, and one prover felt more tired

EMOTIONAL SYMPTOMS

PATTERNS OF BALANCE: "I was able to surrender my emotions," "I found the strength to move through my emotional battle and my fears unscathed," "helped me surrender to my desire to have a baby," "I feel uplifted and better about things," "I feel higher," "I am able to feel emotionally detached if I need to," "I feel better and stronger," "I feel loved, loving, and love," "I feel a light, fanciful, free feeling," "I feel rejuvenated, energetic, and positive," "this essence gave me a boost of energy at all levels"

PATTERNS OF IMBALANCE: "I have an impending surgery and feel fear of having my face cut into while I'm awake," "felt fear," "I feel shut down," "fear of surgeon's knife," "felt protective of myself"

MENTAL SYMPTOMS

PATTERNS OF BALANCE: "I experienced more clarity," "the essence gave me more energy to work through emotional issues," "I felt more grounded in my ability to see through things better"

PATTERNS OF IMBALANCE: "anxiety, apprehension, and loss of focus; worry"

SPIRITUAL REFLECTIONS

"I was spiritually challenged to connect to the Source under difficult conditions," "I had to confront my mortality, my impending physical battle, and how I am living my life," "I feel embraced by loving arms," "the essence helped me feel connected to Great Spirit"

DREAMS/NIGHTMARES

"In my dream, I was verbally fighting with an angry male who pinned me to the floor with his sword and was going to kill me when he noticed a light by my head. He was then going to kill my light when all of a sudden Divine Mother stepped out of my body and said she loved him. He fell to his knees crying and she held him."

"I dreamed I was sleeping outside and looked up in the sky and saw an angel. The angel had a baby in her arms, and I wondered why I hadn't seen her the other times I looked up. She said it was because I was looking with the wrong kind of eyes. Then she came down and put the baby in my arms. The angel made me become very aware of my suppressed desire to have a child."

YELLOW MONKEYFLOWER

(Mimulus guttatus)
PRIMARY QUALITY: OVERCOMING FEAR

FAMILY: Snapdragon or Figwort (Scrophulariaceae)
OTHER NAMES: Common Monkey Flower, Seep-Spring Monkey Flower, Spotted Monkey Flower, Yellow Monkey Flower, Mimulus
WHERE FOUND: Along mountain brooks, streams, wet meadows, marshy places, springs, and seeps with preference to the shade and flowing waters, from Montana to Alaska and throughout the West. Native to North America.
ELEVATION: 500' to 9,500'
ENERGY IMPACT (CHAKRA CORRESPONDENCE): first, second, third, and fifth chakras
BACH FLOWER REMEDY: One of the first three flower essences discovered by Dr. Bach, Mimulus is used to treat those who have known conditions of fears and anxieties, such as fear of darkness, life, other people, heights, death, being alone, illness and pain, animals, insects, accidents, and lack of physical security. Mimulus types tend to be physically sensitive, timid, and shy, or they may appear cheerful or extroverted and hide their fears.
KEY RUBRICS FOR POSITIVE HEALING PATTERNS: cleansing, confidence, courage to communicate, self-expression, self-assertiveness, self-respect
KEY RUBRICS FOR SYMPTOMS AND PATTERNS OF IMBALANCE: abandonment, doubt, fear, restlessness, timidity, unworthiness, lack of confidence to communicate needs
OTHER RUBRICS: anger, anxieties, avoidance, burden, calm, challenge, change, community, conscious, courage, criticism, darkness, defensiveness, emotions, expression, family, flow, focus, frustrated, mental, moodiness, overcome emotions, release, root chakra, self-confident, shy, solar plexus chakra, sorrow, spleen chakra, strength, support, throat chakra, uncertainties, water, worthiness, voice

traditional use

The roots were used as an astringent. The leaves taste somewhat buttery and were included in the diet of Native Americans, who also crushed the raw leaves and stems to use as a poultice to treat rope burns and wounds. The fresh plants can be eaten raw for salad and greens; the leaves can also be cooked as potherbs.

homeopathic use

Unknown to author.

positive healing patterns

- Offers a gentle kindred spirit, giving courage to believe in oneself.
- Helps us identify, understand, and face our fears and emotions.
- Gives the strength to focus mental

faculties and to feel and act creatively in thoughts, feelings, and communication.

- Nurtures our communication skills and teaches us courage and honesty in everyday expression of ourselves, without fear of others. Gives us the confidence to speak our truths.

symptoms and patterns of imbalance

Yellow monkeyflower may be an appropriate flower essence for those who

- Need to overcome known fears or emotions
- Have difficulty expressing their fears to others
- Tend to be timid, shy, and fearful of expressing themselves, or who hide behind false masks to cover their fears and their true expression of self
- Need courage and strength to know and understand themselves in order to fully embrace their fears and express their fears to others.

features of the original flower-essence water

ODOR: subtle mellow smell, difficult to identify

TASTE: subtle, smooth, mellow taste, more noticeable at the palate than the roof or opening of the mouth

SENSATIONS: tingling on palate and back of tongue that moves downward

WATER COLOR: clear

physical makeup

ROOT, STEM, LEAVES/LEAFLETS, HEIGHT: The root is easily pulled and develops from fallen stems where they contact the soil. The smooth, hollow, bending stems root at the nodes and develop clumps on cliffs and along rocks in wet places. The stems grow from 2 inches to 3 feet tall. The dark-green, oval, veiny leaves have toothed margins and grow in opposites. The smooth rubbery leaves grow up to 4 inches long, and the upper leaves are sessile.

FLOWER COLOR: Yellow with reddish orange spots

FLOWERS: The yellow flower with its red spots resembles a monkey's face, which is how the name of the flower was derived. The two-lipped slightly fuzzy flower is about $1^{1}/_{2}$ inches long and $1^{1}/_{4}$ inches wide, with five petals or lobes. The upper lip has two broad lobes that join to form a tunnel and point upward, and the lower lip has three broad lobes that point downward. Both the calyx and the corolla have reddish orange spots, with larger spots toward the outside and smaller spots toward the inside of the flower. Two pairs of threadlike stamens with yellow anthers emerge from the center.

BLOOMING PERIOD: March to September

doctrine of signatures

- One signature of the plant is that it grows in or near flowing waters. Water represents emotions, moods, and gentle nurturing. Since the plant prefers waters that flow, this is an indication of the capability to move out of or flow with moods, thoughts, and feelings without staying stuck in them.

- The plant's ability to root at the stem's nodes and to develop clumps where it contacts the soil is a signature that demonstrates the connection made with earth, air, fire, and water. It also shows a strong desire to live near each other, in need of family and community support.

- The yellow color of the flower refers to the third or solar plexus chakra and mental faculties; it deals with thought patterns associated with feelings, such as uncertainties, fears, emotional upsets, and mood changes. The reddish orange spots indicate a connection with the earth as well as with fire and water, and demonstrate strength and courage. The spots get smaller as they go deeper inside the tunnel and eventually become hidden, resembling how we have to seek deep within ourselves to gather our courage and strength.

- The name of the plant has a legendary meaning of fear as related to the monkey. If you look at the monkeyflower from a side view, you will see that the flower petals express a mouthlike opening that appears shy and fearful, as if it is a monkey gaping with fear. The funnel-like part of the petals resembles a throat that opens into a mouth. I see these signatures as offering the ability to speak freely and to speak one's truths, without fear of shyness or dread.

- The flower petals are mildly flavored, yet they taste noticeably stronger at the palate. This signature refers to the throat and communication from deep within.

- During a plant study of the yellow monkeyflower with one of my students, Gloria Couyancy, she offered her insight about this flower: "The snapdragon is like its name: When you snap to talk, your words can burn like a dragon. You can hurt others' feelings when you speak impulsively."

Helpful suggestions

Take several drops of Yellow Monkeyflower essence and ask yourself, "What am I the most fearful of?" As you identify your most prominent fear, close your eyes and do this visualization exercise — or go sit by some flowing waters to do it.

Imagine yourself lying on the bank of a stream on a warm, sunny day with your head propped up on a smooth rock or up against a grassy bank. Your bottom, elbows, thighs, ankles, and heels all touch soft, muddy soil. Feel the link between the earthy soil and the calmly flowing waters as you breathe in the fresh air and feel the warmth of the sun shining on your face.

Now place the fear that you have identified on top of your solar plexus so that if you lift your head a bit you can see it. What is it that you see? Turn it around, look it over thoroughly, then take it back inside your solar plexus and feel it for a while. What do you feel? Get in touch with the feeling this fear gives you, stay with it, and then put it aside and let it know that you'll be back to deal with it.

Now remember a time in your life that required you to act in great courage and strength. Replay that incident in your mind, remembering how you felt when you were feeling strong and confident. Hold the feeling and the image. Keep them both with you. Open your mouth and, from the deepest part of your gut possible, let out an "Ohhhmmmm." Keep your eyes closed and your head propped up. Stretch out the note as long as possible and then start over. Ohhhmmmm long and deep, holding your strength and confidence. Now take the fear image that you first had, and continue to Ohhhmmmm and chant into that image and feeling of fear that you held deep in your solar plexus. Continue to Ohhhmmmm. Go deeper and longer than ever before. Stay with your breath; sink your bottom, elbows, thighs, ankles, and heels deeper into the muddy soil; feel the flow of the waters moving over your entire body. With each Ohhhmmmm, take the fear and move it from your solar plexus to your heart, and then to your throat. Keeping your mouth gently open, with each Ohhhhmmmm let the fear be released from your mouth and taken away by a gentle breeze.

When you feel you have drawn out the fear and let it go, discontinue the Ohhmmmm and simply relax in the water. How do you feel now? When you're ready, slowly open your eyes, thank Great Spirit, and remember to take this new feeling and image with you as you leave the water.

Affirmations

- "I face my fears with strength and confidence."
- "I allow myself to express my feelings and fears with those whom I know I can trust."
- "I allow the water of my body to cleanse away my fears.

Case History

A woman came to a homeopathic study group that I attend and brought her baby, who had fallen off a changing table the day before. The woman feared for his safety, though she didn't tell anyone about this. I passed out the Yellow Monkeyflower essence to members of the group, who each took several drops, including the baby and his mother. This mother then stood up and told us her story, then said she had to leave to take the baby to a doctor. She said, "I now have the courage and confidence to do this," and she left.

Luke, age eleven, consistently had great fears and insomnia each night, and his mother, Sherri, felt that they were related to watching an episode of *X-Files* (about aliens) two years ago. He had fears of the unknown, wars, and the condition of the world. Sherri called me and asked what flower essence to give him. I immediately thought of the Yellow Monkeyflower essence because I had used it successfully with my own daughter in relation to her nighttime fears. I suggested that Sherri explain to Luke that the Monkeyflower would help him get rid of his fears, and that each night when he takes it he should include the Monkeyflower in his prayers.

Sherri followed my advice and told Luke about the Monkeyflower. She handed him the flower-essence bottle, and as Luke held the bottle in his hands, he closed his eyes and said, "Mom, it's already working." That night Luke slept soundly without waking. Luke has been sleeping throughout the night ever since, and he attributes this change to the Monkeyflower essence. Sherri has done several "rechecks" with Luke about his sleep and fears, and he comments that the Monkeyflower helped him and he rarely has nighttime fears anymore.

LFE's Research Provers' Project Findings

Physical Symptoms

CRAVINGS: Water, protein
SENSATIONS: Twitching in body
PAIN: None
MODALITIES:
  BETTER: None
  WORSE: Difficulty sleeping, restless at night
HEAD: Pressure at head
EYES: None

FACE: None
EARS: None
STOMACH: Upset stomach
ABDOMEN: Heaviness in abdomen
BOWEL CONDITION: Passed gas
URINE: None
FEMALE: None
MALE: None
EXTREMITIES: None
BACK: None
SKIN: None

Emotional Symptoms

PATTERNS OF BALANCE: "calm," "hidden emotions were released and I felt a cleansing take place," "I didn't feel inhibited or keep my emotions inside of me; I said everything I was feeling," "need to transform these emotions through prayer," "had powerful emotional releases," "more self-assertive, felt stronger and more worthy," "helped me face my doubts and darkness"

PATTERNS OF IMBALANCE: "I felt grumpy and I deeply struggled with my issues in the way many humans behave without regard to others; it seems that I am always expected to be kind and loving with my words, but I'm supposed to overlook it when others are not that way to me," "had intense energy around the heart, with intense emotions," "felt sorrow and anger," "was drawn into emotional upsets and anger by others," "I feel this essence deals with emotional shadow work in some way," "I exploded with rage and anger," "felt nervous and guilty in expressing my anger, which resulted in an upset stomach," "self-pity," "I didn't like myself while taking this essence; I was mean and nasty to other people," "frustration and restlessness; frustrated that I'm not trusting myself and that I need to be more self-confident"

Mental Symptoms

Patterns of Balance: "became more conscious of myself," "helped me to analyze reactions and situations in myself, and to figure out what I could do differently," "observation of self and others; became more reflective," "gained self-respect," "allowed myself to know what is true," "helped me remember who I am"

Patterns of Imbalance: "mental confusion about how to say what I think or feel and not think that I should always hold back for fear of hurting or offending," "intensified issues I've always struggled with in regard to injustices and uncaring behaviors in people," "lack of clarity," "actively trying to figure things out and having difficulty with thoughts and words," "critical"

Spiritual Reflections

"Helps me see my stuff and myself more clearly as I continue more surely upon my spiritual quest — that of being more conscious of self and Self," "increased meditation and prayer," "much thought of Good vs. Evil in relation to honoring my true self (the light) and doubt (the dark)"

Dreams/Nightmares

"I had two human-like bears approach me. I was moving away from them because they weren't real bears. They were personified, hyper-bears. Then I shifted my attitude and stopped to hear what they had to tell me. One came forward and told me that I need to practice introspection."

Some provers noted more dreams; some provers had none.

YERBA SANTA

(Eriodictyon angustifolium)
Primary Quality: The Sacred Within

Family: Waterleaf (Hydrophyllaceae)

Other Names: Holy Herb, Sacred Herb, Mountain Balm, Bear Plant, Consumptive's Weed, Gum Bush

Where Found: Dry plains and hills, slopes and ridges of Arizona, Utah, Colorado, New Mexico, and Texas. Other species, *E. Californica* and *E. Tomentosum,* are native throughout California, Oregon, Nevada, and Mexico.

Elevation: 2,000' to 7,000'

Energy Impact (Chakra Correspondence): seventh chakra (indirectly fifth chakra)

Key Rubrics for Positive Healing Patterns: cleansing, inner loving, receptivity, renewal, reverence for all of life, self-discovery, spiritual guidance

Key Rubrics for Symptoms and Patterns of Imbalance: anxiety, impurities, inferiority, out of touch with self, psychic toxins

Other Rubrics: ambition, appreciation, bronchial, chest, clarity, confidence, coughing, crown chakra, follow-through, healing, heart, lungs, outer patience, phlegm, psychic toxins, purifier, receptivity, renewal, sacredness, self-discovery, self-empowerment, self-esteem, throat, understanding

---

traditional use

Yerba santa's history of use includes Indians of Old California and the Spanish, Mexican, and American settlers. Yerba santa, or "holy herb," was adopted by Spanish forefathers who learned of the plant through the American Indians. The fresh or dried leaves of yerba santa were boiled and made into a tea, and are still used today to expel phlegm, restore the liver, clear the urinary tract, and treat chest colds, sore throats, bronchitis, head congestion, asthma, hay fever, chronic alcoholism, poor digestion with no appetite, bladder infections, and even some forms of tuberculosis. Other

conditions, such as stomachaches, vomiting, diarrhea, kidney ailments, and hemorrhoids, can also be treated with yerba santa.

Yerba Santa has a reputation as a woundwort remedy, based on the leaf's shape as a cutting instrument (sword/blade shape). The leaf is actually sticky enough to act as a "natural Band-Aid." The Indians also used the fresh and dried leaves to make a poultice for abrasions and pain associated with rheumatism, swelling, sores, and fatigued limbs. The poultice can be used for broken or unbroken skin and for both people and animals.

Herbalists today use yerba santa for the above conditions, and also as a douche and for steam inhalation for bronchial congestion. Yerba santa contains cerotonic acid and a resin called pentatriacontane. A delicious amber honey made from yerba santa pollen tastes slightly spicy.

Homeopathic use

Yerba santa *(Eriodictyon)* is a remedy used to relieve asthma by expectoration and to treat bronchial disorders with night sweats and emaciation. Symptoms are poor appetite and digestion, whooping cough, dizziness in head, ear pain, burning in throat, foul morning breath, wheezing, inflammation of the mucous membranes of the nasal cavities, chronic bronchitis and bronchial tuberculosis, and dull pain in the right lung. Male patients have sore testicles that cannot withstand pressure.

Positive Healing patterns

- Helps us get rid of "psychic toxins." It works as a cleanser, a purifier, and a means to bring us to a full presence that we can own and honor.
- Helps us sort out our impurities from within to without, reaching into the depths of our dysfunctions and helping us find ourselves.
- Rebuilds energy and strength within our "temple spaces," filling us with Spirit's love and light-filled radiance.

- Builds strength of character, acceptance, willingness, and determination to look and work from within in order to heal the whole person.
- Gives us the spiritual guidance to follow through with our outer tasks and our inner intuition.

symptoms and patterns of imbalance

Yerba Santa may be an appropriate flower essence for those who

- Understand their true needs, yet lack follow-through by not honoring them or carrying them out
- Demonstrate the paradox of two different personalities, such as in one instance being overly naive and trusting, and in another instance lacking trust without a cause
- Seem to have a healthy perspective toward life (have it together), yet don't see their own flaws
- Lack understanding or knowledge to survive their deep, inner, personal work, and who lack follow-through at any level in life
- Have weak resistance to and need cleansing of "psychic toxins."

features of the original flower-essence water

ODOR: slightly sweet; more subtle than the leaves
TASTE: just like the leaves and flowers smell; very strong, powerful, and resinlike

SENSATIONS: a warm tingling sensation and an opening in the heart to the crown chakra that is gentle yet persuasive

WATER COLOR: yellowish, not entirely clear

physical makeup

ROOT, STEM, LEAVES/LEAFLETS, HEIGHT: Yerba santa is a woody bush that grows to between 2 and 6 feet tall. Yerba santa's outer leaves have a sticky, shiny, resinous substance with a smooth top. The lower, slightly woolly leaves are dull green and have a marked central vein with eloquent and numerous small veins. The leaves are sweet-smelling with lanceolate, slightly notched edges, and they grow up to 4 inches long. They have a slightly astringent and mucilaginous property, and they stick to the teeth when chewed. The stem of yerba santa is also resinous, and the entire plant gives off a powerful aroma.

FLOWER COLOR: White

FLOWERS: Yerba santa's flowers are white and funnel-shaped, and they grow in loose terminal clusters at the end of the branches. Each flower has five tiny petals and five tiny stamens with dark yellow anthers. The flower is about 3/8 inch wide and carries a subtle sweet fragrance. It is difficult to tell how strong the actual flower blossoms smell because the leaves and plant are so fragrant.

BLOOMING PERIOD: April to May

doctrine of signatures

- The sticky, astringent, mucilaginous, resinous qualities of yerba santa's leaves strongly indicate the plant's use for chest colds, bronchitis, asthma, hay fever, and so on. If you look closely at the underside of the leaves, you can also see that the tiny veins look like bronchioles. This signature suggests the plant's practical and physical uses, and it also demonstrates the powerful cleansing effect that yerba santa has upon both the inner and outer body. Yerba santa actively cleanses the bronchial tract and works to preventing damage to the internal organs. Matthew Wood describes a characteristic of yerba santa: "The inner spaces defined by the body linings are 'sanctuaries' from which impurities must be kept. Perhaps it was an intuitive recognition of this that gave the plant its name: 'yerba santa' means 'sacred herb' in Spanish. The internal body linings correspond with 'psychic body linings.' Sanctity of psychic space is the internal property which yerba santa guards."[8] Yerba Santa flower essence is a wonderful healer and teacher that helps us to sort out our impurities from within to without. When we feel closed and shut down, it's as if we have shut out everything within us and everything that surrounds us. Yerba santa helps us to discover what it is that we shut down and to find a way to move whatever is stuck. Yerba santa, the "holy herb," renews energy and strength in the "temple space" of the crown chakra, filling our body/mind/soul with Spirit's love and light-filled radiance.

- In association with the above signatures, yerba santa also builds strength of character, acceptance, willingness, and determination to work from within to heal the whole person. Through this process, we begin to truly understand ourselves and to find out who we are. The "holy herb" gives us spiritual guidance in our ability to follow through with our outer tasks and our inner intuition.

- Yerba santa's signature as a wound-wort remedy is indicated by the leaf's shape as a cutting instrument (knife or sword-blade shape) and by the two different sides of the leaf, with the outer-side leaf smooth and shiny (relating to the skin), and the underside leaf dull and veiny (relating to the veins). This signature also demonstrates the plant's natural ability as a Band-Aid, holding both sides of the wound together. Again, we are shown the duality of healing what is on the inside and what is on the outside.

Helpful suggestions

Prepare some time to be with yourself. Take three to four drops of Yerba Santa flower essence and choose one or all of the following exercises:

1. Imagine yourself in a special place in nature with only your closest, most intimate friends and family. You are lying on a blanket of velvety soft green grass, and each person is gently holding or touching you, as if in laying-on of hands. In total trust, you close your eyes. You feel so completely embraced by the loving energy you are receiving that you feel a space in your heart begin to open. The space gets bigger and bigger. The love and compassion for yourself grows bigger in that space and rises all the way to the top of your head. As you feel your heart energy unfold, and as it reaches your crown chakra, you see a beautiful funnel-shaped flower that beckons you to come inside. You step inside the flower, breathe in its pleasant aroma, and touch its soft, delicate petals. You're able to grasp onto that part of you that cries for help, and you hold that part close to your heart as you lean against the delicate flower and take in its entire embrace. Talk to the part of you that cries for help and ask what you can do for it and how you can nurture it when you're back in "the world." Continue to hold it as you stand up and step back outside the flower and reenter the embrace of your friends and family. Gradually open your eyes, still holding that part close to your heart as you feel the entire group

give you one big gigantic hug all at once.

2. Think of one thing about yourself that you might call an "impurity," such as something that goes very deep and probably feels buried. Try to pick it up and look at it carefully. Feel it, touch it, and listen to what it has to say. Ask what you can do for it. The more you can get in touch with it, the better you'll be able to move it around, give it a shove, and throw it out the door.

3. Choose one thing you'd like to follow through until it is complete. Decide what tools you'll need to help you follow through and what method of follow-through would be the most achievable. Go gather your tools, and begin the steps A to Z.

Affirmations

- "I give thanks to myself and my ability to rediscover my lost parts."
- "I pray that I will heal in body, mind, and soul and that all impurities will come out in the open and be seen, heard, and touched."
- "I take full responsibility to follow through with life's tasks (name a particular task for you) and to make an achievable goal of completion."
- "I honor the sacred within myself."

Case History

Grace came for flower essence therapy because she wanted a stronger spiritual connection with and understanding of herself. She was feeling lost, without spiritual guidance and support, and weakened within herself. She had recently experienced a major relationship crisis that brought up deep abandonment issues and much grief. Grace needed a connection with herself and yearned for an unfoldment of self-discovery.

Grace began taking Yerba Santa flower essence and found very quickly that she was rediscovering herself. She felt that she regained some lost parts of herself and through this experience she also felt stronger. "I felt a deeper love for myself, which helped me gather my strength and directed me toward meeting some special personal goals, led by my higher guidance. I feel that Yerba Santa flower essence helped me to not hold on so tight, because I felt more complete and strong within myself."

Life's Research Provers' Project Findings

PHYSICAL SYMPTOMS

CRAVINGS: Bread, hot soup

SENSATIONS: Lightness in the top of the head

PAIN: None

MODALITIES: Inconsistent

HEAD: Lightness in the top of the head

EYES: None

FACE: None

EARS: None

STOMACH: None

ABDOMEN: None

BOWEL CONDITION: Harder bowel movements

URINE: None
FEMALE: Decreased sexual drive
MALE: None
EXTREMITIES: Discomfort in shoulder
BACK: None
SKIN: None
OTHER: One prover developed bronchial pain, postnasal drip, dry cough, and a sore throat. Another prover had had surgery due to an old injury in which the left ankle became swollen and fluid-filled; the left leg and knee were also sore.

EMOTIONAL SYMPTOMS

PATTERNS OF BALANCE: "felt good, sound, peaceful, and happy," "this essence helps me feel provided for," "this essence boosted my self-esteem," "gave me a feeling of ambition, confidence, and self-empowerment," "I felt better and stronger," "my emotions moved from fear to surrender," "felt calm"

PATTERNS OF IMBALANCE: "I was angry and defiant about the way I have acted in my life and have not allowed myself to be me," "I realized how I have felt inferior to others for no good reason," "I felt a sadness from deep within," "restlessness and lack of concentration," "was argumentative," "moderate irritability," "off-balance feelings"

MENTAL SYMPTOMS

PATTERNS OF BALANCE: "I have gained some insight about how much I have not expressed myself in the past," "I am more clairvoyant," "I felt mentally connected to myself emotionally," "I have more clarity and am more creative," "I am more clear," "I felt quiet and introspective," "more calm and inward," "more grounded," "more contemplation"

PATTERNS OF IMBALANCE: "I became clearly aware of how much I don't express myself, how I judge myself, and how much I worry about what other people think of me," "nervous tension, anxiety and worry," "confusion"

SPIRITUAL REFLECTIONS

"I am more loving and patient with myself," "I appreciated being alone," "I felt a big return to my center," "I feel called by the ancestors, but I don't know the meaning of this; they are telling me it is time 'to do the work,'" "I felt new gateways opening," "this was a very healing essence"

DREAMS/NIGHTMARES

Some dreams reported, but none documented.

yucca (soaptree)

(Yucca elata)
Primary Quality: Spear of Destiny

Family: Agave (Agavaceae) or Lily (Liliaceae)
Other Names: Soapweed, Whipple Yucca, Palmalla, Spanish-Dagger, Spanish-Bayonet, Narrowleaf Yucca, Mesa Yucca, Indian Cabbage, Pamilla, Our Lord's Candle
Where Found: deserts, mesas, sandy plains, grasslands, and dry mountain slopes in Arizona, New Mexico, Texas, California, and Colorado
Elevation: 1,500' to 6,000'
Energy Impact (Chakra Correspondence): seventh chakra
Key Rubrics for Positive Healing Patterns: higher consciousness, focus, perseverance, ability to act toward and stay focused on life's goals
Key Rubrics for Symptoms and Patterns of Imbalance: emptiness, feeling lost in the darkness, lacking spiritual direction, purpose, and guidance
Other Rubrics: balance, calm, change, clarity, consciousness, crown chakra, determination, devotion, endurance, feminine, focus, grace, groundedness, guidance, healing, light, meditation, moon, perseverance, prayer, radiance, relaxed, release, sacredness, spiritual purpose, strength, understanding, wisdom

traditional use

The yucca was depicted in several petroglyphs in prehistoric times by the Pueblo Indians in Boca Negra Canyon in New Mexico. Southwest Indians ate the flowers, buds, and young stalks, which are rich in sugar and vitamin C. The saponin-rich yucca root is also known for its ancient use in cleansing and was made into a shampoo by the Southwest Indians to stimulate hair growth and prevent dandruff. It was also used as a soap for cleansing before ceremonies and dances.

A root poultice or salve was made to treat skin disorders, skin eruptions, sprains and breaks, and rheumatism. The root was also made into a tea to treat pain, such as arthritis, and is still used as a laxative. The root, when soaked in water, was given to a woman having a long labor, and the suds mixed with sugar were given to the mother to facilitate the afterbirth. An infusion of the tea is known today to treat urethral and prostate inflammation. The bark is generally removed for medicinal use and left on for making shampoo or soap.

The root has a high content of vitamin A, the B-complex vitamins, vitamin C, calcium, potassium, phosphorus, manganese, copper, and iron. The immature seedpods are quite tasty when eaten steamed. The seeds can also be ground into meal, and the large, juicy fruits can be eaten raw, roasted, cooked, or dried.

The hairy, fibrous leaves were used by the Southwest Indians to make sandals, baskets, mats, cloth, cordage, belts, rope ladders, toe cords, head rings for carrying water, fish nets, cradle lashings, hoops, prayer sticks, chant arrows, and paintbrushes for decorating pottery. Yucca's fibrous leaves are still used today by the Southwest Indians, especially to make baskets.

Yucca was harvested for cattle fodder from 1916 to 1919 during the drought. During World War I, yucca leaves were made into 80 million pounds of fiber to replace jute for covering cotton bales. During World War II, the U.S. Navy used yucca leaves to make a heavyweight paper, and for twine and rope. The stalks of yucca have more recently been used to make surgical splints because they are light and sturdy.

Yuccas have a multitude of natural healing properties that are used today to treat a variety of conditions. At over one hundred research institutes and universities, leading doctors and chemists are conducting research and collecting testimonials about the effectiveness of the yucca plant. The plant's primary ingredients, steroid saponins, are even used at sanitation plants because of their ability to speed up the breakdown of organic waste. Successful clinical research has also shown that the plant, made into a food supplement, can decrease intestinal symptoms and disorders and reduce the tendency to develop toxic waste in the colon. Patients are declaring that yucca supplements in the form of herbal

tablets and a yucca herbal drink have helped them relieve constipation, diarrhea, cramping, intestinal gas, abdominal pains, and migraine headaches, and reduced stress and joint swelling, especially associated with arthritis. Abnormal cholesterol levels of patients have been lowered, as studied through their blood test analysis. Yucca supplements used by veterinarians, pet owners, and dairy farmers are also reportedly helping to restore motion in arthritic animals.

Homeopathic use

Yucca filamentosa (bear-grass) is a homeopathic remedy used to treat symptoms associated with bile and the liver. The patient tends to be despondent and irritable, with severe headaches and throbbing of the forehead. Symptoms are red nose, yellowish face, taste of rotten eggs in mouth, pain in right side of abdomen, yellowish brown stool with bile, reddish skin, and burning and swelling of the foreskin in males.

positive Healing patterns

- Shines its light to help us see where we're going, stay focused on our life's journeys, and become our life's work.
- Encourages strength, endurance, groundedness, and determination, with softness and gentleness.
- Gives a feeling of fullness, satisfaction, and the energy needed to move forward in life.
- Helps us tap into our infinite storage banks and to become our highest good.

- Offers guidance toward devotion, meditation, and prayer.

symptoms and patterns of imbalance

Yucca may be an appropriate flower essence for those who

- Feel lost in the darkness, and need direction to the Light
- Lack strength, endurance, groundedness and are out of touch with their feminine nature
- Feel empty and strive for a fuller, richer way of living and being
- Lack spiritual direction, purpose, and guidance.

features of the original flower-essence water

ODOR: very sweet, full fragrance
TASTE: thick, full, rich, potent, and sweet
SENSATIONS: warmth in feet to the top of the head
WATER COLOR: clear

physical makeup

ROOT, STEM, LEAVES/LEAFLETS, HEIGHT: The high saponin content of the root helps the yucca to flourish in the desert terrain and climate. *Yucca elata* has numerous spiny-tipped, yellowish green leaves that are long and narrow; they rise in a rosette from a central stem. The narrow leaves have fibers that protrude in threadlike margins. The leaves grow up to $2\,^1/_2$ feet long, and they have sharp spines at the terminal end. The upright flower stalk is sturdy, with a light purplish hue, and can reach a height of up to 30 feet. More commonly, the flower stalks range from 5 to 15 feet tall.

FLOWER COLOR: Creamy white
FLOWERS: The cream-colored lilylike flowers open at night and close in the daylight. They have a soft, subtle, sweet yet bitter smell. The petals are thick and rubbery, yet they also carry a softness. The petals grow alternately, upright, and closely together along the stem. Each flower has six petals and is bell-shaped in the daylight and somewhat star-shaped at nighttime or in a bowl of water. The flower grows up to 2 inches long. There are six very full, fuzzy, creamy-white stamens with yellow heads protected inside the flower. The pistil inside the flower is somewhat thick and crunchy, and tastes like a green vegetable. The flower is followed by a symmetrical three-celled cylindrical seed capsule and a large succulent fruit. The entire flower tastes good.
BLOOMING PERIOD: May to July

doctrine of signatures

- Yucca is a night-blooming plant. The flower essence is best made at night and under a full moon. If made in the daylight, the flowers open in the water and look like a star, which is more like how the flower looks at night. In the daytime, the flower closes and is more bell-shaped; it symbolizes the plant's ability to protect itself when in need. The spiny-tipped leaves, shaped like a warrior's spear, are another example of the plant's protection. The clustered flowers offer a glow in the moonlight and are like a soft candle burning. This important signature represents the light that this plant offers, even in the darkness. Like a shining star, the yucca shines its light to help us see where we're going and stay focused on our life journeys. Another feature of yucca's light is the warmth it provides when drinking the flower-essence water, from the bottom of the feet to the top of the head.

- Yucca has great strength, endurance, groundedness, and determination. The plant's sprout grows upright, and when it reaches maturity it stands tall and rises like a spear to meet the sky. Its high saponin content gives the yucca the ability to depend on itself and be nurtured by Mother Earth. It also offers a powerful cleansing effect, signifying humbleness and surrender as well as strength and determination. I see the yucca as a female version of the century plant. Another example of these signatures is in the flower petal. Although the petals are thick, rubbery, and strong, they also carry a soft and gentle nature.

- The taste of the flower is divine. It gives a feeling of fullness, satisfaction, and the energy needed to move forward in life.

- The medicinal qualities described previously, as well as the practical nature of the yucca, show the plant's diversity and its multiple uses. It is like the infinite storage bank within ourselves that allows us to be nowhere yet everywhere at once.

- The cluster of flowers at the top of the plant, in addition to the creamy-white color of the flower, corresponds to the seventh chakra at the top of the head. By working with the Yucca flower essence, we are directed to the Light that guides us to become the purpose of our life's work. We begin to consciously devote time each day to the sacred, and we better understand who we are and how we operate as a system of powerfully focused energy.

Helpful suggestions

Before you go to bed, take several drops of the Yucca flower essence, close your eyes, and take this journey. Take several long, deep breaths into the darkness of your closed eyes. Imagine that you are walking on an old road that winds through the desert. It is a warm, quiet night. A gentle breeze caresses your body. Mother Moon has just shown herself over the peak of a mountain and is lighting your path in the darkness. You don't know where you're going, but you have a sense that by following your intuition you will be led to where you need to go. Although you are faced by your fears of the nighttime silhouettes, you feel an incredible purpose and determination to stay focused on your path.

Off in the distance, you see a soft white glow in the moonlight. You are attracted to its light, and you move in its direction. As you get closer to the soft white light, you realize that it has a long body with a circle of spears around its base. It now stands tall before you. Carefully you walk up to the light and look up. You see that a cluster of flowers makes up the light you are drawn to. You look down at the base of the moonlit, spiny-tipped leaves and you intuitively know not to get to close to them. You realize you have found a soaptree yucca plant, and you graciously give thanks to the yucca and say a blessing to this special plant as you walk in a circle and sprinkle cornmeal around its base.

Then you find what seems to be a safe spot near the light of the yucca in which to lie down. You remove a light sleeping bag from your backpack and crawl into it. You lie under the open sky, breathe in the nighttime air, and feel the moon shining on your face as you are drawn to the light of the yucca. Focusing on the yucca's light and taking in its gentle, yet enduring energy, you gradually let your eyes close and fall off to sleep.

Affirmations

- "May the seeds of my dreams guide my path and destiny."
- "I have the strength, endurance, determination, and wisdom to stay focused on my life's path."
- "I hold the Light energy within me."

Case History

Heather tells the story of her experience with the Yucca flower essence: "I was a young twenty-two at the time when I pulled at the yucca: Spear of Destiny. My life at that time was somewhat chaotic, and I lacked direction and guidance. I took the Yucca flower essence often; every time I did, I prayed that I would be led to do what was 'right' for me. I was definitely looking for the answers that would lead me to happiness, but what I focused on even more was being true to myself and my needs. I took more chances and I risked more. I also was given a sense of direction that helped me take more responsibility in my life. I found courage and strength. I became more conscious of my own needs and became more aware of my limitations. These insights helped me make wiser choices, and I felt more in tune with myself. Taking the Yucca became a conscious activity in my life that led me on a path of purpose."

Life's Research Provers' Project Findings

PHYSICAL SYMPTOMS

CRAVINGS: Chocolate cake

SENSATIONS: Warmth and release of tension, "I felt my aura soften, beginning around my head until it went all the way down to my feet, which felt tingling"

PAIN: None

MODALITIES: Inconsistent

HEAD: None

EYES: None

FACE: None
EARS: None
STOMACH: None
ABDOMEN: None
BOWEL CONDITION: None
URINE: Slight burning
FEMALE: None
MALE: None
EXTREMITIES: None
BACK: None
SKIN: None
OTHER: Some provers wanted to sleep more often and take time to rest, while other provers had an energy boost. "Able to monitor daily intake better, have returned to taking apple cider vinegar and honey daily; I had the urge to eat better and to start cooking again."

EMOTIONAL SYMPTOMS

PATTERNS OF BALANCE: "felt more at peace after returning from a health crisis," "I experienced a release of emotional build-up and balancing," "I felt a healing in the heart-center area," "sense of balance and relaxation," "feel more loving and grateful for all that is in my life," "feel a warmth toward others," "release of tension," "I felt less disturbed by the demands of others," "I was able to set better boundaries," "I feel very balanced and extremely relaxed," "felt calm, relaxed, and secure," "this essence calmed my anger and fears"

PATTERNS OF IMBALANCE: "I felt a strange sadness," "depression," "tension," "anger," "fear"

MENTAL SYMPTOMS

PATTERNS OF BALANCE: "I felt a strong desire and focus to take care of loose ends and remove old clutter," "I wanted to organize and get clearer," "increased awareness and ability to study," "ease of tension and sense of well-being," "mental calmness," "mental direction"
PATTERNS OF IMBALANCE: None reported

SPIRITUAL REFLECTIONS

"I must clear the old to allow room for the new," "if I could stay in this place all the time, my life would appear as a blessing," "felt an opening in the seventh chakra," "became more prayerful," "I was shown more of my spiritual purpose," "I felt more connected and relaxed, which allowed more spiritual grace to enter my life," "more feelings of love"

DREAMS/NIGHTMARES

Several provers reported an increase of dreams. Due to the level of involvement of some dreams, they are not documented here.

CONCLUSION

I am thankful for the wondrous bounty the plant kingdom gives us. Like people, plants embody many mysteries, stories, personalities, and expressions, and they each have their own modes of survival. They are great teachers and great healers. I thirst for the knowledge they give me and the ways in which they fill my soul. Being a student of the plant kingdom is a lifelong journey; there are always new plants to discover, to be with, and to experience. Even the plants that are familiar to me continue to surprise me with new awareness and a deeper understanding of their value and their gifts.

I am also thankful for the wonderful herbalists, homeopaths, gardeners, and plant teachers I've met along my path. They have made my journey lighter and more joyful, and they have filled me with their wisdom and their insights into the vast, powerful world of plants.

I hope that you will join us in discovering the healing qualities and the essences of the plant kingdom. This adventure will open new doorways along your life's path and will reveal to you the parts of yourself that require inquiry, healing, and nurturing. This exploration will change the way you view and live life, and it will remain dear to your heart forever.

APPENDIX
Living Flower Essences' Products, Training, and Retreats

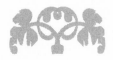

The forty-eight flower essences featured in this book are available from Living Flower Essences in half-ounce cobalt-blue glass bottles and in one-ounce bottles upon request. Our flower essences can be purchased singly, as Specialty Formulas, or in a Practitioner's Kit. All our bottles are prepared with healing prayers and love. You will find our flower essences to have a delightfully soothing taste.

The labels on the bottles indicate the following contents: brandy and vegetable glycerin as a preservative, pure water, and an infusion of flowers in water. Special orders may specify a nonalcohol base, and requests can be made for organic apple cider vinegar and/or vegetable glycerin as preservatives. These will contain minute amounts of alcohol, which is present in the Mother Essence tincture. Unless you request otherwise, the flower essences will be shipped to you with the original contents listed on the label.

practitioner's kit

This kit contains the forty-eight flower essences featured in this book and represents the complete line of flower essences found in the professional display unit. The bottles are secured in two separate boxes that hold twenty-four bottles each, with a reference guide included. This kit is an indispensable tool for flower-essence practitioners or for anyone interested in working in greater depth with flower essences.

You may also purchase a sturdy canvas bag with forty-eight sections that hold the bottles. The bag is designed for carrying and traveling. Color choices for the canvas may vary, and they are lined with colorful material on the inside.

chakra healing kit

Flowers, like chakras, embody colors and vibrations of light and sound. This kit contains seven flower essences that correspond to the seven chakras, packaged colorfully and including directions. The flower essences in this kit are Indian Paintbrush, Pomegranate, Sunflower, Wild Rose, Desert Larkspur, Aster, and Saguaro.

specialty formulas

Each formula is designed to fully embrace the qualities represented by its name. The formulas are very effective and offer a blend of complementary flower essences.

ABUNDANCE FORMULA: This great-tasting formula is prepared with prayers for abundance and plenty. For those whose intention is to receive the blessings of harvest and to eliminate any feelings or concerns of lack, try this delightful blend. The formula is made up of the flower essences of Desert Willow, Paloverde, Pomegranate, and Purple Robe.

ADDICTION FORMULA: For those who are addicts (including mental and emotional addictions as well as physical addiction), try this formula to bring insight and heal addictions and old wounds. The essences included in this energizing formula are Black-Eyed Susan, Blue Flag, California Poppy, Century Plant, Crimson Monkeyflower, Mexican Hat, and Onion.

CHILDREN'S EMPOWERMENT FORMULA: These essences are chosen specifically for children (infants to adolescents). This formula provides a doorway through which children can enhance their awareness. The flower essences include Bells-of-Ireland,

Chamomile, Cliff Rose, Onion, Sweet Pea, and Yarrow.

TEEN'S EMPOWERMENT FORMULA: These essences are chosen to work with the challenging emotions and issues faced by today's teenagers. The formula includes Chicory, Cliff Rose, Indian Paintbrush, Mullein, Onion, and Yarrow.

MEN'S EMPOWERMENT FORMULA: The flower essences in this formula focus on the needs of men. Included are Century Plant, Mullein, Sage, Scarlet Penstemon, Sunflower, and Yarrow.

WOMEN'S EMPOWERMENT FORMULA: These flower essences are chosen especially for a woman's needs. They are Chamomile, Desert Willow, Pomegranate, Sage, and Yarrow.

LIFE TRANSITIONS FORMULA: These flower essences are combined to provide guidance and strength when facing life changes or passages. They include Century Plant, Desert Larkspur, Lupine, Sage, Saguaro, Yarrow, and Yucca.

FATIGUE FORMULA: This uplifting mix of flower essences is made especially for those who experience a chronic state of exhaustion and weariness. The essences included in this formula are Blanketflower, Chamomile, Echinacea, Sunflower, and Yarrow.

NIGHT FREEDOM FORMULA: This soothing blend of essences can help you or your child sleep better and experience freedom from nighttime fears such as fear of the dark, fear of being alone, or nightmares. The essences included are Calendula, Yellow Monkeyflower, Saguaro, and Yarrow.

LOVERS' SPECIAL FORMULA: This is a

unique blend of essences that promote love and harmony in discovering and maintaining all aspects of true intimacy. The essences include Bouncing Bet, Desert Willow, Honeysuckle, Mullein, Pomegranate, Scarlet Penstemon, and Strawberry Hedgehog.

MEDITATION FORMULA: This powerful blend of flower essences offers deep inner peace, balance, and silence. It is a great formula for meditation and for those seeking a peaceful, gentle flow of energy throughout their being. This formula also helps release tension and nervousness. The essences included are Chamomile, Indian Paintbrush, Lupine, Saguaro, and Yerba Santa.

STRESS FORMULA: This calming blend of flower essences offers peace and relaxation and for anyone who is experiencing post-traumatic stress or the emotional and mental stresses of daily life. The essences in this formula are Calendula, Century Plant, Chamomile, Lupine, Saguaro, and Yarrow.

SECRET PLEASURES FOR MEN: This spectacular, well-loved blend of flower essences is prepared to help men discover their hidden sexual pleasures and desires. The extraordinary formula includes Bouncing Bet, Mullein, Pomegranate, Scarlet Penstemon, and Strawberry Hedgehog.

SECRET PLEASURES FOR WOMEN: This wonderful blend of flower essences was created to help women discover their hidden sexual pleasures and desires. This formula is a well-loved favorite! The essences include Bouncing Bet, Desert Willow, Pomegranate, and Strawberry Hedgehog.

DEPRESSION-LIFTING FORMULA: A unique combination of Aster, Peace Rose, and Wild Rose. Roses open the heart to help us give and receive joy, love, and compassion. Wild Rose is for apathy caused by depression, and Aster offers a boost by helping us understand and accept the cause of the depression. Aster also helps us embrace higher spiritual principles in ordinary living.

YARROW FORMULA ENERGY SHIELD: This is a special combination of pink, yellow, and white Yarrow flower essences for those who feel "bone-tired," exhausted, overworked, and run down. The blend of these three essences offers protection, harmony, and insight about how to take action and redirect ourselves without being drained by others. Yarrow is a soothing, soft, protective flower essence that is recommended for everyone.

Living flower essences' salves

In addition to preparing flower essences, we also make herbal salves that are included in our product line. These salves make great gifts and are a helpful addition to the family first-aid kit. Each formula is the result of thorough research and careful selection. Most plants in the salves are wildcrafted by Living Flower Essences (LFE) staff or grown in organic gardens free of toxins and picked for highest quality. The essential oils used in the salves are pure and of the highest concentration. These salves are well liked by our customers.

ARNICA SALVE: "The Sports Remedy" — for sprains, injuries, and blows to the limbs, especially if accompanied by aching. Ingredients: extra-virgin olive oil, arnica leaves and flowers, beeswax, cocoa butter, and oils of clove, rosemary, marjoram, and cedarwood.

BLUE VERVAIN SALVE: "Massage Therapy for Muscles" — to release muscle tension and muscle spasms. Ingredients: extra-virgin olive oil, blue vervain leaves and flowers, beeswax, cocoa butter, and oils of basil, cypress, ginger, marjoram, and lemongrass.

CALENDULA/COMFREY SALVE: "All-Healing Salve" — for cuts, chapped skin, and skin abrasions. Ingredients: extra-virgin olive oil, calendula flowers, chaparral flowers and leaves, comfrey leaves, beeswax, cocoa butter, aloe vera, and oils of lavender, rosemary, sage, and yarrow.

CHI SALVE: "The Reflexology Salve" — for massaging the reflexology areas of the hands and feet. This salve directly affects the glands, nerves, and organs of the body and is great for all your aches and pains. Ingredients: almond oil, beeswax, cedarwood, frankincense, ginger, hot pepper oil, lemon, marjoram, nutmeg, oil of birch, sandalwood, sesame, and benzoin as a preservative.

STINGING NETTLE SALVE: For ant bites, bee or wasp stings, and unusual itchy sores or pains caused by bites. Ingredients: extra-virgin olive oil, stinging nettle leaves, goldenseal, beeswax, cocoa butter, and oils of basil, lavender, and lime.

GOLDENSEAL SALVE: Helps prevent and heal infections in wounds. Ingredients: extra-virgin olive oil, goldenseal root, beeswax, cocoa butter, and oils of bergamot, thyme, cinnamon, and oregano.

PLANTAIN SALVE: For mild skin abrasions and for drawing out splinters. Ingredients:

extra-virgin olive oil, plantain leaves, thyme leaves, beeswax, and oils of thyme, lemon thyme, and lavender.

THE TRIAD SALVE: "The Skin Salve" — for warts or fungus-like skin growths. The word "triad" in this salve's name refers to the three trees that contribute to it: thuja, oak, and pine. Ingredients: extra-virgin olive oil, thuja occidentalis leaves, oak bark, pine bark, pine sap, beeswax, cocoa butter, and oils of frankincense, sage, and vitamin E.

YARROW SALVE: "Massage Therapy for Bones" — for broken bones, bruises, and deep cuts. Ingredients: extra-virgin olive oil, yarrow flowers and leaves, beeswax, cocoa butter, and oils of birch, cypress, and lemongrass.

YUCCA SALVE: "Massage Therapy for Joints" — for inflammation of the joints, including pain, stiffness, swelling, and redness. Ingredients: extra-virgin olive oil, arnica leaves and flowers, yucca root, yerba santa leaves, yarrow leaves, horsetail, cocoa butter, and oils of birch, cedarwood, chamomile, fir ginger, and nutmeg.

Bottled water: A gift from Nature

Living Flower Essences offers two kinds of Living Flower Bottled Water infused with flower essences. All active ingredients are produced by Living Flower Essences.

CHILL OUT: A relaxing blend of fresh purified water; flower essences of Calendula, Chamomile, and Lavender; and raw organic apple cider vinegar as an imperceptible natural preservative.

Rev Up: An energizing blend of fresh purified water; flower essences of Blanketflower, Echinacea, and Sunflower; and raw organic apple cider vinegar as a natural preservative.

Living Flower Essences' Handmade Display Units

LFE offers two basic styles of handmade custom display units. Displays are made of oak or spruce, and will add beauty and elegance to any display counter. These displays can be freestanding or mounted on a wall.

Professional Display: The first style, designed for professional use, contains three shelves. The entire display cabinet holds three each of forty-eight $^1/_2$-ounce individual essences, totaling 144 bottles. This display is approximately 24 inches long and 14 $^1/_2$ inches tall and 4 inches deep.

Economy Display: The second style is a smaller display and also contains three shelves. This display holds a maximum of thirty-nine $^1/_2$-ounce bottles of your choice. The display is approximately 15 $^1/_2$ inches long, 15 $^1/_2$ inches tall, and 3 $^1/_2$ inches deep.

Living Flower Essences' Flower Essence and Chakra Healing Practitioner Course

This 200-hour program is offered through Living Flower Essences, sponsored by the Arizona School of Integrative Studies (A.S.I.S.), and approved by the State of Arizona. It includes 125 correspondence hours and 75 experiential hours. This course for 240 contact hours has also been approved by the American Holistic Nurses Association, which is accredited as an Approver of Continuing Education in Nursing by the American Nurses Credentialing Center's Commission on Accreditation.

75-Hour Experiential Portion: This portion of the course includes two full weeks of hands-on experiences in nature, taught one week at a time. Students will learn both practical and intuitive approaches to using flower essences for themselves and others, including study of the chakras and their relationship to plants, healing, and personal balance.

In Verde Valley's natural surroundings, we will gather, collect, and journey with various plants and make mother essences from them. The course will address preparation of stock bottles, ordering supplies, and marketing. Health and safety issues will also be practiced and discussed.

125-Hour Correspondence Portion: This portion of the course will cover the history, integration, and basic therapeutic practices of herbalism, homeopathy, and flower essences. Special emphasis will be placed on the use and study of the chakra system and the corresponding essences. Students will be involved in provings and in working with essences personally and professionally.

For further information about this course, call: (928) 639-3614 or (928) 639-3455 or e-mail asis@wildapache.com or info@livingfloweressences.com.

plant Healers and Life celebrations women's Healing Retreats and Mother/Daughter Retreats

Join us for weekend retreats, co-facilitated by Rhonda PallasDowney and Veronica Vida, in the serene, rustic setting of a private hot springs near Safford, Arizona. Retreat activities and free time are offered to nurture both body and soul. Soak and play in the many natural hot-spring pools as you let your spirit soar.

Through ceremony, guided imagery, art, flower essences, aromatherapy, lotions, and potion-making, we will invoke and awaken healing energy. Using fruits, flowers, and plants to create body wraps and treatments, we will nourish and rejuvenate mind, body, and soul.

For more information, call (928) 639-3614 or visit www.livingfloweressences.com.

consultations

Telephone

If you are interested in a consultation, please telephone to schedule an appointment. You will receive your own personalized flower essence formula in a $^1/_2$ oz. cobalt bottle. Consultations are 45 minutes long and the fee is $55.00 which includes your own personalized formula. Add $5.50 to cover shipping and handling costs.

In person

If you are interested in a direct consultation that includes an interview and light energy/body work, please telephone to schedule an appointment.

These consultations are 1 to 1 $^1/_2$ hours long and take place in an office. The fee is $75, and includes your own personalized formula in a $^1/_2$ oz. cobalt bottle.

Living Flower Essences collects anecdotal case studies of clients and conducts ongoing provings of flower essences. Feedback regarding LFE is always welcome and appreciated. If you would like to participate in a provers' project, please contact LFE at (928) 639-3614.

Living Flower Essences
P.O. Box 1492 • Cottonwood, AZ 86326
Phone/Fax: (928) 639-3614
E-mail: info@livingfloweressences.com • www.livingfloweressences.com

Name: _____

Address: _____

City: _____ State: _____ Zip: _____

Telephone: _____ E-mail: _____

item description	price each	total cost
Individual Flower Essences: $^1/_2$ oz. cobalt-blue bottle	$10.95	
Specialty Flower Essences: $^1/_2$ oz. cobalt-blue bottle	$12.95	
Practitioner's Kit: 48 $^1/_2$ oz. cobalt-blue bottles (w/15% discount)	$446.76	
Set One: 24 $^1/_2$ oz. cobalt-blue bottles (w/12% discount)	$231.50	
Set Two: 24 $^1/_2$ oz. cobalt-blue bottles (w/12% discount)	$231.50	
Chakra Healing Kit: 7 $^1/_2$ oz. cobalt-blue bottles in colorful box	$69.95	
Practitioner's Canvas Bag: Call for available stock and colors	CALL FOR PRICING	
Chi Salve Only: 1 oz.	$6.50	
2 oz.	$12.95	
All other Salves: 1 oz.	$5.50	
2 oz.	$10.50	
4 oz.	$18.50	
Put together your own First Aid Kit: Choose 7-1 oz. salves (except Chi)	$35.95	
Bottled Flower-Essence Water: Chill Out or Rev Up (16.95 oz.)	CALL FOR PRICING	
Professional Display (holds up to 144 $^1/_2$-oz. cobalt-blue bottles)	$159.00	
Economy Display (holds up to 39 $^1/_2$-oz. cobalt-blue bottles)	$89.00	

Domestic Shipping and Handling Fees:
$25.00 or less $6.75
$25.00 to $69.00 $8.50
$70.00 to $150.00 $12.50
$151.00 and more   9% of order

Gift certificates available
Gift wrap: call for pricing
For Arizona orders, please add 8.5% sales tax

Special Discount: Choose any ten flower essence bottles and subtract 10%

Method of Payment: Check _____ Money Order _____ Visa _____ Mastercard _____

Make check or money order payable to Living Flower Essences

Credit Card Account Number: _____ Expiration Date: _____/_____

Credit card orders must include a signature.

Signature:_____ Date: _____/_____

CHAPTER NOTES

chapter 2

1   Manly P. Hall, *Paracelsus* (Los Angeles: The Philosophical Research Society Inc., 1964), p. 2.

2   Matthew Wood, *The Magical Staff* (Berkeley: North Atlantic Books, 1992), p. 25.

3   Ibid., p. 18.

4   Ibid., p. 19.

5   Ibid., p. 21.

6   Trevor Cook, *Homeopathic Medicine Today: A Modern Course Of Study* (New Canaan, Conn.: Keats Publishing Inc., 1989), p. 1.

7   George Vithoulkas, *The Science of Homeopathy* (New York: Grove Press, Inc., 1980), p. 96.

8   Nora Weeks, *The Medical Discoveries of Edward Bach, Physician* (New Canaan, Conn.: Keats Publishing, Inc., 1973), p. 35-3.

9   Gary Zukav, *The Seat of the Soul* (New York: Simon & Schuster, 1985), p. 31.

Resources Referenced:
Weeks, Nora, *The Medical Discoveries of Edward Bach, Physician.* New Canaan, Conn.: Keats Publishing, Inc., 1973.

chapter 3

1   *Metaphysical Bible Dictionary* (Unity Village, Mo.: Unity School of Christianity, 1931), p. 585 in reference to Exodus 25:31–39 and II Chronicles 13:11.

2   Ibid.

3   Holy Bible, King James Version (Wichita, Kans.: Fireside Bible Publishers, 1970), Genesis 9:12 & 13.

4   Barbara Brennan, *Hands of Light* (New York: Bantam Books, 1988), p. 31. The material in this section, "A Brief Historical Perspective on Chakras and the Human Energy Field," is also based on Brennan's book.

5   C.W. Leadbeater, *The Chakras* (Wheaton, Ill.: The Theosophical Publishing House, 1927, 5th Printing 1987).

6   Brennan, p. 33.

chapter 4

1   John Bradshaw, *The Family* (Deerfield Beach, Fla.: Health Communications, 1988), p. 45.

2   The International Network for Esoteric Healing, *Esoteric Healing, Part 1* (Hampshire, England: International Network for Esoteric Healing, 1993), p. 14.

3   Anodea Judith and Selene Vega, *The Sevenfold Journey* (Freedom, Calif.: The Crossing Press, 1993), p. 260.

4   Carolyn Myss, Ph.D., *Energy Anatomy* cassette tapes, (Boulder, Colo.: Sounds True Publishing, 1996).

5   David Sunfellow and James Gregory, *The NewHeaven, NewEarth News Brief,* Jan 10, 1997.

Resources Referenced:
    Kaptchuk, Ted J., *The Web That Has No Weaver.* New York: Congdon & Weed, Inc., 1983.

chapter 7

1   Muscle testing and pendulum dowsing material in this section is based on Ted Andrews, *The Healer's Manual* (St. Paul Minn.: Llewellyn Publications, 1996).

chapter 11

1   Matthew Wood, *Seven Herbs: Plants as Treachers* (Berkeley, Calif.: North Atlantic Books, 1986), p. 57.

2   Mabel Burkholder, *Before the White Man Came* (Plattsburgh, N.Y.: McClelland & Stewart, 1923).

3   *Culpeper's Complete Herbal* (Hertfordshire, England: Wordsworth Editions, Ltd. 1995), p. 248.

4   Harriette Lanner, *The Pinyon Pine: A Natural and Cultural History* (Reno, Nev.: University of Nevada Press, 1981), p. 62.

5   Christine Downing, *The Goddess: Mythological Images of the Feminine* (New York: Crossroad Publishing, 1984).

6   Edward Bach, *The Collected Writings of Edward Bach* (Bath, England: Ashgrove Press, 1994), p. 39.

7   Matthew Wood, Unpublished lecture in Cottonwood, Arizona, 1993.

8   ———, *Seven Herbs: Plants as Teachers* (Berkeley, Calif.: North Atlantic Books, 1986), p. 49.

GLOSSARY

ACHENE: A small, dry, hard one-seeded fruit that does not split open.

ACIDULOUS: Moderately tart, sour, or acidic.

ACUTE: Sharp or severe in its effect; a sudden onset of a condition that is short-acting and temporary in nature.

ALKALOID: Nitrogenous organic substances of vegetable origin, having alkaline properties.

ALTERNATE: A pattern of leaf growth on a stem, alternating from one side to another; not opposite.

ANTHER: The top of the stamen, which bears pollen.

ANNUAL: A plant that grows for only one season.

ANTISEPTIC: Having properties that prevent the growth of bacteria.

AREOLE: A small cavity from which spines develop on a cactus.

ASTRINGENT: A substance that decreases discharge of mucus from the nose, intestines, vagina, and draining sores by increasing the tone and firmness of the tissue.

AUTONOMIC NERVOUS SYSTEM: A part of the nervous system that functions independently of the will.

AUTONOMOUS: Self-governing.

AXIL: The angle between a leaf and the stem from which it arises.

AYURVEDA: An ancient system of healing from India, based on an integrative approach to health.

BASAL: Near the base or bottom of the plant.

BIENNIAL: A plant that completes its life cycle in two years, producing vegetation in its first year and flowers and seed in its second year.

BRACT: A modified leaf or leaf-like part that grows at the base of the flower head or fruit, resembling additional layers of sepals.

BROW CHAKRA: An energy center located slightly above and between the eyes; associated with the pineal gland and the entire endocrine system, the immune system, and the synapses of the brain. Also known as the sixth chakra, third eye, or ajna chakra.

CALYX: The usually green outer circle (whorl) of a flower, consisting of sepals.

CARMINATIVE: A plant composed of volatile oils that activate the expulsion of gas from the gastrointestinal tract, increasing muscle tone and relaxation of bowel movements.

CAROLIS, LINNAEUS (1707–1778): A Swedish botanist known as the "Father of Taxonomy." He developed the foundation for a system of naming, ranking, and classifying living organisms that is still in use today. He established the modern binomial system of nomenclature (genus name plus specis name) for plants and animals.

CATARRH: Inflammation of the mucous membranes, typically of the nose and throat, accompanied by watery discharge.

CATKINS: Small petalless flowers that grow in a long cluster; usually unisexual.

CELLULAR DROPSY: A disease in which bodily fluids collect in the body tissues.

CHAKRA SYSTEM: An ancient, universal concept of the human energy system as composed of subtle life-force energy centers; each center, or chakra, is represented by a color and a frequency vibration that includes sound and light.

CHI: See "Qi."

CHRONIC: Having an underlying cause that is of a more or less permanent nature. Chronic diseases are deep-seated and have no definite onset, direction, or end; either recovery is not possible, or there is lifelong suffering, or the condition reappears.

CLASPING LEAF: A growth pattern wherein the leaf stalk is wrapped around the stem.

COLIC: Pain associated with the abdomen or bowels.

COMPOSITE: A plant of the sunflower family (Compositae).

CONCENTRIC: A pattern of flower-petal growth in which each circle of petals has the same center.

COROLLA: The inner envelope of a flower, consisting of fused or separate parts.

CORONA: A trumpet-shaped appendage on the inner side of flower petals.

CORPUS CALLOSUM: A part of the brain of higher mammals that unites the left and right hemispheres.

CROWN CHAKRA: Located on the top of the head, this energy center is associated with the cerebral cortex, the central nervous system, the pituitary gland, and all the pathways of the nerves and electrical synapses within the body. It represents the two hemispheres of the brain and both conscious and unconscious thoughts. Also known as the seventh chakra.

CULPEPER, NICHOLAS (1616–1654): A physician and astrologer who believed that herbs and their uses should be available to everyone. He was a firm believer in the Doctrine of Signatures. Culpeper published two books, *The*

English Physician's: A People's Herbal and an English translation of the later *Pharmacopeia.* Culpeper also opened an apothecary that sold low-cost herbs to the public to further his goal. These actions gained him the enmity of the English medical community, which desired to control botanical knowledge and usage.

DECIDUOUS: A plant that sheds or drops its leaves each year.

DECOCTION: A process of extracting the healing qualities of the stronger parts of the plant, such as its bark, nuts, roots, and nonaromatic seeds, by one of two methods: either bringing water to a boil, adding the plant parts, and letting them simmer for fifteen to twenty minutes, or by placing the plant parts in a pan of cold water on low heat for fifteen to twenty minutes.

DIAPHORETIC: An herb that induces perspiration and affects the entire circulatory system.

DIOSCORIDES, PEDANIUS: A Greek physician and pharmacologist with the Roman armies of the first century A.D. His *De Materia Medica* provided the use and description of about 1,000 herbs known during his time. His manuscript served as the source for all books on the subject of herbs for at least the next 1,500 years.

DISK: The center of a flower that consists of tiny tubular petals.

DISSECTED: Leaves that are divided into numerous narrow sections.

DIURETIC: An herb that activates the flow of urine.

DYSCRASIA: An abnormal or undefined blood disease.

DYSMENORRHEA: Painful cramping in the lower abdomen associated with menses.

EMETIC: An herb that induces vomiting.

EMMENAGAGUE: An agent that promotes the menstrual discharge.

EXPECTORANT: An herb that releases mucous discharge or phlegm from the throat or lungs, often by coughing.

EXTRACTION: Preparation of herbs by aging them in alcohol or apple cider vinegar.

GERARD, JOHN (1545–1612): Author of *The Herball or General Historie of Plantes,* which was an important compilation of the work of previous and contemporary herbalists and authors. He also included new information about plants arriving from the New World. Gerard was a medical man, apprenticed at an early age to a warden of the Barber-Surgeon Company, of which he later became chairman. However, his main interests lay with his gardens and herbal research.

HEART CHAKRA: The energy center that relates to the functions of the heart, the thymus gland, the immune system, and the circulatory system. This center is also associated with the right hemisphere of the brain and with tissue regeneration. Also known as the fourth chakra.

HEMOSTATIC: An herb that alleviates internal bleeding or hemorrhaging.

HERING'S LAW (LAW OF HEALING): This law, named for homeopath Constantine Hering, states that, in order for true healing to take place, it must first begin at the deepest parts of the person and proceed to the less vital parts. It is the process of sorting out impurities, from within to without, observing that symptoms leave the body in the reverse order of how they began. This law teaches us the importance of selecting the remedy that will take us in the direction of cure.

HYDROCEPHALUS: A condition of the brain in which excessive cerebrospinal fluid accumulates within the cavities of the brain, resulting in mental deficiency.

INFUSION (HERBS): A process of steeping the more delicate parts of the plant, such as its leaves, stems, blossoms, or powdered herb, by pouring boiling water over the plant parts and steeping them for fifteen minutes or bit longer, making it into a tea.

INVOLUCRE: Bracts and leaves that encircle or support a flower head.

IRREGULAR: Flower parts that are unequal in size and shape.

JOINT: A plant node or a section of a stem.

KUNDALINI: A Hindu word referring to the vital energy at the base of the spine that is channeled upward through the body in a spiral pattern to the brain; this is called an "awakening" of energy.

LANCEOLATE: A lance-like leaf shape: long, narrow, and tapering to the tip.

LAW OF HEALING: *See* "Hering's Law."

LEAFLET: One section of a compound leaf.

LEAFSTALK: The part of a plant that attaches a leaf to the main stem.

LINEAR: A leaf shape that is long and narrow and has parallel margins or edges.

LIP: Two folds that form the upper or lower segment of an irregular flower.

LOBED: A leaf shape that is roundish with marginal indentations dividing the leaf less than halfway.

MANDALA: A round geometric design that is often used in meditation.

MODALITIES: As related to LFE's Research Prover's Project, refer to any kind of modifying influences that either aggravate (worsen) or ameliorate (improve) a patient's symptoms. Modalities influence the choice of a homeopathic medicine and are demonstrated in various forms, including physical (touch, rest, exercise, position of the body), temperature (cold, damp, warmth, climate), time (day, night, hour of the day, season), dietary (food, drink, alcohol), localized (right- or left-sided symptoms), and other miscellaneous modalities. Very few modalities were given by providers and the ones that were pertained mostly to sleep patterns.

MUCILAGINOUS: Full of or secreting mucus.

NEURALGIC: A sharp, intermittent pain that occurs along a nerve, especially in the head or face.

NODE: The joint or part of the stem from which a leaf or bud sprouts.

OBLANCEOLATE: A leaf shape that is roundish and somewhat short.

OPPOSITE: A pattern of growth in which leaves grow in pairs opposite each other on a stem.

OVAL: A leaf shape like an egg.

OVARY: The hollow lower region of the pistil containing the female germ cells, which are fertilized by pollen and develop into seeds.

PALMATELY COMPOUND: A leaf shape in which leaves are divided or lobed from the same point, extending outward like fingers on a hand.

PARASYMPATHETIC NERVOUS SYSTEM: One of two portions of the autonomic nervous system. This system consists of nerves and ganglia that arise from the cranial and sacral regions and functions opposite but in harmony with the sympathetic nervous system. It controls the involuntary activities of the organs, glands, blood vessels, and other tissues in the body.

PATHOGENIC AGENT: A bacteria or virus that causes disease.

PERENNIAL: A type of plant that lives longer than two years.

PERITONEUM: The membrane lining the stomach.

PETAL: A segment of the corolla of a flower.

PETIOLE: A leaf stem.

PINNATELY COMPOUND: A leaf shape in which leaves are divided and lobed along each side of a leafstalk and appear similar to a feather.

PISTIL: The female organ of a flower, including the ovary, a thin style, and a stigma.

PLINY (A.D. 23–A.D. 79): The Roman Pliny (or Pliny the Elder), best known for his massive thirty-seven-volume *Natural History,* part of which is devoted to botany and medicinal plants. It is speculated that the information in these volumes may not have been well researched, leading to some bizarre uses of herbs by common people.

POLLEN: Male germ cells that grow in the anthers of a flower.

POTENTIZE: A homeopathic term referring to the steps of dilution and succussion in the preparation of remedies. The more potentized a remedy becomes, the greater its therapeutic effect.

POTHERB: An herb prepared to eat as food or as seasoning for food.

POULTICE: A soft, heated mix of chopped, grated, blended, or powdered herbs wrapped in a cloth and applied directly to the skin to treat external swellings such as inflammations, wounds, stings, bites, or chest colds.

PSOAS: A muscle of the loin.

QI (OR CHI): The energy or vital life-force energy of a human being.

RACEME: A group of flowers attached to a main stem by short stalks, with newer flowers forming at the top.

RAY FLOWERS: Flat, straplike flowers that form a ring around the disk flowers in a composite head.

REGULAR: A growth pattern in which the petals or sepals of a flower are radially symmetrical and of equal size and shape.

RIBS: The main veins of leaves or the ridges of cacti.

ROOT CHAKRA: The energy center located between the tailbone (the coccyx) and the pubic bone. It includes the entire pelvic area and the functions of the anus, rectum, circulatory system, kidneys, and reproductive system (including the testicles and ovaries), and the lower extremities (feet and legs). Also known as the physical, base, or first chakra.

ROSETTE: A cluster of leaves growing in a circle at the base of a plant.

RUBRICS: Keynotes, symptoms, or main features that correlate with a flower essence remedy.

SAPONINS: Substances in a plant that have soaplike qualities.

SEPAL: One of the modified leaves that form the calyx of a flower.

SESSILE: A manner of leaf attachment without a stalk or stem.

SMUDGE: A Native American method of cleansing and purifying the body/mind by burning herbs such as sweetgrass or sage.

SOLAR PLEXUS CHAKRA: The energy center that includes the functions of the adrenals, stomach, digestive system, assimilation process, liver, and gall bladder. This center is also associated with the left hemisphere of the brain and its activities. Also known as the third chakra or mental chakra.

SPINE: A sharp needle-like outgrowth on a plant stem or cactus.

SPLEEN CHAKRA: The energy center that encompasses the lower back, the muscles, and the reproductive system, including prostate and sex organs and the production of estrogen, progesterone, sperm, and testosterone. It also includes the partial functions of the adrenal glands, the lymphatic glands, the spleen, the bladder, the pancreas, and the kidneys. This center also affects the process of elimination and detoxification of the body. Also known as the second chakra or emotional chakra.

SPUR: A hollow tubular projection from the base of a petal or sepal, which usually produces nectar.

STAHL, GEORG ERNST (1659–1734): Believed the "soul" was seated in the stomach and was in charge of life's activities.

STAMEN: The pollen-bearing male organ of a flower, consisting of a filament and an anther.

STEM: The stalk that supports a leaf or flower.

STIGMA: The top part of the pistil, which receives pollen during pollination.

STYLE: The narrow part of the pistil, where the ovary and stigma join.

SUCCULENT: A plant or part of a plant that is fleshy and juicy.

SUCCUSS: A homeopathic term referring to a method of vigorous shaking with impact in each sequential step of the dilution process. Succussion creates a mechanical action within the smallest particles of a substance by shaking it with an inactive substance in order to separate the particles. Succussion creates a noticeable change in the quality of a substance, thereby releasing its power to heal and influencing the vital force of the inert substance.

SYMPATHETIC NERVOUS SYSTEM: One of the two portions of the autonomic nervous system, consisting of nerves and ganglia that arise from the thoracic and lumbar regions of the spinal cord. It functions opposite but in harmony with the parasympathetic nervous system and controls many of the involuntary activities of the glands, organs, and other parts of the body.

SYNAPSE: The region of contact between two nerve cells across which a signal passes. A single nerve cell may form thousands of these connections with adjacent nerve cells.

TAPROOT: A main root that stores food, with descending branches that draw nutrients.

TENDRIL: A modified stem or leaf that allows a plant to attach itself to and climb up another plant or a structure.

TERMINAL: The end of a branch or stem.

THROAT CHAKRA: The energy center that includes the throat, larynx, tongue, mouth, lips, teeth, esophagus, thyroid, and parathyroid glands. It also includes the activities of the respira-tory system, bronchial and vocal functions, and the processing and absorption of nutrients. The throat chakra is associated with the upper extremities, neck, shoulders, arms, and hands. Also known as the fifth chakra and the communication chakra.

THYMUS: A gland situated in the upper part of the chest, behind the breastbone, consisting of two lobes that join in front of the trachea (windpipe). This gland acts as a vital part in the body's defense against viruses and other infections.

TINCTURE: A highly concentrated liquid extract consisting of herbs aged in alcohol or apple cider vinegar.

TUBULAR: A form of flower in which the petals unite to form a tube.

UMBEL: A flower cluster shaped like an umbrella, with flowers spreading from a common center.

VOLATILE OIL: An oil that evaporates quickly, usually made from plant tissue.

WHORL: A circular arrangement of three or more leaves or flower parts shaped like a coil and radiating outward from a point on an axis of the stem.

WILDCRAFTED: Plants picked in their natural environments, such as in mountain meadows, along streams, or in desert canyons.

WOOLLY: Having fuzzy, soft, wool-like hairs.

WOUNDWORT: A remedy used to treat wounds, such as cuts, burns, sprains, inflammatory conditions, or broken bones.

BIBLIOGRAPHY

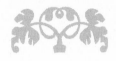

Abbey, Edward. *Desert Solitaire: A Season in The Wilderness.* New York: Ballantine Books, 1968.

Andrews, Ted. *Animal-Speak.* St. Paul, Minn.: Llewellyn Publications, 1993.

———. *The Healer's Manual.* St. Paul, Minn.: Llewellyn Publications, 1996.

Arnberger, Leslie P. *Flowers of the Southwest Mountains.* Salt Lake City: Southwest Parks and Monuments Association, 1982.

Bach, Edward, M.D. *The Collected Writings of Edward Bach.* Bath, England: Ashgrove Press, 1994.

Bach, Edward, M.D., and F. J. Wheeler, M.D. *The Bach Flower Remedies.* New Canaan, Conn.: Keats Publishing, Inc., 1977.

Bailey, Alice A. *The Soul and Its Mechanism.* New York: Lucis Publishing Company, 1930.

Barnard, Julian. *Patterns of Life Force.* Hereford, England: Flower Remedy Programme, 1987.

Barnette, Martha. *A Garden of Words.* New York: Times Books, a Division of Random House, Inc., 1992.

Blunt, Wilfrid and Sandra Raphael. *The Illustrated Herbal.* New York: Francis Lincoln Publishers Ltd., Thames and Hudson, Inc., 1979.

Boericke, W., M.D. *Homoeopathic Materia Medica and Repertory.* New Delhi, India: B. Jain Publishers, Limited, 1995.

Bowers, Janice Emily. *100 Desert Wildflowers of the Southwest.* Salt Lake City: Lorraine Press, 1989.

———. *100 Roadside Wildflowers of Southwest Woodlands.* Salt Lake City: Lorraine Press, 1987.

———. *Shrubs and Trees of the Southwest Deserts.* Salt Lake City: Southwest Parks and Monuments Association, 1993.

Bradshaw, John. *The Family.* Deerfield Beach, Fla.: Health Communications, Inc., 1988.

Bremness, Lesley. *The Complete Book of Herbs.* London: Dorling Kindersley Limited, 1988.

———. *Herbs.* New York: Dorling Kindersley, Inc., 1994.

Brennan, Barbara Ann. *Hands of Light.* New York: Bantam Books, 1988.

Brewster, J. L. *Onions and Other Vegetable Alliums.* Oxford, U.K: Cab International, 1994.

British Institute of Homoeopathy Diploma Coursework, Surrey, England: Homoeopathic Studies Ltd., 1996.

Bruyere, Rosalyn L. *Wheels of Light.* New York: Fireside, 1994.

Burkholder, Mabel, *Before White Man Came.* Plattsburgh, N.Y.: McClelland & Stewart, 1923.

Chancellors, Philip M., M.D. *Bach Flower Remedies.* New Canaan, Conn.: Keats Publishing, Inc., 1971.

Chevallier, Andrew. *The Encyclopedia of Medicinal Plants.* New York: DK Publishing, Inc., 1996.

Christopher, John R., M.D. *School of Natural Healing.* Provo, Utah: BiWorld Publishers, Inc., 1976.

Clarke, John Henry, M.D. *A Dictionary Of Practical Materia Medica.* New Delhi, India: B. Jain Publishers, Limited, 1994.

Coats, Alice M. *Flowers and Their Histories.* New York: McGraw-Hill Book Company, 1971.

Cook, Trevor. *Homeopathic Medicine Today: A Modern Course of Study.* New Canaan, Conn.: Keats Publishing, Inc., 1989.

Cousens, Gabriel, M.D. *Spiritual Nutrition and the Rainbow Diet.* Boulder, Colo.: Cassandra Press, 1986.

Cowan, Eliot. *Plant Spirit Medicine.* Newberg, Ore.: Swan Raven & Company, 1995.

Craighead, John J., Frank Craighead, Jr., and Ray J. Davis. *A Field Guide to Rocky Mountain Wildflowers.* Cambridge, Mass.: The Riverside Press, 1963.

Culpeper's Complete Herbal. Hertfordshire, England: Wordsworth Editions, Ltd., 1995.

Cunningham, Donna. *Flower Remedies Handbook.* New York: Sterling Publishing Co., Inc., 1992.

Dalichow, Irene and Mike Booth. *Aura-Soma.* Carlsbad, Calif.: Hay House, Inc., 1996.

Desert Botanical Garden Staff. *Desert Wildflowers.* Phoenix, Ariz.: *Arizona Highways,* 1988.

Devi, Indra. *Yoga for Americans.* Englewood Cliffs, N.J.: Prentice-Hall, Inc., 1959.

Dodge, Natt N. *Flowers of the Southwest Deserts.* Tucson, Ariz.: Southwest Parks and Monuments Association, 1985.

Dorson, Richard M. *Folklore and Folklife.* Chicago: University of Chicago Press, 1972.

Downing, Christine. *The Goddess: Mythological Images of the Feminine.* New York: Crossroad Publishing, 1984.

Dunmire, William W. and Gail D. Tierney. *Wild Plants of the Pueblo Province.* Santa Fe, N. Mex.: Museum of New Mexico Press, 1995.

Elmore, Francis H. *Shrubs and Trees of the Southwest Uplands.* Tucson, Ariz.:

Southwest Parks and Monuments Association, 1976.

Encyclopaedia Britannica. *The New Encyclopaedia Britannica.* Chicago: Encyclopaedia Britannica, Inc., University of Chicago, 1993.

Epple, Anne Orth. *A Field Guide to the Plants of Arizona.* Helena, Mont.: Falcon Press Publishing Company, Inc., 1995.

Epstein, Ron. *Making and Using Flower Essences.* Los Angeles: Self-published, 1986.

Erichsen-Brown, Charlotte. *Medicinal and Other Uses of Native American Plants: A Historical Survey with Special Reference to the Eastern Indian Tribes.* Toronto: General Publishing Company, Ltd., 1979.

————. *Medicinal and Other Uses of North American Plants.* Minneola, N.Y.: Dover Publications, 1989.

Evans, Mark. *A Guide to Herbal Remedies.* Essex, England: The C. W. Daniel Company Ltd. and Wigmore Publications, 1990.

Forey, Pam. *Wildflowers of North America.* San Diego, Calif.: Thunderbay Press, 1994.

Gerber, Richard, M.D. *Vibrational Medicine.* Santa Fe, N. Mex.: Bear & Company, 1988.

Gibbons, Euell. *Stalking the Healthful Herbs.* New York: David McKay Company, Inc., 1966.

Gimbel, Theo, D.C.E. *Healing Through Color.* Essex, England: The C.W. Daniel Company, Ltd., 1980.

Gladstar, Rosemary. *Herbal Healing for Women.* New York: Simon & Schuster, 1993.

————. *The Science and Art of Herbalism.* E. Barre, Vermont: Sage Mountain, 1984.

Grieve, M. *A Modern Herbal.* 2 vols. New York: Dover Publications, Inc., 1971.

Gunther, Bernard. *Energy Ecstasy and Your Seven Vital Chakras.* Van Nuys, Calif.: Newcastle Publishing Company, 1983.

Gurudas. *The Spiritual Properties of Herbs.* San Rafael, Calif.: Cassandra Press, 1988.

Hahnemann, Samuel. *Organon of Medicine.* 6th ed. New Delhi, India: Homeopathic Publications, 1921.

Hall, Manly P. *Paracelsus.* Los Angeles: The Philosophical Research Society Inc., 1964.

Hayfield, Robyn. *Homeopathy for Common Ailments.* Berkeley, Calif.: Frog Limited, 1993.

Heline, Corinne. *Color and Music in the New Age.* Marina del Rey, Calif.: DeVorss and Company, 1985.

————. *Healing and Regeneration through Color.* Marina del Rey, Calif.: DeVorss and Company, 1983.

Hermann, Matthias. *Herbs and Medicinal Flowers.* New York: Galahad Books, 1973.

Hill, Lewis and Nancy Hill. *Successful Perennial Gardening.* Pownal, Vt.: A Garden Way Publishing Book, Storey Communications, Inc., 1988.

Hodge, Carle. *All About Saguaros.*

Phoenix, Ariz.: *Arizona Highways* Magazine, 1991.

Hoffmann, David. *The Holistic Herbal.* The Park, Forres, Scotland: Findhorn Press, 1983.

Holmes, Peter. *The Energetics of Western Herbs.* 2 vols. Boulder, Colo.: Artemis Press, 1989.

Holy Bible, King James Version. Wichita, Kans.: Fireside Bible Publishers, 1970.

Howard, A. B., M.D. *Herbal Extracts.* Berkley, Mich.: The Blue Goose Press, 1983.

Hutchens, Alma R. *Indian Herbalogy of North America.* Boston: Shambhala Publications, Inc., 1973.

Jacobs, Betty E. M. *Growing and Using Herbs Successfully.* Pownal, Vt.: A Garden Way Publishing Book, 1976.

James, William R. and Wilma Roberts James. *Know Your Poisonous Plants.* Happy Camp, Calif.: Naturegraph Publishers, Inc., 1973.

Johnson, Steve M. *Flower Essences of Alaska.* Homer, Alaska: Alaskan Flower Essence Project, 1992.

Joshi, Sunil, M.D. *Ayurveda and Panchakarma.* Twin Lakes, Wisc.: Lotus Press, 1997.

Judith, Anodea. *Wheels of Life.* St. Paul, Minn.: Llewellyn Publications, 1988.

Judith, Anodea and Selene Vega. *The Sevenfold Journey.* Freedom, Calif.: The Crossing Press, 1993.

Kaptchuk, Ted J., O.M.D. *The Web That Has No Weaver.* New York: Congdon & Weed, Inc., 1983.

Katz, Richard and Patricia Kaminsky. *Flower Essence Repertory.* Nevada City, Calif.: Flower Essence Society, 1994.

Keith, Velma J. and Monteen Gordon. *The How to Herb Book.* Pleasant Grove, Utah: Mayfield Publishing, 1984.

Kent, J. T. *Kent's Repertory.* New Delhi, India: B. Jain Publishers Limited, 1988.

Kent, James Tyler, M.D. *Lectures on Homoeopathic Philosophy.* Berkeley, Calif.: North Atlantic Books, 1900.

Kirk, Donald. *Wild Edible Plants of the Western United States.* Healdsburg, Calif.: Naturegraph Publishers, 1970.

Kowalchik, Claire and William Hylton. *Rodale's Encyclopedia of Herbs.* Emmaus, Penn.: Rodale Press, 1987.

Kroeger, Hanna. *Instant Herbal Locater.* Boulder, Colo.: Self-published, 1979.

Kruger, Anna. *An Illustrated Guide to Herbs, Their Medicine and Magic.* Surrey, England: Dragon's World Limited, 1993.

Lanner, Harriette. *The Pinyon Pine: A Natural and Cultural History.* Reno, Nev.: University of Nevada Press, 1981.

Leadbeater, C. W. *Man Visible and Invisible.* Wheaton, Ill.: The Theosophical Publishing House, 1971.

———. *The Chakras.* Wheaton, Ill.: The Theosophical Publishing House, 1927.

Leek, Sybil. *Book of Herbs.* Nashville, Tenn.: Thomas Nelson Inc., 1973.

Lemmon, Robert S. and Charles L. Sherman. *Flowers of the World.* Garden City, N.Y.: Doubleday & Company, Inc., 1964.

Lockie, Andrew, M.D. and Nicola Geddes, M.D. *Homeopathy: The Principles and Practice of Treatment.* London: Dorling Kindersley Limited, 1995.

Lommen, Ursula K. E. *Essential Oils Reference Manual.* Maple Plain, Minn.: Una Publishing, 1994.

Magley, Beverly. *Arizona Wildflowers.* Billings, Mont.: Falcon Press Publishing Company, 1991.

Mansfield, Peter. *Flower Remedies.* Boston: Charles E. Tuttle Publishing, 1995.

Mark-Age. *Twelve Spiritual Systems.* 2 vols. Fort Lauderdale, Fla.: Mark-Age Inc., 1981.

Mason, Charles, Jr., and Patricia B. Mason. *Mexican Roadside Flora.* Tucson, Ariz.: The University Press, 1987.

Mayes, Vernon O. and Barbara Bayless Lacy. *Nanise': A Navajo Herbal.* Tsaile, Ariz.: Navajo Community College Press, 1989.

McHoy, Peter and Pamela Westland. *The Herb Bible.* London: Barnes & Noble Books, 1994.

McPherson, Alan and Sue McPherson. *Edible and Useful Wild Plants of the Urban West.* Boulder, Colo.: Pruett Publishing Company, 1947.

Meuninck, Jim. *The Basic Essentials of Edible Wild Plants and Useful Herbs.* Merrillville, Ind.: ICS Books, Inc., 1988.

Mindell, Earl. *Earl Mindell's Herb Bible.* New York: Simon & Schuster, 1992.

Moore, Michael. *Medicinal Plants of the Desert and Canyon West.* Santa Fe, N. Mex.: The Museum of New Mexico Press, 1989.

———. *Medicinal Plants of the Mountain West.* Santa Fe, N. Mex.: The Museum of New Mexico Press, 1979.

Muktananda, Swami. *Play of Consciousness.* South Fallsburg, N.Y.: SYDA Foundation, 1978.

Myss, Caroline, PH.D. *Energy Anatomy.* Louisville, Colo.: Sounds True Publishing, 1996.

Nada-Yolanda. *Birth of the Light Body.* Fort Lauderdale, Fla.: Mark-Age Inc., 1995.

———. *Seven Rays of Life.* Fort Lauderdale, Fla.: Mark-Age Inc., 1980.

Nelson, Ruth Ashton. *Plants of Zion National Park.* Springdale, Utah: Deseret Press, 1976.

Noble, Vicky. *Motherpeace: A Way to the Goddess through Myth, Art, and Tarot.* San Francisco: HarperSanFrancisco, 1994.

Ody, Penelope. *The Complete Medicinal Herbal.* New York: Dorling Kindersley, Inc., 1993.

O'Reilly, Aleia. *Rainbow Warriors Awake.* Flagstaff, Ariz.: Little Hummingbird Publishing, 1994.

Panos, Maesimund B., M.D. and Jane Heimlich. *Homeopathic Medicine at Home.* Los Angeles: J. P. Tarcher, Inc., 1980.

Pesman, Walter M. *Meet Flora Mexicana.* Globe, Ariz.: Dale S. King, Publisher, 1962.

Phillips, Arthur M., III. *Grand Canyon Wildflowers.* Salt Lake City: Lorraine Press, 1990.

Quillin, Patrick. *The Wisdom of Amish Folk Medicine.*: North Canton, Ohio: The Leader Company, Inc., 1984.

Rain, Mary Summer. *Earthway.* New York: Pocket Books, 1990.

Raphaell, Katrina. *Crystal Enlightenment.* New York: Aurora Press, 1985.

Ray, Richard and Michael R. MacCaskey. *Roses: How to Select, Grow, and Enjoy.* Los Angeles: Horticultural Publications Company Inc., H P Books, 1981.

Ritchason, Jack. *The Little Herb Encyclopedia.* Orem, Utah: Biworld Publishers, 1982.

Roberts and Nelson. *Mountain Wild Flowers of Colorado and Adjacent Areas.* Denver: Denver Museum of Natural History, 1967.

Rodale Press. *Field Guide to Wild Herbs.* Emmaus, Penn.: Rodale Press, Inc., 1987.

————. *Rodale's Illustrated Encyclopedia of Herbs.* Emmaus, Penn.: Rodale Press, 1987.

Scheffer, Mechthild. *Bach Flower Therapy.* Rochester, Vt.: Healing Arts Press, 1988.

Schneck, Marcus. *Cacti.* Avenel, N.J.: Crescent Books, 1992.

Scully, Virginia. *A Treasury of American Indian Herbs.* New York: Bonanza Books, 1970.

Selby, John. *Kundalini Awakening: A Gentle Guide to Chakra Activation and Spiritual Growth.* N.Y.: Bantam Books, 1992.

Spellenerg, Richard. *National Audubon Society Field Guide to North American Wildflowers.* Toronto: Chanticleer Press, Inc., 1994.

Sri Aurobindo Ashram. *The Mother: Flowers and Their Messages.* Aspiration, India: Sri Aurobindo Ashram Publishers, 1984.

Strehlow, Dr. Wighard and Gottfried Hertzka, M.D.. *Hildegard of Bingen's Medicine.* Santa Fe, N. Mex.: Bear & Company, 1988.

Stubendieck, J., Stephan L. Hatch, and Kathie J. Hirsch. *North American Range Plants.* Lincoln, Nebr.: University of Nebraska Press, 1945.

Sunfellow, David and James Gregory. *The NewHeaven NewEarth News Brief,* Jan 10, 1997.

Sunset Books and *Sunset Magazine. Sunset Western Garden Book.* Menlo Park, Calif.: Lane Publishing Co., 1995.

Sweet, Muriel. *Common Edible and Useful Plants of the West.* Happy Camp, Calif.: Naturegraph Publishers, 1976.

Tenney, Louise. *Today's Herbal Health.* Provo, Utah: Woodland Books, 1983.

Thomas, Lalitha. *10 Essential Herbs.* Prescott, Ariz.: Hohm Press, 1996.

Unity School of Christianity. *Metaphysical Bible Dictionary.* Unity Village, Mo.:, 1931.

University of Wyoming. *Weeds of the West.* Jackson, Wyo.: Pioneer of Jackson Hole, 1996.

Venning, Frank D. *Wildflowers of North America.* Racine, Wisc.: Golden Press, New York and Western Publishing Company, Inc., 1984.

Vida, Veronica. "The Stranger." Unpublished poem, 1997.

Vithoulkas, George. *The Science of*

Homeopathy. New York: Grove Press, Inc., 1980.

Vlamis, Gregory. *Bach Flower Remedies to the Rescue.* Rochester, Vt.: Healing Arts Press, 1986.

Ward, Harold. *Herbal Manual.* London: L. N. Fowler & Co., Ltd., 1969.

Weber, Ruth and Heinz Weber. *The Dictionary of Healing Plants.* London: Blandford Press, 1989.

Weeks, Nora. *The Medical Discoveries of Edward Bach, Physician.* New Canaan, Conn.: Keats Publishing, Inc., 1973.

Weiner, Dr. Michael. *Weiner's Herbal: The Guide to Herb Medicine.* Briar Cliff Manor, N.Y.: Stein & Day Publishers, 1982.

————. *Earth Foods.* Toronto: Collier-MacMillan Limited, 1972.

Wherry, Edgar T. *Wild Flower Guide.* New York: Doubleday & Company, Inc. and The American Garden Guild, Inc., 1948.

Wood, Matthew. *The Magical Staff.* Berkeley, Calif.: North Atlantic Books, 1992.

————. *Seven Herbs: Plants as Teachers.* Berkeley, Calif.: North Atlantic Books, 1986.

————. *The Book of Herbal Wisdom: Using Plants as Medicine.* Berkeley, Calif.: North Atlantic Books, 1997.

Wren, R. C., F.L.S. *Potter's New Cyclopedia of Botanical Drugs and Preparations.* Essex, England: The C. W. Daniel Company Limited, 1994.

Zimmerman, James H. and Booth Courtenay. *Wildflowers and Weeds.* New York: Simon & Schuster, 1978.

Zukav, Gary. *The Seat of the Soul.* New York: Simon & Schuster, 1985.

INDEX

Main entries appear in bold type.

A

abandonment: Indian Paintbrush, 114, 228, 229; Mexican Hat, 242; Mullein, 254; Sweet Pea, 116, 346, 347; Yellow Monkeyflower, 117, 384, 385

abundance: Desert Willow, 113, 206, 207; Pomegranate, 115, 300, 302; Purple Robe, 115, 308, 309; Saguaro, 320; Wild Rose, 364

abuse, physical: Bells-of-Ireland, 127, 129; Black-Eyed Susan, 131; Mexican Hat, 114, 242; Sweet Pea, 346

abuse, verbal: Crimson Monkeyflower, 113, 192, 193; Palmer's Penstemon, 115, 273, 274

accomplishment: Vervain, 117, 357, 358

addiction.7; Black-Eyed Susan, 131; Blue Flag (Iris), 144; Mexican Hat, 114, 242

agitation: Scarlet Penstemon, 116, 327, 328

aggression: Crimson Monkeyflower, 113, 192, 193; Mullein, 254; Strawberry Hedgehog, 116, 333, 334

amend-making: Paloverde, 115, 278, 279

anger: Crimson Monkeyflower, 113, 192, 193, 195; Indian Paintbrush, 114, 228, 229; Mexican Hat, 114, 242; Palmer's Penstemon, 115, 273, 274; pink flower essence and, 76–77; red flower essence and, 76; Scarlet Penstemon, 116, 327, 328; second chakra, 36, 37, 38; sixth chakra, 53; Sunflower, 116, 339, 341; transforming, 38

anxiety: Calendula, 112, 152; Chamomile, 112, 167, 168; Chicory, 173; Honeysuckle, 223;

Paloverde, 279; sixth chakra, 53; Thistle, 116, 351, 352, 354–55; Yarrow, 117, 376, 379; Yerba Santa, 117, 390, 391

apathy: Wild Rose, 117, 362, 363, 366. *See also ennui*

appreciation: Blue Flag (Iris), 142; Columbine, 113, 182, 183; Desert Willow, 113, 206, 207; Pinyon, 115, 291, 293

arcana, 6

Aristotle, 6, 10

assertiveness: Sunflower, 341; Yellow Monkeyflower, 117, 384, 385

Aster (Desert Aster), **120–25;** affirmations, 123; case history, 123–24; color, 121, 122; Doctrine of Signatures, 121–22; dreams/nightmares, 125; emotional symptoms, 125; features of the original flower-essence water, 121; helpful suggestions, 122–23; Key Rubrics Guide, 112; mental symptoms, 124; patterns of imbalance, 124; physical makeup, 121; physical symptoms, 124; positive healing patterns, 54, 120–21; quality: illumination, 107, 120; sixth chakra, 120, 122; spiritual principles, following, 54; spiritual reflections, 124–25; symptoms and patterns of imbalance, 121; third chakra, 41, 120, 122; traditional use, 120; sixth chakra (third eye), 51, 54, 122

attachments, 37; Century Plant, 162; Honeysuckle, 114, 222, 223; Mexican Hat, 114, 242, 243

auras, 28–29

Aurobindo, Sri, 47

avoidance: Black-Eyed Susan, 112, 131–32, 134; Paloverde, 115, 278, 279; Wild Rose, 117, 362, 364

C

H

I

J

K

L

M

S

ACKNOWLEDGMENTS

Many people have generously given their time and talents to the birth of this book. I am fortunate to have received loving support and dedication throughout this work, which began sixteen years ago when I met herbalist Matthew Wood. As a mentor and friend, Matthew inspired me to explore the vast world of plants and their flowers. He also provided valuable feedback on early versions of this book. I also give thanks to Alana Marie Davis for pursuing with me the profound healing qualities of flower essences.

I am truly grateful for my husband, Curt PallasDowney. He has lovingly encouraged my work throughout the years. Curt's knowledge of and passion for religious mystery have contributed significantly to this book, especially in the chapters related to the chakras. He has also shared with me his deep insights, understanding, and magical experiences of nature's plant kingdom.

I extend heartfelt appreciation to Roby Nelson and Veronica Vida for their unconditional friendship, wisdom, and support; for all the time they spend with me in nature; and for their incredible insights into the plant world.

I give great thanks to Charlie McGuire and Wendy Wetzel for their friendship, direction, and assistance with this book, and for directing me and supporting me to pursue nursing contact hours with the American Holistic Nurses Association in relation to my Living Flower Essences' "Flower Essence and Chakra Healing Practitioner Course." I extend my appreciation to Joseph and Jamie Rongo, owners of the Arizona School of Integrative Studies (A.S.I.S.) in Clarkdale, Arizona; they facilitated the State of Arizona's approval for the Flower Essence and Chakra Healing Practitioner Course sponsored by A.S.I.S. (see Appendix). This book is the foundation for that course. I gratefully acknowledge Nancy DePuy for her friendship and support. She has a special relationship with the plant kingdom and she devoted endless hours of work to this book.

I deeply thank Joy Wilson Loerger for her financial support in assisting this project to manifest. I give warm appreciation to Dr. Trevor Cook, one of my mentors and the Director of the British Institute of Homoeopathy, for his kind support of my work. I am grateful to Steve Stubenrauch, Doctor of Oriental Medicine (OMD), for his expertise and assistance with "The Eight Principle Patterns of Chinese Herbal Medicine" and with the discussion of plants in chapter 4: The Seven Chakras.

I extend my gratitude to Dr. Gail Derin Kellogg, OMD and Classical Homeopath, for her guidance and review of the homeopathic descriptions listed in the Materia Medica and for her general critique of this book. I thank Eileen Nauman, DHM, for providing direction and for generating the original Provers' Research Diary, which I modified for my Research Provers' Project. I am also deeply grateful to Karen David and her staff at Mystic Farms in Glen Willow, Ohio, who helped facilitate the Research Provers' Project.

Dr. Michael Edmiston, Professor of Chemistry and Physics at Bluffton College in Bluffton, Ohio, generously assisted me in developing the essence formulas and performed laboratory evaluation of the essences and herbal tinctures that I make. James Gregory kindly provided computer assistance with this book. Soma Clifton and Jeffrey Neugebauer made beautiful handcrafted wood displays that hold the flower essence bottles (see Appendix), and Reverend Selina Clifton nurtured me with massage and wonderful food while I wrote this book.

I deeply thank David Holladay for my time with him in nature, and for teaching me the ways of indigenous life and plant medicines. I also am grateful to Julie Smelzer for her friendship, dedication, and support of this work.

I am deeply grateful for the friendship and support of John Alden and Don Giacobbe. I also express my appreciation to Cory Vandemoer for her consultations and input to this book. And I am very thankful to Dr. Vasant Merchant for providing me with her insights, support, and guidance.

I thank Andrea and Rennie Radoccia, who generously shared their beautiful organic flower garden with me over fourteen years ago, and the following people who shared their land and organic flower gardens with me: Linda and Dave Burkholder, Norm and Lin Reichenbach, Elaine DeVore and Marlys Morgan, Jean Sumney, Harriet Loker, Veronica Vida, and Jeffrey Neugebauer. I also give my appreciation to Ron Marvin and Karen Reider for designing the chakra/flower diagram.

I also want to acknowledge the following authors and their books: Ted Andrews, *The Healer's Manual;* John Selby, *Kundalini Awakening;* Anodea Judith, *Wheels of Life;* Anodea Judith and Selene Vega, *The Sevenfold Journey;* Rosalyn Bruyere, *Wheels of Light;* Barbara Brennan, *Hands of Light;* Dr. Gabriel Cousens, *Spiritual Nutrition and the Rainbow Diet;* Dr. Caroline Myss, *Energy Anatomy* (cassette tapes); and Ted Kaptchuk, *The Web That*

Has No Weaver. These books, in addition to those listed in the bibliography, have inspired me and helped me understand my relationship with the chakras. (See part II, Chakras and Flower Essences, for an explanation of the chakra system.)

I extend special gratitude to the people at New World Library for their immeasurable support and assistance with this book. I especially give warm thanks to Georgia Hughes for her kind advocacy of this book; to Katharine Farnam Conolly, my editor, for her friendly disposition and efficiency; to Carol Venolia, my copyeditor, who drew me out with her incredible insights and perspective; to Monique Muhlenkamp for her publicity and marketing savvy; and to Tona Pearce Myers, Mary Ann Casler, and Katie Blount for making the book look so beautiful. They were each a pleasure to work with.

And in loving memory, I give my deep and heartfelt appreciation to my dear artist friend Vera Louise Drysdale, who passed on to the "other world" in January 1993. It was Vera Louise who nurtured my seeds of inspiration and encouraged me to believe in myself enough to follow through on my dreams.

I deeply thank each of the provers who dedicated their time and energy to the extensive Research Provers' Project. I am especially appreciative of the quality of their responses and their sincere intention to live life to its fullest. I especially thank my stepdaughter, Jenny Dawn Downey, for her diligent assistance with this project. The following people participated in all of or part of the Research Provers' Project: Craig Bacharach, Cameron Bazzill, Anne Boyle, Linda Burkholder, Selina Clifton, Soma Clifton, Lei Lani Cochran, Karen David, Nancy DePuy, Ashley Dixon, Gina Emanuel, Mary Fackler, Ann Flinn, James Gregory, Laura Harness, Bennett Harris, John Harris, Forrest Hayes, Lori Kalina, Kumari, Jo Ann Kuruc, Carol Luhman, Shannon Lynch, Bob Maxey, Marlys Morgan, Delisa Myles, Robyn Nelson, Jeffrey Neugebauer, Curt PallasDowney, Donna Parker, Shea Patridge, Lauren Patridge, Laura Pax Piper, Sherri Ricker, Terri Roberts, Berenice Sara Romero, Keena Rowe, Marianne Shaefer, Jade Sherer, Steve Stubenrauch, Veronica Vida, and Amy Williams. There are many others who participated in one or several provings, and I am grateful for their feedback and involvement with the project.

I also extend my gratitude to Cleona Ellis, Ruth Hutchinson, and Linda Nanez for their financial contributions to the Research Provers' Project, which helped make this project possible.

ABOUT THE AUTHOR

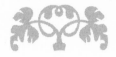

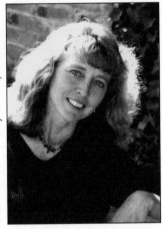

Photo Credit: Tere Ireys at Benjemax Studio

Rhonda PallasDowney's integration of flower essences, herbalism, and homeopathy, coupled with her understanding of the whole plant, the chakra system, flower colors, and psychology of plants, makes her a pioneer in the realm of plant medicine. Rhonda is a flower essence practitioner, herbalist, and photographer of flowers, specializing in indigenous flora. She has a diploma in Homeopathic Medicine (DiHom) from the British Institute of Homoeopathy and

is a member of the National Center of Homeopathy. Rhonda has studied herbalism with Matthew Wood and is a student of Rosemary Gladstar. She has B.S. and M.A. degrees in Special Education and vast experience in counseling and coordinating services for people who have developmental disabilities and their families. Rhonda is a staff member at the Arizona School of Integrative Studies (A.S.I.S.) in Clarkdale, Arizona, where she teaches herbal studies, plant life, and her Flower Essences and Chakra Healing Practitioner Course, which has been approved by the American Holistic Nurses' Association, which is accredited as an Approver of Continuing Education in Nursing by the American Nurses Credentialing Center's Commission on Accreditation. Rhonda also cofacilitates various groups, specializing in women's groups with ceremony, music, and council.

Rhonda owns and operates Living Flower Essences in Cottonwood, Arizona, where she prepares essences and provides consultations nationwide. She also gives workshops internationally, is a tutor at the British Institute of Homoeopathy, and continues to expand the knowledge base about flower essences by conducting testings and collecting case studies. Ms. PallasDowney is a Reiki practitioner, and she has practiced various healing arts over the past twenty-five years, including neuro-linguisitic programming, yoga, Tai Chi, polarity, massage, applied kinesiology, and Touch for Health acupressure. Her articles have appeared in various national publications.

Rhonda lives in Cottonwood, Arizona.

New World Library is dedicated to
publishing books and audio programs that inspire
and challenge us to improve the quality
of our lives and our world.
Our books and cassettes are available
at bookstores everywhere.
For a complete catalog, contact:

New World Library
14 Pamaron Way
Novato, California 94949
Phone: (415) 884-2100
Fax: (415) 884-2199
Or call toll free: (800) 972-6657
Catalog requests: Ext. 50
Ordering: Ext. 52
E-mail: escort@nwlib.com
newworldlibrary.com